# Health
# Psychology
# in Global
# Perspective

# Cross-Cultural Psychology Series

**SERIES EDITORS**

*Walter J. Lonner*
*Western Washington University*

*John W. Berry*
*Queens University*

Many of the basic assumptions contained in standard psychology curricula in Western universities have been uncritically accepted for many years. The volumes in the **Cross-Cultural Psychology** series present cultural perspectives that challenge Western ways of thinking in the hope of stimulating informed discussions about human behavior in all domains of psychology.

**Cross-Cultural Psychology** offers brief monographs describing and critically examining Western-based psychology and its underlying assumptions. The primary readership for this series consists of professors who teach, and students who take, the wide spectrum of courses offered in upper-division and graduate-level psychology programs in North America and elsewhere.

**EDITORIAL BOARD**

John Adamopoulos
*United States*

Fanny Cheung
*Hong Kong*

Pierre R. Dasen
*Switzerland*

Rolando Diaz-Loving
*Mexico*

Cigdem Kagitcibasi
*Turkey*

Yoshihisa Kashima
*Australia*

Kwok Leung
*Hong Kong*

Bame Nsamenang
*Cameroon*

Ype Poortinga
*The Netherlands*

T. S. Saraswathi
*India*

Gisela Trommsdorff
*Germany*

Fons van de Vijver
*The Netherlands*

Books in this series:

1. **Methods and Data Analysis for Cross-Cultural Research,** Fons van de Vijver and Kwok Leung
2. **Health Psychology in Global Perspective,** Frances E. Aboud
3. **Masculinity and Femininity: The Taboo Dimension of National Cultures,** Geert Hofstede

# Health Psychology in Global Perspective

Frances E. Aboud

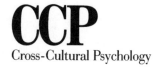
Cross-Cultural Psychology

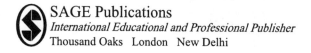
SAGE Publications
*International Educational and Professional Publisher*
Thousand Oaks  London  New Delhi

Copyright © 1998 by Sage Publications, Inc.

All rights reserved. No part of this book may be reproduced or utilized in any form or by any means, electronic or mechanical, including photocopying, recording, or by any information storage and retrieval system, without permission in writing from the publisher.

*For information:*

SAGE Publications, Inc.
2455 Teller Road
Thousand Oaks, California 91320
E-mail: order@sagepub.com

SAGE Publications Ltd.
6 Bonhill Street
London EC2A 4PU
United Kingdom

SAGE Publications India Pvt. Ltd.
M-32 Market
Greater Kailash I
New Delhi 110 048 India

Printed in the United States of America

*Library of Congress Cataloging-in-Publication Data*

Aboud, Frances E.
 Health psychology in global perspective / by Frances E. Aboud.
  p. cm. — (Cross-cultural psychology ; vol. 2)
 Includes bibliographical references (p.   ) and indexes.
 ISBN 0-7619-0940-0 (cloth : acid-free paper). — ISBN 0-7619-0941-9 (pbk. : acid-free paper)
  1. Clinical health psychology. 2. World health. 3. Clinical health psychology—Developing countries. I. Title. II. Series: Cross-cultural psychology series ; v. 2.
 R726.7.A26  1998
 362.1—dc21                                  97-33937

98  99  00  01  02  03  10  9  8  7  6  5  4  3  2  1

| | |
|---|---|
| *Acquisitions Editor:* | Jim Nageotte |
| *Editorial Assistant:* | Fiona Lyon |
| *Production Editor:* | Sanford Robinson |
| *Production Assistant:* | Lynn Miyata |
| *Designer/Typesetter:* | Danielle Dillahunt |
| *Cover Design:* | Ravi Balasuriya |
| *Print Buyer:* | Anna Chin |

# CONTENTS

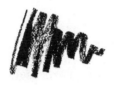

| | |
|---|---|
| Series Editors' Introduction | ix |
| Preface | xi |
| **1. What Is International Health Psychology?** | **1** |
| The History of a Salt Solution | 5 |
| How Many Hats Can You Wear? | 6 |
| Student Activity | 28 |
| **2. Social Science Measures for Health Research** | **29** |
| Social Science Variables | 30 |
| Qualitative and Quantitative Methods | 32 |
| Focus Group Discussion | 35 |
| Systematic Nonparticipant Observation | 42 |
| Participant Observation | 47 |
| Key Informant Interviews | 51 |
| Structured Self-Report Measures | 57 |
| Student Activity | 66 |
| **3. Family Planning and Contraceptive Use** | **67** |
| The Case in Favor of Family Planning | 69 |

|  |  |
|---|---|
| How Couples Weigh the Costs and Benefits of Children | 75 |
| The Prevalence of Contraception Use | 78 |
| What Makes a Family Planning Program Effective? | 85 |
| Student Activities | 92 |

## 4. The AIDS/HIV Pandemic — 94
*Michaela Hynie*

|  |  |
|---|---|
| Modes of HIV Transmission | 97 |
| Measuring the Magnitude of AIDS and HIV | 99 |
| International Prevalence Rates and Patterns | 101 |
| Prevention Strategies: Whom and What to Target | 105 |
| Interventions to Prevent HIV Infection | 116 |
| Student Activity | 122 |

## 5. Community Participation and Agency Involvement — 123

|  |  |
|---|---|
| What Does It Mean to Participate? | 125 |
| Benefits and Costs of Participation | 128 |
| Ways to Raise Community Participation | 130 |
| Two International Participation Schemes | 136 |
| Frameworks for Evaluating Community Participation | 140 |
| NGOs Who Promote Participation | 150 |
| Student Activity | 153 |

## 6. Nutrition for Child Growth and Development — 154

|  |  |
|---|---|
| Measuring Malnutrition | 156 |
| Prevalence of Malnutrition | 160 |
| Causes of Malnutrition | 162 |
| Health and Psychosocial Consequences of Malnutrition | 169 |
| Treatment and Community Prevention Programs | 180 |
| Student Activity | 184 |

## 7. Alcohol Use and Abuse — 185

|  |  |
|---|---|
| Definitions and Measures of Problem Drinking | 187 |
| International Rates of Alcohol Use and Abuse | 193 |
| Personal and Social Consequences of Alcohol Abuse | 199 |
| Risk Factors for Alcohol Abuse | 203 |
| Alcohol Prevention Programs | 205 |
| Student Activity | 209 |

| | |
|---|---|
| **8. Health Education and Promotion** | **210** |
| Concepts and Components of Health Education | 211 |
| Case 1: Family Planning in Ethiopia | 214 |
| Case 2: Community Norms for Face Washing in Tanzania | 216 |
| Case 3: Interactive Radio for Children in Bolivia | 220 |
| Case 4: Dyadic Problem Solving on Child Feeding in the Philippines | 223 |
| Case 5: Mobilizing Students for Sanitation in Bangladesh | 225 |
| Case 6: Home Management of Diarrhea in Gambia | 227 |
| Case 7: School Feeding Programs | 230 |
| Learning From Successes and Mistakes | 232 |
| Taking Theories into the Field | 233 |
| The Case for Education | 239 |
| Student Activity | 243 |
| **9. Mental Health and Illness** | **244** |
| Definition and Classification | 245 |
| Community Measurement Instruments | 246 |
| Is Mental Illness Universal or Culture Specific? | 251 |
| Prevalence of Mental Illness | 256 |
| Social and Personal Consequences | 258 |
| Risk Factors | 260 |
| Prevention and Treatment | 264 |
| Student Activity | 269 |
| A Final Note: Where Do You Go From Here? | 271 |
| Glossary | 275 |
| References | 289 |
| Author Index | 311 |
| Subject Index | 322 |
| About the Author | 327 |
| About the Contributors | 329 |

*This book is dedicated to my partner in life,
Charles,
and to the children who make our life exciting,
Charles and Leila.*

# SERIES EDITORS' INTRODUCTION

The comparative study of thought and behavior across cultures has been one of the most interesting and productive developments in psychology during the past quarter century. We believe, as do many others, that psychology can mature into a valid and global discipline only to the extent that it incorporates paradigms, perspectives, and data from an ever-widening circle of both cultures and ethnic groups. That was the general guiding philosophy behind the **Cross-Cultural Research and Methodology** series that was started in 1975, in which 20 volumes were published. Like the CCRM series, this new series offers books describing and critically examining Western-based psychology and its underlying assumptions. Most of the basic assumptions contained in standard psychology curricula in the many universities of the highly industrialized Western world have been unchallenged. The volumes in this new series present cultural elements that challenge Western ways of thinking in the hope of stimulating informed discussions about human behavior in all domains of psychology. Books in this series are written for use as core texts or as supplements, depending on the instructor's requirements. We believe that the cumulative totality of books in this series will contribute to the development of a much more inclusive psychology and will lead to the formation of the interesting, testable hypotheses about the complex relationships between culture and behavior.

As series editors, we are fortunate to have an international panel of experts in cross-cultural psychology to help guide us in the selection and evaluation of manuscripts. The 14 members of the editorial board represent 11 different countries and many of the domains within psychology.

This volume in the series is written by a cross-cultural social psychologist who has spent her professional career teaching and studying the topics included in the book. Using McGill University as her base, Frances Aboud has been involved in social psychological applications to health and education, with an interest in countries in the developing world. She is particularly knowledgable about Ethiopia, where she has been involved for many years in a variety of research projects. An energetic and creative researcher, her passionate interest in health psychology is timely and efforts like hers are sorely needed throughout the world. Covering critical areas such as family planning, nutrition for proper child growth and development, uses and abuses of alcohol, and mental health and illness, the breadth of the book will be of great interest to psychologists, many in medical fields, educators, and others who are interested in the parameters of international health. The book also contains solid material on certain methodological procedures and perspectives that are critical to the gathering of reliable data.

All things considered, the scope and tone of this volume make it attractive as a text for classroom use, as a guide for research, and as solid background material for a wide assortment of field projects. We are pleased that it appears in the **Cross-Cultural Psychology** series, and we believe it will become an influential book in an interesting and growing field. We thank Frances E. Aboud for writing it with her characteristic clarity and unbridled enrhusiasm.

—Walter J. Lonner
—John W. Berry

# PREFACE

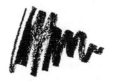

The title of this book combines *global health* and *psychology*, two disciplines that have come together in my life. As a psychologist, teaching and researching in Ethiopia, I tried to bring all my understanding of human existence to bear on the health problems of rural people. Fortunately, there were many colleagues, students, and acquaintances willing to fill me in on the details of health and illness in a developing country. I hope to pass on to you, the reader, what I learned from them.

The field of international health attracts many people, each with his or her own motivation and own orientation: the medical profession, the social scientists, the humanitarians. Professional and academic writings are full of their contributions as well as their quarrels. Each has a unique contribution to make, but it can best be made by working closely with others. Community health work, in particular, demands a collaborative effort. My experience and my nature tend to be inclusive, to avoid fights over who can and can't do what. Regardless of your major discipline, I am sure you can learn to develop a qualitative and a quantitative measure or help develop an intervention for a health problem.

I have taken a biopsychosocial approach to international health by discussing the biological, psychological, and social contributions to health and illness. As a social and developmental psychologist, my strength lies in explaining the middle factor, without excluding the other two. Although there is a thriving group of health psychologists, they have not been particularly visible in developing countries, where people are more likely to recognize the social science work of anthropologists. However, the field of psychology includes topics that range from physiological and developmental mechanisms to social and educational applications. It also has developed and used a wide range of measurement techniques not only to assess personality but also to examine learning, attitudes, and group problem solving, to name but a few. My work in cross-cultural psychology has taught me that a different nation or cultural group sometimes sees their lives from a different perspective, although we all have much in common. I know that there are many right ways to reach our common goals of health and development, and I hope we will explore these together through discussions generated by my text. Without glossing over the differences, I have taken a broad psychological perspective while including the published ideas and research of people from other disciplines. Whatever region of the world you live in, and whatever your particular interest in health, I hope this book provides some impetus for pursuing your own personal and collective goals.

## ACKNOWLEDGMENTS

I would like to thank colleagues and students from the following places for their intellectual and financial support: the McGill-Ethiopia Community Health Project, the International Development Research Center, the Canadian International Development Agency, the Jimma Institute of Health Sciences, Addis Ababa University, Concordia University, and especially McGill University. I am grateful to colleagues who gave me feedback on earlier versions of chapters: Will Boyce, Judith Graeff, Catherine Hankins, Morton Mendelson, Joyce Pickering, Robert Pihl, and Lisa Serbin.

*Preface* xiii

I am grateful to Dr. Michaela Hynie, a psychologist, for writing the complete chapter on AIDS and HIV (Chapter 4) and to Dr. Charles P. Larson, an epidemiologist and physician, for writing the epidemiology section in Chapter 1.

Copyright permission was granted by the following:

- The Canadian University Consortium for Health in Development for extensive borrowing from my chapter in their book, *Health Research for Development: A Manual*, edited by Joyce Pickering, for Chapter 2 here.
- Carfax Publishing Ltd., P.O. Box 25, Abingdon, Oxfordshire OX14 3UE, United Kingdom, for Table 7.1, which was adapted from an article by Saunders, Aasland, Amundsen, and Grant in the journal *Addictions*, 1993, 88, 349-362.
- The *Guardian Weekly* for referencing in Chapter 4 an article from the March 25, 1997, issue by P. Brown titled "And Now for the Bad News About AIDS."
- The *Washington Post* for quoting from two articles published in the *Washington Post* section of the *Guardian Weekly:* The quote in Chapter 3 was written by B. Vobejda in an article titled "U.S. Aid Cut 'Will Increase Abortions' " in the March 17, 1996, issue of the *Guardian Weekly*; the quote in Chapter 9 was written by J. Mathews in an article titled "Population Control That Really Works" in the April 10, 1994, issue of the *Guardian Weekly*.
- UNAIDS for the rates and numbers shown in Figure 4.1, which were taken from their web site www.us.unaids.org.

# 1

# WHAT IS INTERNATIONAL HEALTH PSYCHOLOGY?

International health is both a serious concern and an exciting discipline. Around the world every year, 585,000 mothers die giving birth, 2.7 million young adults contract human immunodeficiency virus from unprotected sex, and 7 million children die of diseases such as diarrhea and pneumonia that could have been prevented. Many others become disabled—physically, intellectually, and emotionally—because of malnutrition, injury, infection, and trauma. To these people and their families, health is a serious and constant concern. To their communities and nations, especially those of the developing world, managing meager resources to provide needed health care is a serious and often frustrating business.

The international community sustains its concern, for the most part, by proxy, that is, by means of organizations created by governments and citizens to provide needed resources. Some of our taxes and volunteer donations go to government agencies (e.g., British Overseas Development, USAID, CIDA, SIDA) and to nongovernmental organizations (e.g., CARE, World Vision, Save the Children, Hope, Oxfam), but we let their planners decide where and how to spend the money. As an agency of the United Nations, the United Nations Children's Fund (UNICEF), for example, spent hundreds of millions of dollars on our behalf to immunize children. Experts from around the world who work with UNICEF led the campaign to immunize children by providing a coordinated blueprint for action along with funds for vaccines, refrigerators, manpower, and gasoline. Any interested person can find out how their money was spent, why it was spent on immunization, and whether the campaign was successful—it was (see LaFond, 1994).

Attempting to combine these two perspectives is the field of international health. As a discipline, **international health** takes a multination perspective on the state of people's health, seeking knowledge and effective action strategies through a systematic examination of health problems, their determinants, and their solutions around the world (definitions of words in **bold** print can be found in the Glossary at the back of the book). The term **health** is defined as physical, mental, and social well-being, an important resource for a satisfying and productive life. Therefore, the focus is on good health or well-being as well as poor health or disease, and on mental and social health in addition to physical health. The international perspective makes at least two powerful and unique contributions. It reminds us that as members of the international community, we have a responsibility at least to be informed about the quality of life and the struggles of people who live in other countries. Second, we have come to realize that we can learn from each other; we gain greater understanding about our own problems and their solutions when we build on ideas and information coming from many different sources.

So where is all the excitement? you might ask. Many of us who work in the field of international health find the challenges exciting. One day the problem appears as a statistic and the next day as concrete reality. The challenge is to translate back and forth from global problems to local problems, from local solutions to global solutions. Sometimes concrete reality presents simpler solutions than we ever dreamed were possible, and sometimes it complicates solutions that appeared neat in the planning stages. For example, one day we surveyed a village to find that only half of the households had a latrine; the next day I became part of a latrine-digging team. A simple solution—but only for the short term, I remind myself. Another problem was the number of children with diarrhea and malaria during the rainy season; then I heard mothers insist that the larger-than-life-size virus and mosquito drawn on the flip chart did not exist there. "The consumer is always right" is a sales motto that can complicate the work of a health educator; it can complicate the goals of international health work if we unthinkingly apply it to all aspects of life (see Box 1.1).

Experiences like this touch us at the professional and the personal levels. Health problems that could once be put into neat flowcharts become as complicated and intriguing as a diagram of the brain. Professional growth therefore comes from expanding our framework to include other perspectives as well as the daily details. A mosquito or virus can be studied at many levels—from the biochemical (effects on body functioning), to the psychological (mothers' understanding of its effects), to the social (a community's efforts to give oral rehydration salts to every needy child). Although our expertise may be in only one area, solutions come from coordinating the expertise of different areas. Personal growth is not easily described but is best captured by phrases used by people when they return from an international venture: "My life will never quite be the same." "Problems at home seem so petty and mundane in comparison." "The friends we made will be part of us forever."

To those who work in the field of international health, excitement also comes from the small successes: teaching enthusiastic health workers, watching a mother mix the salt-sugar solution for her sick child, helping the people in a village organize themselves to build safe water wells. There are also many disappointments: latrines built but left unused, fruit sold to passersby rather than fed to family members, health workers trained but unappreciated and underused by their community. To cope with the pain of failure, someone coined the phrase *lessons learned*, which refers to reasons for the failure that we identify after much reflection and evaluation, and that we hope not to repeat in subsequent attempts. There are lessons to be learned not only from failures but from successful activities in that and other cultures. There is no one winning formula for success in international health, and no single explanatory theory. Social scientists and biomedical scientists are still in the process of putting the pieces together, as the following example of oral rehydration clearly demonstrates.

## BOX 1.1.
## ARE YOU AN ADAPTER OR AN ACTIVIST?

Some social scientists are adapters and some biomedical scientists are activists, but regardless of your training, you must come to terms with this question. It is a fundamental dilemma for all change agents: Do you have the right to try to change the lives of other people? Is there a universal set of values for determining a better life, or are all values relative to a culture?

*Adapters* take the position that we should be working for social cohesion and the survival of the community. Events that are common in a community may have a useful purpose, namely, to help the community function and survive within its given context. Even practices that lead to the death, disease, and disability of individuals may help the community as a whole thrive. If ecological adaptation is the engine driving human behavior, then outsiders should not interfere with the traditional practices followed in a community. Attempts to change people's behavior might interfere with the social bonds that are essential for the community's survival. The role of a change agent is to study the physical and social context in which the behavior occurs to understand its ecological significance. Change agents should promote the adaptation of the group, not solely the health of an individual.

*Activists* take the position that health is a universal standard to be pursued even at the cost of radical change and some disruption. They assume that people value the health of their family more than the long-term survival of their community. Attempts to change people's behavior and the environment are actively pursued if they promise to result in better health for a number of people. Thus change agents should promote healthy behaviors regardless of their effect on traditional bonds.

Cassidy (1987) describes the positions well with respect to child malnutrition. Adapters feel that the well-being and productivity of the kin group may be enhanced by letting the malnourished and sickly children die. Activists believe that malnutrition is a health problem and that community and family changes must be made to eliminate the problem. There are two similar positions with respect to female circumcision (Armstrong, 1991; Dorkenoo, 1996; Macklin, 1996).

There are certain pitfalls in both positions. Adapters mistakenly assume that the status quo is the best adaptation to that context, that practices in a

> kin group or community are homogeneous, and that survival of the group motivates people to act the way they do. None of these is correct. Activists assume that health is a priority value for most people, that others share their sense of control over themselves and the environment, and that active efforts on their part will bring about change for the better. These are self-centered views. Although my views are more compatible with the activists', I can see that the change they advocate needs to be user-friendly, that is, geared to the competing values, resources, and sense of control held by people. Perhaps each of us has different goals with respect to the balance of physical, mental, and social well-being we seek.

## THE HISTORY OF A SALT SOLUTION

The history of oral rehydration salts is a good example of how we have integrated successful contributions from different fields. Diarrhea has many causes, the important ones being the rotavirus, *E. coli* bacteria, and cholera, but it leads to death mainly because it dehydrates the body. Within a few days or hours, young children can die unless they receive water. The problem is that microorganisms prevent villi, or folds of tissue in the small intestines, from doing their usual job of absorbing sodium and, with it, water. As a result, water leaves the body as watery stools, and the blood that would normally pick up water from the villi and carry it to other parts of the body has no new supply. Biomedical researchers in England and the United States discovered in the 1940s and 1950s how to get sodium (and with it water) absorbed into the villi blood vessels. They called it the cotransport system because they found that sodium was absorbed if it went hand-in-hand with glucose. Adding electrolytes such as potassium and salt helped retain even more water. Clinical research with people followed in the 1960s, this time in a region of the world where diarrhea was killing millions of people. Researchers at the International Center for Diarrheal Diseases in Dacca, Bangladesh, found that the sodium-glucose transport system worked with patients suffering from diarrhea. At first, the glucose-electrolyte solution was used only in hospitals, given intravenously. But researchers continued to work on producing a solution that could be drunk. Its initiation by fire came during the Bangladeshi war of independence in 1971, as refugees were pouring into India with cholera and other types of diarrhea. The Indian doctor recruited children of the sufferers as medical volunteers and told them how to give the fluid to their parents. Deaths were reduced from 50% to 3%.

The World Health Organization (WHO) then set a standard recipe of dry ingredients—sodium chloride, potassium chloride, trisodium citrate, and glucose—in specific quantities to be added to one liter of water. Sachets of oral rehydration salts (ORS) are now manufactured in many countries and prevent millions of deaths around the world. The story has not yet ended. Despite strong promotion by UNICEF, many children do not receive ORS. There are a number of possible reasons, most having to do with people's expectations and behavior. For example, even when the package is free and accessible, mothers and sometimes health workers are reluctant to try an innovation. Mothers want to stop their children's watery stools, and ORS does not do that. Health workers want to give medicine such as antibiotics, but most diarrhea in children is caused by a virus that does not respond to antibiotics. ORS prevents dehydration until the virus become ineffective, usually in 4 or 5 days. With this feedback, social scientists realized that they would have to explain why more, not less, fluid was needed, and simplify instructions. They realized that behavioral strategies were needed to help mothers and health workers remember the mixing formula. Some even suggested that a homemade soup or porridge, with the right ingredients, would be easier to learn, more acceptable to mothers, and more nutritious for the child. Biomedical researchers are working on improved concentrations of salts and glucose as well as the addition of grains such as rice and maize to reduce stool output and shorten the duration of the diarrhea. Efforts on many fronts have helped to make ORS a revolutionary advance in community-level prevention of childhood death (Greenough & Khin-Maung-U, 1991; Hamilton, 1997; Hirschhorn & Greenough, 1991).

## HOW MANY HATS CAN YOU WEAR?

Because international health integrates the perspectives of many disciplines from the social and biomedical sciences, one needs to under-

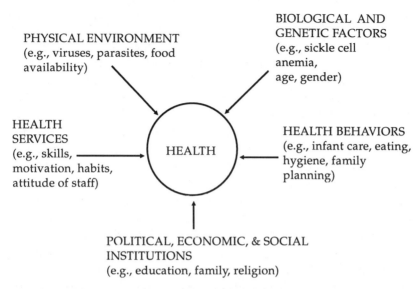

**Figure 1.1.** A Framework for Picturing the Different Components of Community Health

stand something about the concepts and the approach of each. Many people use the **biopsychosocial framework,** which seeks to understand health and illness in terms of three components: biological, psychological, and social (Schneiderman & Tapp, 1985). The framework offered in Figure 1.1 proposes five major inputs to the health of people living in a community: biological and genetic factors within the person, the physical environment, health services, social institutions, and health behaviors. Some inputs may circle around the wheel and enter the hub of health through several spokes. For example, being male or female is a genetic endowment that influences health directly as well as indirectly by way of institutions such as education and status within the family. Likewise, our adoption of recommended health behaviors will influence how we are treated by health service workers, and vice versa.

The remainder of this chapter is organized into the professional hats you will need to wear to understand material on international health. In addition to the psychosocial hat and the biomedical hat, you will need to know the statistics used to describe the health of communities as well as the geographic organization used by world health bodies.

The Psychosocial Hat

*Health* is defined by the World Health Organization as a state of physical, mental, and social well-being. Thus mental and social well-being are recognized to be important in their own right and in their effect on physical well-being. The mental and social health of people can affect not only their own productivity and enjoyment of life but also the development of their children, the quality of their marriages, and the safety of their communities. Psychologists have developed ways of measuring mental and social well-being, in addition to the better known measures of psychopathology. The *mentally healthy* person shows development and maturity in cognitive, emotional, and social capacities, for example, problem solving, positive emotions, and mutually satisfying social relationships (see Box 1.2 for some useful definitions).

Figure 1.1 points to another contribution of psychology to international health. Behaviors influence physical health directly and indirectly (behavioral medicine). **Health behaviors** are actions that directly influence one's own and others' health. They include behaviors that promote physical well-being (e.g., good eating habits, family planning), prevent illness (e.g., getting infants immunized and washing with soap), manage or eliminate illness (e.g., giving a child oral rehydration and taking tuberculosis medication regularly), and those that demote or reduce health (e.g., eating too much junk food, drinking too much alcohol).

These health behaviors are acquired, maintained, and changed with the help of other psychosocial factors, such as one's values, attitudes, knowledge, and personality; social institutions like one's family and school; and health professionals. Psychologists are therefore interested in how people learn health behaviors from their parents, teachers, peers, and the media, and why they perform only some of the behaviors they learn. They are particularly interested in why some health behaviors are maintained and others change. To this end, they examine influences inside as well as outside the person. Inside influences include attitudes, automatic habits that are performed without much thought, perception of personal risk, knowledge of the consequences, expectations of reward from others, and problem solving to overcome obstacles. Outside influences include other people who serve as models for behavior and attitudes, and who give approval and disapproval as well as instructions and reminders. Psychologists give as much weight to the psychological as to the social influences because they see that even people from the same family are not carbon copies of their social environment. For various reasons, people consciously and unconsciously select from what they see and hear. The attitudes, knowledge, and motivation already possessed by a person partly determine what he or she selects.

Not all health problems are influenced by behaviors. Hubley (1993) suggests that first we conduct a **behavioral diagnosis** of the health problem, meaning the process by which we look at the causes of a health problem and find out whether human behavior is involved in its prevention or treatment. Health psychologists in industrialized countries have identified a number of important health behaviors such as overeating, cigarette smoking, and infrequent exercise. Because the pressing health problems are different in developing countries, other health behaviors may be more prevalent and causal. However, there will be many areas of overlap: the method of studying health and health behaviors, the concepts used to describe psychosocial forces, and the explanations, for example, the process of learning health behaviors.

In summary, the psychology perspective contributes to an understanding and explanation of mental and social health, both of which are part of the definition of health. It also contributes to an understanding of how and why people perform various health behaviors, which in turn influence their physical health.

The Biomedical Hat

Doctors, nurses, health assistants, and community health workers spend their days working on preventive and curative services and research to reduce the burden of disease. For this book, I selected only those health problems that entail a large behavioral component. These and many others have special significance in developing countries because they disable or kill millions of people. Children are vulnerable to certain diseases. Others, such as tuberculosis and schizophrenia, strike during the productive middle years. The biomedical perspective contributes knowledge on common diseases and how they are treated and prevented. A description of common diseases in the developing

## BOX 1.2.
## WHAT DOES THIS PSYCHOLOGY JARGON MEAN?

Some readers may not be acquainted with the psychology terms I have used. Here are some brief definitions of the terms used in the preceding section (see Reber's dictionary, 1985).

*Mental and social health* refers to growth and maturity in cognition, emotion, and interpersonal relations.

*Cognition* refers to interpreting the world, memory, learning, thinking, reasoning, problem solving, and knowledge.

*Emotion* refers to states of affect (e.g., happiness, anger, fear), moods (a brief positive or negative emotion), and attitudes (long-term evaluations of people, objects, and events).

*Relational* refers to actual interactions with other people that involve participation in friendship, family, and community life as well as the mental processes involved in relationships with others, such as emotional attachments and realistic interpretations of others.

*Health behaviors* are actions that directly influence the well-being of oneself and others, through promotion or demotion, illness prevention and treatment, and rehabilitation. A *habit* is a set of actions that have become automatic, fixed, and easily and effortlessly carried out, as a result of repetition.

*Learning* is the process of acquiring a relatively permanent mental or behavioral response as a result of rewarded practice or observation of someone performing the behavior. The reward may take the form of a biologically satisfying object or it may be social approval and recognition. The observed model is likely to be a parent, older sibling, or teacher.

*Values* are relatively enduring preferences for certain end states, such as health and social recognition, and the means for achieving them, such as through self-control or obedience. Rokeach measured the values of a person and culture by asking people to rank in importance to them a list of 18 values. A traditional culture is one that values ways of living that have been passed down through many generations.

> *Attitudes* are predispositions to respond in a positive or negative manner toward a person, object, or event.
>
> *Knowledge* refers to all the information possessed by a person or group, however it was acquired (i.e., a form of cognition).
>
> *Personality* refers to relatively enduring ways of behaving, thinking, and feeling that characterize a person and that to a certain extent distinguish that person from others.
>
> *Skills* are capacities for carrying out complex, well-organized patterns of behavior smoothly and adaptively to achieve a goal.
>
> *Motivation* refers to energized, goal-directed behavior, influenced by need, the value of the goal, and expectations of reward.

world follows (Jamison, Mosley, Measham, & Bobadilla, 1993). The number of people who acquire the diseases was obtained from a world progress report (World Health Organization, 1995).

**Acute respiratory infection** affects the tract from the nose to the lungs. The most fatal, pneumonia, is an infection of the lungs that usually follows an upper tract infection such as influenza or cold. There are many different causal agents and many different symptoms, some of which are fever, cough, and shallow breathing. The infection is caused by bacteria or virus and is treated with antibiotics. It is prevented by maintaining good nutrition, full immunization, and indoor air ventilation. Annually, 2,000 million episodes occur in children and 4.1 million die.

**Diarrheal diseases** in children are caused by many microorganisms, the most common of which are rotavirus and *Escherichia coli* (*E. coli*). Virus and bacteria enter the body through contaminated water and food, contaminated milk bottles, or dirty fingers. For this reason, the best prevention is to drink clean water and to be vigilant about hygiene. The child is considered to have diarrhea when it passes three or more loose, or one watery, stools in 1 day. Typically it lasts for 5 days. The best treatment involves preventing dehydration by giving the child oral rehydration. Annually, 1,500 million episodes of diarrhea occur, resulting in 3 million deaths in children under 5 years. Cholera is the most deadly form of diarrhea; 78 countries report cholera, with a total of 400,000 cases.

**Leprosy** has been around for centuries and has the reputation of being a contagious, disfiguring disease. It is caused by *Mycobacterium leprae*, and symptoms are worse for those with a weak immune response. A mild form results in depigmentation of a patch of skin that spontaneously heals, whereas a more severe form damages nerves, bones, and muscles. If the severe form goes untreated for a long time, the person may suffer deformity of the face, hands, and feet. Hands and feet may become injured as a result of nerve damage, which then makes people unaware that they are exposing their body to injury. Some forms of the disease are highly contagious and others less so. Symptoms generally appear several years after infection and so gradually that the person may not be aware. The multidrug therapy now in use has reduced treatment to a few years, with few deaths. Currently 2.4 million people have leprosy, although millions of others may have undetected infections.

**Malaria** results from infection by a parasite of the *Plasmodium* genus. It is transmitted by the Anopheles mosquito, in which the parasite lives. The mosquito picks up the parasite from one infected person and passes it on when biting an uninfected person. The main symptom is fever. Repeated infections lead to some immunity, but young children do not yet have this immunity and so may die from severe bouts. Half the world is exposed to malaria, resulting in about 2 million deaths annually. Drugs are available to prevent malaria and to treat it, but normally the strategy is to control the mosquito vector through insecticide sprays, to fill water bodies where they breed, and to encourage the use of chemically treated bed nets.

**Malnutrition** in its extreme can take two forms, marasmus and kwashiorkor. Marasmus is the result of insufficient calories due to diet or illness. The child's body lacks the layer of fat normally seen under the skin and the muscles are wasted. Kwashiorkor is the result of insufficient protein due to diet. The child's legs and sometimes face are swollen with edema, the skin becomes flaky, and the hair turns a red color. The child is treated with a protein-calorie-electrolyte fluid sent directly to the stomach and then with active feeding. All infections are simultaneously treated. Malnutrition in a community takes a different form (see Chapter 6).

**Measles** is a highly contagious viral disease transmitted from person to person through simple respiration. The main symptoms are rash and fever. Without immunization, all children would be infected and 1% to 5% of those in developing countries would die from pneumonia because of complications due to poor nutrition. Breast-fed infants are protected for a time, but most must receive vaccination by the end of their first year to prevent the disease. In recent years, 45 million children have had measles and annually 1 million have died.

**Neonatal tetanus** is acquired when the tetanus bacteria, present in the soil and dust, enter an open wound. In the case of newborns, the bacteria enter from unsterile razors or other sharp objects used to cut the umbilical cord or from improper dressing or cleaning of the stump. Mothers can also become infected after an unsterile delivery. Tetanus manifests with rigidity of the mouth and lips, and finally in the second week of life the child dies from respiratory failure. In recent years, 580,000 newborns have died annually from neonatal tetanus. It can be treated but it is much more cost effective to vaccinate infants and mothers and to use sterile delivery instruments.

**Poliomyelitis** is a viral infection; only 1% of those infected have symptoms. Muscles may become sore and lower limbs paralyzed. There is no cure. In time, a paralyzed limb becomes wasted from lack of use and the person may need crutches. The best prevention is immunization. The United Nations hopes to eradicate polio soon; at the moment, 141 countries have no cases of polio and 46 countries have under 8,000 new cases.

**Tuberculosis** is caused by the bacillus *Mycobacterium tuberculosis*, which is transmitted from one person to another through coughing or sneezing. This infects the lungs. Another route of infection is from the contaminated milk of cows with tuberculosis in places where milk is not pasteurized. The lung infection leads to inflammation and then a calcified lesion that can be detected on an X ray. The infection may take up to 2 years or more to produce symptoms, so it is difficult to eliminate in a community. Treatment requires taking two drugs over 6 months. Thus one means of preventing the spread of tuberculosis is the early detection and treatment of infected people by routine examination of sputum for the bacilli. Another is through vaccination at birth with the BCG vaccine (bacillus of Calmette and Guérin), which may be anywhere from 40% to 70% effective. One third of the world's population is thought to be infected, with 8 million new cases each year and 3 million deaths. Tuberculosis is on the rise.

## Primary Health Care Services

Health services are organized to receive people at the primary health care level, where preventive and curative services are offered. Only if resources are not available at the local level will patients be referred to a regional hospital. **Primary health care** has eight major components, which can be remembered with the French acronym MEDECINS, coined by Charles Larson.

- **M** Maternal and child health, including antenatal care, weighing, delivery
- **E** Education for health
- **D** Essential drugs, referring to the subset of those needed for common diseases
- **E** Endemic disease control, such as malaria control
- **C** Curative services
- **I** Immunization of children for six diseases and mothers for tetanus
- **N** Nutrition
- **S** Safe water and sanitation, such as protecting water sources and using latrines

Future goals have been set to reduce or eliminate most of the major diseases and promote healthy lives through primary health care. One goal is to immunize 90% of infants each year. Another is to make ORS accessible to more than 80% of the population and reduce death from diarrhea by 50%. One cost-effective intervention proposed by the *World Development Report* (World Bank, 1993) would cost $12 per capita per year in a low-income country and reduce the effects of disease by 31% (Mosley, 1994). The package includes immunization, micronutrient supplements, family planning and delivery care, along with treatment of worm infections, tuberculosis, and sexually transmitted diseases. As yet, no concerted action has been taken to adopt this as a policy.

## The Epidemiologist's Hat[1]

Anyone who follows the international health literature must deal with a virtual gauntlet of statistics. These include data on mortality, disease occurrence, important risk factors, and health services use and coverage. How are these figures derived and what do they tell us? To answer these questions and begin to make some sense of the vast quantity

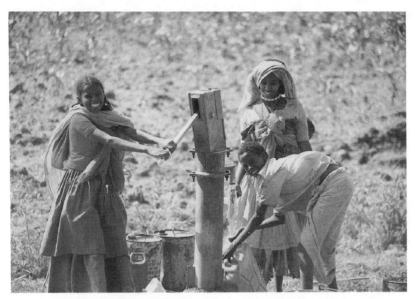

*An important part of preventive health care is the installation of pumps that supply uncontaminated water.*

of published statistical information, a rudimentary knowledge of epidemiological measures is needed. These measures will be grouped under four headings: demographic, mortality, morbidity, and coverage statistics.

*Demographic Statistics*

Let us begin by considering a hypothetical rural district in a Third World country with a population of around 200,000. One of our first requirements as a district health manager will be to put together a health profile that describes the health of the population, identifies important determinants of health and disease, and assesses what resources we have at our disposal to maintain or improve the people's health. Relevant data might already exist in reports. Lacking these, as health manager, we may chose to allocate some of our precious resources to collect the information through a survey, focus group, or observational study.

First, we will need a description of the district's population, usually beginning with a breakdown by age and sex. In most developing countries, there is neither the money nor capacity to carry out a census at the

**TABLE 1.1**  Age and Sex Distribution of a Hypothetical District

| Age | Males Number (%) | Females Number (%) | Total Number (%) |
|---|---|---|---|
| 0–1 | 4,401 (2.20) | 4,443 (2.22) | 8,844 (4.4) |
| 1–4 | 14,555 (7.28) | 15,099 (7.55) | 29,654 (14.8) |
| 5–14 | 28,244 (14.1) | 28,476 (14.2) | 56,720 (28.4) |
| 15–49 | 44,196 (22.1) | 45,366 (22.7) | 89,562 (44.8) |
| 50+ | 6,446 (3.22) | 8,774 (4.39) | 15,220 (7.61) |

district level. Nevertheless, based upon representative **sampling** of the population, we can obtain an **estimate** of the age and sex distribution. We may never know the true distribution; however, if the data sources are taken from samples truly representative of the population as a whole and are adequate in number, then we can have a reasonable **level of confidence** in the estimates provided.

From Table 1.1 it can be seen that nearly half the population is under 15 years of age. If one considers ages 15 to 49 to be the productive years, then a ratio of nonproducers to producers, known as the **dependency ratio,** is 110,438:89,562 = 1.23:1. For every productive member of the population, there are another 1.23 to support.

Other relevant demographic data would include births and deaths. The **crude birthrate (CBR)** is expressed as the number of live births per 1,000 population per year. In Table 1.1, we see that nearly 20% of the population is under 5 years of age. Based on these figures, we can confidently assume that the CBR is high. CBRs will vary within and between countries, ranging from 20 (low) to 50 (high) live births per 1,000 population per year. As a general rule, rural rates will be higher than urban. A closely related figure is the **total fertility rate (TFR).** The TFR estimates the average number of live births a woman can be expected to have during her reproductive lifetime (15 to 49 years of age), assuming that current age-specific rates remain unchanged during that time. In developing country settings, TFRs typically range from 3 (low) to 7 (high) expected live births over a woman's reproductive lifetime. Where CBRs are high, TFRs will also be high.

The **crude death rate (CDR)** is an estimate of the number of deaths per 1,000 population per year. The CDR typically varies between 10 (low) and 20 (high) deaths/1,000 population/year. Assuming there is little in- or out-migration, the *crude growth rate (CGR)* is simply the difference between the CBR and the CDR. Returning to the above example, let us assume that the CBR and CDR estimates from our survey are 48 and 18/1,000 population/year. Thus the CGR = 48-18 = 30/1,000 population/year. This means the population is increasing by 3% per year. The **population doubling time** can be estimated by dividing the CGR into 75, which in this instance equals 25 years. The population of our district will double in 25 years and we will need to plan ahead to cope with such an increase.

*Mortality Statistics*

If the mortality surveys carried out in the district have recorded the age at death, then it is possible to determine several important mortality rates that are used to compare the health of populations. Let us begin with the **infant mortality rate (IMR)**. This is the number of deaths in infants 0 to 12 months of age per 1,000 live births. Using the above figure of 48 as the CBR, we can estimate the number of live births occurring in the district during 1 year to be $48 \times 200{,}000/1{,}000 = 9{,}600$. If, during the same period of time, there were an estimated 936 deaths in children under 12 months of age, then the IMR = $936/9{,}600 \times 1{,}000 = 97.5$. This is an exceptionally high rate, with international comparisons ranging from 5 (very low) to above 100 (very high).

If we have mortality data at all ages and know the number of people in each age grouping (the denominator), then we can calculate *age-specific mortality rates*. For example, if there are 29,654 children 1 to 4 years of age and 404 children in that age group died during the past year, then the 1-4 age-specific mortality rate is

$$\text{ASMR}_{1 \text{ to } 4} = 404/29{,}654/\text{year} \times 1{,}000$$
$$= 13.6 \text{ deaths}/1{,}000 \text{ children 1-4 years of age/year}$$

Age-specific mortality rates are not frequently reported in the international health literature. A much more frequently cited rate, used for international and between-region comparisons, is the **under-5 mortality rate (U5MR)**. The U5MR is an estimate of the cumulative probability of dying before reaching one's fifth birthday. Conversely, 1-U5MR is the cumulative probability of surviving until one's fifth birthday. If we know the ASMRs, then one approach is to add these for each year. The total represents an estimate, for every 1,000 live births in the population, of the number who will die prior to their fifth birthday. The calculation of the U5MR is based upon the assumption that the ASMR will remain unchanged through time. Taking the above information on IMR and ASMR,

$$\begin{aligned} \text{U5MR} &= \text{sum of each year's ASMR} \\ &= \text{IMR}_{year\,1} + \text{ASMR}_{year\,2} + \text{ASMR}_{year\,3} + \text{ASMR}_{year\,4} \\ &= 97.5 + 13.6 + 13.6 + 13.6 \\ &= 138 \text{ deaths by age } 5/1{,}000 \text{ live births} \end{aligned}$$

Internationally, the U5MR ranges from 10 to more than 200—the latter being found under conditions of extreme poverty plus social disorder.

*Morbidity Information*

What are the most important health problems in the district? The importance of a particular problem or disease can be evaluated in terms of its occurrence, severity, and outcome. Taken together, these are a measure of impact.

$$\begin{aligned} \text{Impact} &= \text{Occurrence} \\ &+ \text{Severity} \\ &+ \text{Outcome} \end{aligned}$$

The occurrence of a disease can be measured in terms of its prevalence and incidence. **Prevalence** tells us what proportion of the population is ill and so is a crude measure of the burden of disease in a population. **Incidence** is a measure of the occurrence of new cases over a specified time interval (frequently 1 year). The two measures are related in that disease prevalence is the product of disease incidence times its duration. Diseases that are relatively uncommon, but of longer duration, are best suited to prevalence estimates. Diseases of short duration may be missed at any one point in time, thus the need to measure incidence. If a disease is very frequent, even if short in duration, both prevalence and incidence estimates may be considered.

If we found that acute childhood diarrhea in children under 5 years of age was a common complaint, we might want to determine its occurrence in our hypothetical district in the following ways: (a) The proportion of children having diarrhea at any point in time would be an estimate of the point prevalence. (b) The proportion of children who have now or have had diarrhea over the past 2 weeks would be an estimate of the period prevalence. (c) The number of episodes of diarrhea per child per year would be an estimate of the incidence. It is important to keep in mind that the occurrence of most communicable diseases is affected by the season of the year. It is therefore important to know if all seasons are equally represented in the data collected or if an adjustment has been made to account for these differences during the course of a year.

Once the occurrence of a disease is established, the next question to consider is severity. This will be reflected by disease duration, lost productivity, and functional impairment. In the case of diarrhea, most children will have a self-limiting illness of less than 7 days' duration. Between 5% and 10% will continue to be ill more than 2 weeks. At this point, the illness is defined as persistent (as opposed to acute) childhood diarrhea. Although much less common than acute diarrhea, persistent diarrhea may account for more than one half of all diarrhea-related deaths.

Disease outcomes are assessed in terms of three possibilities: cure, disability, and death. One approach to measuring the relative impact of diseases in a population is to combine disabilities and deaths. Such measures can be further refined by accounting for the age at which death occurs, thus giving greater weight to diseases killing the young (AIDS) as opposed to the old (cardiovascular disease). One example is the measure of **disability adjusted life years (DALYs)** lost, which is the product of two indicators. The first is the number of years lost, calculated by subtracting the age of death or onset of disability from the life expectancy of a healthy person, usually set between 65 and 75. The second is a value from 0 to 1, representing the degree of functional disability, where death receives a maximum value of 1 and minor disabilities are closer to 0. Dementia and blindness receive a disability value of 0.6, while leprosy has a disability value of .22. DALYs provide health planners with an objective measure of the relative impact of specific diseases in the population. The addition of disability to the calculation greatly increases our ability to assess the impact of nonfatal, yet debilitating, diseases such as depression and other mental health disorders (Barker & Green, 1996).

*Health Services Use and Coverage Statistics*

The goal of a health service is to reach people with preventive, curative, and rehabilitative services either by having them visit a health clinic or by having health workers go to rural sites to provide "outreach" services. It is important, then, to know how many people come into contact with our health services. One of the first considerations is to determine what percentage of the population has access. Access will be affected by several factors, including the distance one must travel, the time it takes to reach a health facility, and any costs. Typically, **access** is defined as the percentage of the population living within 10 kilometers (km) of a health facility. In rural districts, access is sometimes very low, with less than 50% of the population within 10 km.

Additional factors affecting use include **acceptability** (satisfaction with the service), **affordability** (direct and indirect costs), **availability** of physical and human resources (e.g., the number of health workers per 1,000 population), and **effectiveness** (Does it work?). **Utilization** rates are measured by determining the number of people who have used the service during a specified period of time. If we tally how many visits were made, we would be inflating the numbers, because some people make many visits. For example, a pregnant mother might come for several prenatal checkups. Consequently, we count only first visits as an index of the number of clients and divide this by the number who have access.

**Coverage** refers to the proportion of the population that has received a particular intervention. It is therefore a measure of how successfully the service has penetrated the population. National and international health organizations use coverage figures to monitor the progress of primary health care. The success of interventions to extend access to safe water, use of oral rehydration, and safe delivery of babies is closely monitored through the indicators seen in Box 1.3.

The most frequently observed example of coverage is estimates of the proportion of children who have received the full complement of vaccinations by 1 year of age (BCG, DPT, + polio × 3, and measles):

$$\text{Coverage}_{\text{under-1 fully immunized}} = \frac{\text{Number fully vaccinated} / \text{year}}{\text{Total children under 1 yr}}$$

Coverage calculations are quite vulnerable to variations in estimates of the denominator, that is, the number of children under 1 year of age eligible to be vaccinated. The most appropriate denominator for international comparisons is the number of births during 1 year (with or

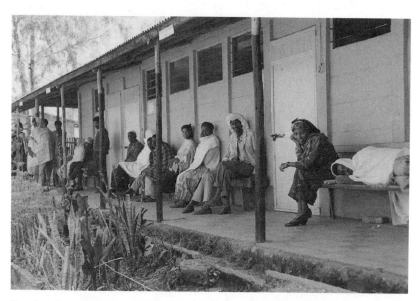

*People who come to a rural health clinic may spend half a day waiting for service.*

without an adjustment for infant mortality). Often coverage calculations are determined on the basis of the number of children with access to health services or relative to a predetermined target population. Obviously, such calculations will result in much higher, more favorable estimates of coverage.

We will be using these measures shortly to evaluate the health of various nations and the success of international efforts to reduce death and disability through childhood immunization. Throughout this book, various health problems will be discussed and it will be important to determine whether or not they are priority problems on which to spend scarce resources. Priority will be given to problems with high impact: those that have high prevalence or incidence, result in pain and suffering, contribute to high mortality rates, and have disabling outcomes. Solutions to these problems must also be evaluated to demonstrate that they work. One of the critical indicators, along with the cost and acceptability of the solution, will be its coverage. It is possible to use the concepts discussed in this section without resorting to their measure-

> **BOX 1.3.**
> **INDICATORS OF HEALTH USE AND COVERAGE RELEVANT TO PRIMARY HEALTH CARE**
>
> *Access to safe water:* Percentage of the population that can reach a protected source of drinking water that is uncontaminated by parasites and bacteria.
>
> *Access to adequate sanitation:* Percentage of the population that has household waste disposal facilities such as a latrine and garbage pit.
>
> *Fully immunized 1-year-old children:* Percentage of all 1-year-old children who have been immunized for tuberculosis, diphtheria, pertussis, tetanus, polio, and measles. (More than 120 million babies born each year need to receive vaccinations on five occasions during their first year.)
>
> *ORT use rate:* Percentage of all cases of diarrhea in children under 5 years of age treated with oral rehydration salts (the UNICEF sachet) or an appropriate household solution of salt, sugar, water, and sometimes porridge.
>
> *Births attended by a trained health worker:* Percentage of deliveries made by someone trained in obstetric care, as opposed to deliveries made by relatives or traditional attendants who do not follow sterile procedures.
>
> *Breast-feeding:* Percentage of children who are exclusively breast-fed from 0 to 3 months, breast-fed along with solid food (6-9 months), and breast-fed for up to 2 years (20-23 months).
>
> *Contraceptive prevalence rate:* Percentage of married women aged 15-49 years currently using contraception.

ment definition; however, if we are to make international comparisons and monitor solutions implemented in different locations, we need to agree on a set of definitions—conceptual and numerical.

The International Organizer's Hat

"Where in the world is PNG?" asked one student. PNG stands for Papua New Guinea and it can be found near Indonesia and Australia. For the sake of organizing information about world health, most people use the regions and categories of the U.N. agencies. The annual UNICEF report on the state of the world's children provides information about each of 150 countries (plus 40 less populous ones in a separate table).

The 150 countries are organized into groups for which summary statistics are also given. One group comprises the 22 industrialized countries, sometimes referred to as the (more) developed countries. Another group, called countries in transition, includes the 27 former Soviet bloc countries, which have seen drastic declines in health since 1990. The largest group consists of the 101 developing countries. These countries are also divided into five regions: sub-Saharan Africa (40), Middle East and North Africa (17), South Asia (7), East Asia and Pacific (15), and Latin America and Caribbean (22). For special attention, data are sometimes aggregated for 36 least developed countries, those in the developing countries group who fit the following criteria: per capita gross domestic product of U.S.$765 or less; low quality of life index based on literacy, school enrollment, supply of calories, and life expectancy; low economic diversification index; and population of 75 million or less.

Does it matter how countries are organized? To develop coherent solutions for health problems, people look at countries with similar problems and similar resources. The organization described uses level of economic development and geography to group countries because these two variables allow for a somewhat crude indication of problems and resources. There are many anomalies within such a system; Singapore and Hong Kong have per capita gross national products (GNP) that are as high as industrialized countries, along with excellent health and education levels, yet they are grouped with developing countries. One way of avoiding complaints about how countries are labeled is to group solely by geography. The problem with this organization is that regional summary figures mask huge differences between countries. For the moment, then, most documents provide summary figures for countries grouped according to development and geography.

Table 1.2 shows how countries are grouped. It also provides information about population (millions) and per capita gross national product (in U.S. dollars) for a few countries (UNICEF, 1996). You might look up information about other countries in the six regions.

The international community contributes money and expertise to promote health around the world. **Official development assistance**

**TABLE 1.2** Regional Groupings Along With Population and GNP Figures for Some Countries

|  | Least Developed | Developing | In Transition | Industrialized |
|---|---|---|---|---|
| **Sub-Saharan Africa** | Ethiopia 53.4 million $100 | Senegal 8.1 million $750 | | |
| **Middle East and North Africa** | Yemen 13.9 million $520 | Egypt 61.6 million $660 | | Israel 5.5 million $13,920 |
| **South and Central Asia** | Bangladesh 117.8 million $220 | India 918.6 million $300 | Uzbekistan 22.4 million $970 | |
| **East Asia and Pacific** | Cambodia 10.0 million $200 | China 1,208.8 million $490 | | Japan 124.8 million $31,490 |
| **Latin America, Caribbean, and North America** | Haiti 7.0 million $370 | Brazil 159.1 million $2,930 | | United States 260.6 million $24,740 |
| **Europe** | | | Ukraine 51.5 million $2,210 | Germany 81.3 million $23,560 |

(ODA) is the amount of money given by a government for aid and development. Although a target of 0.7% of the donor's GNP was set in 1969, most countries continue to give less. Nonetheless, approximately $40 billion in assistance goes from donor governments to recipient governments each year. Add to this $20 billion or so given by the United Nations and nongovernmental organizations. Money and other resources are given for two types of assistance: aid and development. **Aid** refers to emergency, life-saving interventions that are not intended to be sustained whereas **development** refers to interventions that are intended to be sustainable, such as skill training and resource building. Of the $60 billion given in ODA, $48 billion is aid and only $12 billion goes to development. The least developed countries receive $6 billion in assistance for development, as opposed to aid, and only 10% of this goes to health. Of the three major types of organizations involved in disbursing funds and expertise, the United Nations provides only $10-$12 billion, but it often sets the standards and coordinates the action.

*How Is the United Nations Involved?*

Several U.N. bodies have been created to coordinate the goals and activities of health development around the world. The most well known is UNICEF, the United Nations Children's Fund. It has visibility through campaigns to raise money through Halloween boxes and Christmas card sales. It is also very visible in the developing countries where it promotes child health and pays for specific activities such as immunization. The World Health Organization (WHO) is the body that examines world health problems and provides leadership in solving these problems through technical cooperation and technology transfer. In addition, two U.N. agencies are not primarily associated with health but their impact on health is large—namely, the World Bank and the U.N. Development Program. The World Bank has recently seen the development of health as an essential component of social and economic development; consequently, it *loans* money to countries for specific health projects. Finally, the U.N. Development Program (UNDP) tries to coordinate all U.N. funds and projects found in a particular country so that they work toward the development goals set by the country.

*UNICEF.* The United Nations Children's Fund is a U.N. agency with a mandate to improve the lives of children. It has focused on children's health, nutrition, and education in developing countries. Although its headquarters are in New York, each country has a local office staffed by local professionals where "situation analyses" and decisions are made concerning field operations. In this respect, UNICEF works closely with in-country services, specifically the ministry of health and its primary health care priorities. However, for a variety of reasons, UNICEF has recently been focusing on a few short-term goals instead of employing the broad-based approach it took initially. Government and individual donors, for example, want to see that their money is being spent well and is producing results. Of the

U.S.$900 million raised each year by UNICEF (with approximately one third going to health), only 35% is mandated by the United Nations; 35% comes through negotiations with donor governments, and 30% comes from public fund-raising activities (LaFond, 1994). Not everyone is happy with this focused approach, because they feel that political agendas should not override criteria based on humanitarian values. However, scarce resources in developing countries may be more effectively used if focused on a few simple, inexpensive activities.

The focused approach was taken in the 1980s when UNICEF adopted the GOBI strategy (growth monitoring, oral rehydration, breast-feeding, and immunization), and then in the late 1980s it concentrated on immunization alone. The Expanded Program on Immunization (EPI) had the goal of 80% coverage of the world's children by the year 1990. UNICEF's role was to issue general guidelines and targets to national ministries of health, provide a cold chain of refrigerators along with the vaccines, give money for fuel needed to travel to outreach sites, and pay health workers for the time they spent on immunization activities. The name and logo of UNICEF is also sufficiently well known in developing countries to mobilize leaders and communities in a concerted effort to meet the target. During a 10-year period, UNICEF invested U.S.$600 million in immunization activities.

The immunization program was evaluated by Kim-Farley (1993) as a success. The coverage, or percentage of children under 1 year who were fully immunized—meaning three doses of DPT (diphtheria, pertussis, tetanus) and poliomyelitis vaccine—increased from 5% in 1974 to 20% in 1981 to 80% in 1990. Most of the increase took place in the 5 last years of the campaign. The 80% level has been maintained into the mid-1990s even by developing countries. This means that 80% of approximately 100 million infants each year are being immunized. UNICEF claims that this level of coverage saves the lives of 3 million children who would otherwise die from the six diseases. It also claims that if polio is eradicated the way smallpox was, even the developed countries will save hundreds of millions of dollars because there will be no need to vaccinate their own children. The cost-effectiveness of this intervention can be measured in terms of the money we need to invest to gain a disability-free year of life (DALY)—less than $1 per DALY (Kim-Farley, 1993).

There were some major exceptions to this success story. Countries in sub-Saharan Africa immunized 52% of their infants in 1991 and the figure has not increased since. Many countries, such as Chad with 18% and Zaire with 29%, still have very low percentages, while a few such as Kenya, Zimbabwe, Botswana, and South Africa have reached 80%. As a consequence, under-5 mortality has also remained higher in sub-Saharan Africa, where 177 out of 1,000 children die before the age of 5. Some would say that UNICEF was wrong in using a top-down approach and isolating the immunization program from an integrated health system. Others argue that nothing is served, especially not children, by waiting for communities to organize and to see immunization as a priority. Furthermore, in practice, immunization is often integrated with other services; health workers who immunize at an outreach site (receiving money for fuel and time) use the opportunity to do other maternal and child health activities and discuss family planning. The organization needed to get community leaders involved, motivate health workers, mobilize school children to inform mothers, and provide mothers with reminders worked during the campaign years and has remained in place to promote other health activities.

*Local and International
Nongovernmental Organizations*

Nongovernmental organizations (NGOs) are not part of a national government or an international agency but they have some form of permanent organization with a central office. Their goals are to promote development, whether it is economic, education, or health. In the health field, they train community health workers, help to create and monitor the quality of a national pharmaceutical industry, dig safe water sources, and carry out many other activities. Only a few are involved in emergency relief, although, like Doctors Without Borders, they tend to get the most media attention. Institutions such as universities are involved in international work; they have training, as well as development, as one of their objectives. Most people refer to such organizations and institutions simply as NGOs. They operate in one or more developing countries on the basis of a written agreement outlining the purposes and procedures. NGOs spend an estimated U.S.$8 billion a year on long-term development, and the figure has been rising. They raise this through donations, income generation, contracts, and government funding agencies. In the United States alone, there are more than 175 registered NGOs, and one of the largest, CARE US, has more than a million donors. Most NGOs are nonprofit. They conduct their activities in specific villages, often in partnership with a local NGO or a group of citizens who have the same goals. NGOs are therefore the ones who most often are trying to find local solutions for global problems.

In conclusion, there are many international groups involved in health: governments, the United Nations, and nongovernmental organizations. Their efforts and those of people living and working in developing countries will be presented throughout this book.

## STUDENT ACTIVITY

Each student will choose a developing country to research, as if he or she were the health representative for that country. By looking up the relevant WHO and UNICEF documents, each student can complete a table with statistics relevant to the health of the nation. From this, students should be able to identify priority problems, using magnitude and severity figures, and identify solutions that are feasible given the country's resources.

## NOTE

1. "The Epidemiologist's Hat" section was written by Charles P. Larson, epidemiologist and physician.

# 2

# SOCIAL SCIENCE MEASURES FOR HEALTH RESEARCH

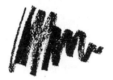

The chapters in this book cover health problems and solutions for which behavior is a critical element. Much of the information described here comes from researchers who used a combination of measures to help them understand the full scope of the problem. On the one hand, to assess people's health and illness, they may use biochemical or clinical techniques. When the goal is to study the health of rural people in developing countries, the measures must be simple, inexpensive, and easy to administer. New techniques that do not require sophisticated training and equipment are continually being developed for these purposes. On the other hand, to assess behavior and the social environment, social science methods of measurement are used. This chapter describes some of the more commonly used ones: focus group discussions, participant and nonparticipant observation, key informant interviews, and structured self-report questionnaires. The goal will be to encourage you, the reader, to become personally involved in learning how to measure social science variables. A tailored version of this chapter, along with others devoted to conducting health research in developing countries, is published in manual form and has been the basis of workshops in several countries (Aboud, 1997).

Certain researchers prefer in-depth data collected through participant observation; others prefer structured survey questionnaires that yield quantifiable data. My preference is for quantifiable data, regardless of the measure. I have seen data from most of these measures put into code and number form for statistical analysis. Not everyone believes this to be feasible or desirable. However, most people believe that there are strengths and limitations to all the measures, and that a good project will include several. Each will have a different purpose. For example, in-depth interviews with focus groups or key informants will be used to collect information on the way people categorize types of childhood diarrhea and the treatment they use for each. A representative sample of people will then be asked specific questions about the nature of the latest episode in their family and the treatment they used, to find out how many mothers use each treatment and in what order. Observation will be used to see how mothers make food and drink for an ill child. That information might then be related to the outcome—whether the child died, got worse, or improved. On the basis of this information, a program to promote oral rehydration salts will be developed and evaluated.

## SOCIAL SCIENCE VARIABLES

At least four types of social science variables are commonly used in international health research. They can be measured through any of the means just mentioned, depending on whether the purpose is to discover details on context and meaning or to discover reliable figures on events, behaviors, and their relation. Here are examples of health-related variables that social scientists might study:

*(1) Psychosocial variables as risk and protective factors.* Psychosocial variables include demographic variables such as education of the mother, socioeconomic status, family size, religion, ethnicity, marital status, family stress, literacy skills, and social support. Many, such as religion, have conventional measures. However, sometimes the conventional measure can be improved. A mother's education, for

example, is an important protective factor for her children's health; this is usually measured as years of school completed. What is perhaps most important is her functional literacy, which can be measured by giving her a text to read, such as a health message, and assessing her reading and comprehension.

Socioeconomic status is more problematic. It can depend on a family's income, the education level of the head of the household, and the social influence of the family. For an unsalaried family, such as one engaged in subsistence farming, the amount of produce or the number of oxen may be a good proxy. An alternative would be to ask key informants in the community to categorize families according to their perceived status in the community.

*(2) Health behaviors.* The term **health behavior** refers to actions that directly or indirectly affect your health or someone else's. This includes exercise, alcohol consumption, protected sex, taking steps to limit or space childbirths, eating well, and using the services of health workers. Not all potential health behaviors actually affect one's health; their impact must be demonstrated by showing a statistical relation to health.

*(3) Psychosocial antecedents and consequences.* We often overlook the fact that our behavior may be sparked by a reminder or incentive, and may furthermore elicit positive and negative reactions from others. Sometimes what is important is the actual event that precedes or follows our behavior; more often it is our interpretation of the event that matters. For example, what young adults think their chances of getting HIV are may differ from what their chances actually are. Thoughts and impulses, not objective probabilities, guide sexual behavior! The consequences of behavior have a particularly powerful effect on whether or not the behavior is repeated. Even expecting disapproval from family and friends might be enough to stop us from trying a behavior in the first place.

Examples of antecedents of health behavior are reminders of vaccination days, advertisements for products such as oral rehydration salts, media messages, knowledge, attitudes, and a community's decision to protect their water. Examples of consequences of health behaviors are respectful treatment by a health worker, criticism from a spouse for talking about contraception, community recognition for families of immunized infants, and recovery from illness after receiving oral rehydration.

*(4) Mental and social well-being.* Mental and social well-being are two important components of health as defined by the WHO. They include not only the absence of problems such as mental disorders, alcohol abuse, antisocial isolation, and violence but also the progress toward fulfilment of work and family role obligations, participation in social activities, and social-emotional competence. Standardized, structured questionnaires have been developed and are discussed in the relevant chapters.

## QUALITATIVE AND QUANTITATIVE METHODS

Overview and Comparison

Both qualitative and quantitative methods are used by social scientists. An example of a qualitative method is a focus group discussion on attitudes toward contraception and reasons that people use or do not use it. An example of a quantitative method is a prevalence survey of contraception use, attitudes toward contraceptives, and the value of children. Although qualitative and quantitative methods are not mutually exclusive, people tend to use the term *qualitative* to refer to, among others, focus group discussions, participant observation, and key informant interviews. They use the term *quantitative* to refer to systematic nonparticipant observation, structured questionnaires, and standardized tests.

As the names imply, qualitative methods emphasize in-depth descriptive information whereas quantitative methods rely on information that can be statistically analyzed. Beyond this simple distinction, one could say that **qualitative methods** provide rich descriptive information about a community or about individuals, usually accompanied by information about the context in which they function. This is particularly useful when the researcher lacks an understanding of the phenomenon or its importance and cannot yet formulate propositions to be tested with statistics. **Quantitative methods** are particularly appropriate when the quantity of a phenomenon is of interest, such as prevalence, severity, distribution across a population, frequency of a behavior, intensity of an attitude, and the norm of a group, especially when the purpose is to evaluate the association between two variables.

Table 2.1 outlines some important characteristics of qualitative and quantitative methods, using participant observation as a typical qualitative method and structured survey questionnaires as a typical quantitative method. The two are compared on a number of dimensions, such as the purpose (i.e., what kind of information is needed), sampling (i.e., from whom), who drives the measurement procedure, the role of the data collector, the locus of bias, and other interpretation issues. Certain methods are similar to qualitative ones when it comes to sampling but similar to quantitative ones in the choice of a standardized measure. Whatever methods you choose, you should ask yourself how they fit each dimension.

Many research questions will require several methods to be satisfactorily answered. Thus qualitative and quantitative methods can be used sequentially, to build on each other, or simultaneously, to support and cross-validate the other's findings. For example, sometimes questionnaires are given to people immediately before they participate in a focus group discussion; answering the questions brings to each participant's mind his or her personal experiences with the topic being discussed. More often, focus group or key informant interviews will precede the development of a structured questionnaire; qualitative data provide the questionnaire developers with information about appropriate terms to use, relevant behaviors, and an exhaustive list of response options (e.g., Bentley et al., 1988; Scrimshaw, Carballo, Ramos, & Blair, 1991). Others use both kinds of methods simultaneously—each measuring what it is best at—to assess different variables. Their relation to each other and to the health outcome is then examined (e.g., Graeff, Elder, & Booth, 1993; Green & Lewis, 1986; Steckler, McLeroy, Goodman, Bird, & McCormick, 1992).

Distinctions between the two methods blur on a number of dimensions. One dimension is quantifiability of the data; a second is generalizability of the data. For example, one of the strengths of quantitative methods is that verbal and behavioral responses can be given a number; this allows for data reduction and statistical analysis. However, it is also

**TABLE 2.1** A Comparison of Qualitative and Quantitative Methods

|  | *Qualitative* | *Quantitative* |
|---|---|---|
| **Purpose** | Discover relevant behaviors | Prediction |
|  | Intelligibility | Prevalence and associations |
|  | Provide context information | Control extraneous information |
|  | Describe terms, process | Evaluate outcome |
| **Synthesis versus analysis** | Holistic understanding | Separate components |
|  | Respondents' perspective | Statistical relation |
| **Sampling** | Small sample | Large sample |
|  | Purposely selected | Representative of demography |
|  | Stop when data repetitive | Preselected to be unbiased |
| **Questions** | Determined by respondent | Predetermined by researcher |
| **Response categories** | Determined by respondent | Predetermined and fixed |
|  | Semi- or unstructured | Structured |
| **Reliable (interobserver)** | Rarely evaluated | Usually very good |
| **Validity of responses** | Usually very good | Must be demonstrated |
| **Role of data collector** | Highly educated | High school educated |
|  | Integrate theory & data | Trained to administer measure |
|  | Personally involved | Attentive, neutral, consistent |
| **Interpretation of responses** | Biased by researcher who writes report | Biased by respondent who interprets question |
| **Locus of researcher bias** | Interpreting responses | Selecting questions and responses |
| **Locus of respondent bias** | Choice of words | Interpreting question |
|  |  | Social desirability |
| **Generalizable** | Only if replicated | Only if proper sampling |
| **Compare with other data** | Difficult unless comparable response categories used | Yes |
| **Quantify for statistical tests** | Generally not done | Yes |
| **Cost, effort, time** | At the end to code and describe responses | At the start to develop, pretest, and revise measure |

possible to assign numbers to the output from qualitative research, using a coding scheme, and to conduct statistical analyses (Huberman & Miles, 1994; Jones & Hunter, 1995; Richards & Richards, 1994). Another strength of quantitative methods is the opportunity to calculate rates and means, because the number and nature of respondents can be specified. This allows one to estimate whether a health behavior is common or rare in the population sampled. If the sample is representative of a larger population, then the rates and means can be generalized to the population. If the sample is not representative, then the study can be replicated with another sample and the rates and means compared. Normally, rates and means are not calculated on data from focus groups; however, it is entirely possible to do so. Sample size can be determined with focus groups by using either the number of groups or the number of people in a group. If, for example, fear of sterility as a result of taking contraceptives is mentioned in 40 out of 50 focus groups, the rate of 80% would be very informative. The other side of the coin is that structured questionnaires have been made more informative by incorporating some of the open-ended questions used by qualitative researchers. Observation of behaviors in their natural context is also recognized by quantitative researchers as a more accurate way to assess health behaviors than self-report surveys. Thus researchers are learning how to incorporate the strengths of one method into the other (see Box 2.1 on the "rapid researcher").

## FOCUS GROUP DISCUSSION

A **focus group** is a group of people with similar backgrounds brought together to talk about a specific topic of interest under the guidance of a moderator. The moderator facilitates discussion among the participants while keeping them on the topic. The moderator encourages participants to express their perceptions and opinions using two strategies: posing open-ended questions and letting people respond to ideas expressed by other group members. The goal is to get as many people as possible to express their different perceptions; the goal is *not* to bring about agreement. Descriptions of this method are found in Fontana and Frey (1994), Morgan (1992), Moulton and Roberts (1993), Rasmuson, Seidel, Smith, and Booth (1988).

## BOX 2.1.
## THE RAPID RESEARCHER

Anthropologists are known for their careful, in-depth study of different cultures. Participant observation has been the tool of their trade, supplemented with key informant interviews. To understand a culture thoroughly, one has to live in it for many years. For example, it might take 5 years to measure the socioeconomic status of people in a community, because you first have to discover the bases of economic, social, and political power. When I asked a friend if it couldn't be measured more quickly, he gave the stock reply, "Garbage in, garbage out," meaning quick and sloppy measures give you useless information. Without intending any disrespect to the community, a health researcher might have another purpose in mind, namely, to see if the health problem is confined to people of lower status so that their particular living conditions can be examined and altered. Some would argue that an in-depth understanding of the basis of status is not necessary to determine whether SES is related to the health problem in a community—although an in-depth understanding might be necessary if you wanted to change it. Another example of a situation that calls for a more focused approach is when an epidemic or an endemic condition is severely affecting many people. Anthropologists have recently devised a number of more rapid techniques for collecting data in the field. These include group interviews, nonparticipant observation, and individual interviews with community members, not just elite, key informants (Manderson & Aaby, 1992). The assessment has become more of a community participation activity in which neighborhood groups gather to identify problems and devise solutions. Local people are trained to coordinate and conduct the assessment, in place of the professional anthropologist. These new directions are more compatible with the methods used by psychologists to measure social and behavioral variables relevant to health (Dasen, Berry, & Sartorius, 1988; Lonner & Berry, 1986; Schneiderman & Tapp, 1985). For their part, epidemiologists have helped speed up the process of identifying representative samples of people, which is called cluster sampling. At this point, it appears that our disciplinary differences have all but disappeared in the area of measurement, for the sake of collecting valid information quickly and efficiently. Following are three examples of Rapid Assessment Procedures (RAP):

> *HealthCom's Child Survival Project* (Graeff et al., 1993): This project used a diverse set of quantitative methods to collect community data on childhood diarrhea and mothers' care of sick children as well as qualitative methods to find out how easily mothers understood the concept of germ and their reaction to new ways of coping with childhood diarrhea. They used the data to develop new strategies for increasing mothers' use of ORS.
>
> *AIDS Rapid Assessment Procedures* (Scrimshaw et al., 1991): The Social and Behavioral Research unit of the World Health Organization's Global Programme on AIDS (now UNAIDS) has prepared materials to collect data on patterns of behavior related to HIV and AIDS. They include most of the methods described in this chapter to gather information on sexual behavior, nonsexual modes of transmission, knowledge, and attitudes.
>
> *BASIC's Toolkit* (Roberts, Pareja, Shaw, & Boyd, 1996): This is a how-to collection of measurement tools for gathering, evaluating, and organizing the information necessary to make decisions about health promotion. The tools have been developed and used in many developing countries. They include tools for identifying problems and solutions, gathering information, using local resources, identifying who and what behavior can be changed, selecting and implementing communication strategies, and evaluating the outcomes.

In contrast to personal interviews, focus group discussions result in respondents being provoked by one another to express their ideas. People may be more willing to elaborate on their opinions and experiences in the presence of supportive peers. In contrast to participant observation, the discussion is more structured because the moderator begins with a specific topic and some questions.

Purpose

What kind of information is usefully obtained from focus group discussions? Focus groups can provide information on the importance, relevance, and range of health behaviors related to a specific issue. Once you have this information, you could use it to develop a structured questionnaire, knowing that you have included all the important and relevant behaviors. You could also use this kind of information to help interpret inconsistent or unexpected data from a survey. For example, after receiving survey results showing that many women like modern contraception but few use it, you might convene a focus group to help you explain the discrepancy. They might tell you that it is valuable only for other women who want to stop having babies but is dangerous for women like themselves who want more children.

Strengths

Focus groups give you information in the language of ordinary people rather than in the language of the researcher. They save time and money because you are interviewing about eight people at one time. People often provide more detailed and honest information when talking with their peers because the discussion puts them at ease, arouses their interest, and jogs their memory, which allows for the emergence of new information that can be pursued with probing questions. In summary, the strengths of focus groups are as follows:

- Laypersons' language is used for terms.
- The process is efficient in terms of time and money.
- The process allows collection of more detailed information.
- The process allows for new insights.

Limitations

The opinions expressed are not necessarily representative of the group, much less the community. People with strong opinions and a strong voice will be heard more often than people who are shy, but this does not mean that their opinions are more common. Conclusions about the prevalence of an opinion are not possible because participants have not been systematically and privately asked if they agree or disagree with the opinion. Another potential problem is the tendency for people to avoid the disapproval of their peers by agreeing with them; steps can be taken to minimize "groupthink." Sensitive, private topics cannot be discussed in a group of familiar people. In summary, the limitations of focus groups are as follows:

- Comments may not be representative of the group.
- Comments may not be representative of the community.

- There may be group conformity.
- There may be reluctance to discuss sensitive topics

Participants

You are advised to include six to ten people in a group, ensure that the members of a group are strangers to each other but homogeneous in demographic characteristics and experience, and convene four to six groups to collect enough information. Participants are purposely selected, often because they are opinionated and articulate, not because they are representative of the community.

These are rules of thumb that should be broken to suit the purpose of the research (Morgan, 1992). Larger groups may be intimidating to some people, although they allow for more opinions to be aired. Smaller groups give each member a chance to say more. Strangers are less reluctant to express disagreement and disclose private experiences, but this may be impossible in a small community. Homogeneity in age, sex, and education often create enough similarity in experience and interest to allow for a stimulating discussion. Similarity in background ensures that members will be provoked by each other's comments. However, you want people to have different opinions and behaviors. The number of groups to convene is highly variable. Some researchers suggest you stop whenever the comments start to become repetitive and no new insights are gained. Others, who want to use the focus group to cross-validate survey data, will collect data from as many as 50 groups. The replication of data across groups and across methods enhances their validity.

Procedure

The group meets in a neutral site so that the context does not constrain people. People usually sit in a semicircle so that everyone feels equally a part. The moderator of the group guides the discussion. The moderator may be the researcher but obviously will be someone who is fluent in the local language yet not too familiar to the participants. The moderator can be less involved and more of an observer if participants are opinionated and articulate and if the purpose of the group is to explore spontaneous ideas. The moderator will be more directive if people are reticent, if the discussion becomes disorganized and digresses from the topic, and if the purpose is to generate information on specific issues. The moderator needs to have certain social skills to manage group dynamics while focusing on issues, such as being attentive, accepting, empathic, nonjudgmental, and flexible. To ensure that all sides of the issue are covered, the moderator needs to encourage all participants to talk openly, discourage certain members from dominating, repeat a person's opinion to ask if others agree or disagree, present alternatives not mentioned to gauge agreement or disagreement, and gently redirect the discussion if it digresses or becomes repetitive. People are not asked to justify or explain their opinions, simply to express them.

The procedure lasts about 60 minutes. It starts with the moderator and participants introducing themselves. The moderator states the reason for inviting people. It should be stated here that the purpose is to hear as many different opinions as possible, as long as they are honest thoughts and feelings. The moderator then begins to guide the discussion with a set of eight or so preplanned questions that cover the topic, then repeats the question, alters the order, and probes for further information if required.

For example, a discussion on family planning might begin with the question: Do you know how many children you and your husband (or wife) want, and do you ever feel you might want to stop? Other questions might be as follows: What do you do when you want to stop for a while or for good? What do you do when you and your spouse disagree on limiting babies? Why might you be afraid to stop having babies? If only a few people answer the question, the moderator can prod others by saying something like the following: Some people have said they don't think about a number; they just have children. What do the rest of you have to say about that? The moderator could also introduce a new opinion and ask participants for their views: Some people I talk to say they want ten children and others say they want two. Why?

Data Collection

The discussion is recorded on an audiotape as well as by an assistant who takes notes. The assistant sits in an unobtrusive position outside the group and takes notes on who says what. Speakers should be identified by code names rather than their real ones to keep the record anonymous. Nonverbal reactions of listeners can also be informative. This is carefully explained to the group before beginning.

Data Analysis

This will depend on what kind of information you want to get from the groups. Here are some possibilities.

*(1) Taxonomies and lists.* You can generate a list of all the different reasons people give for using and for not using contraception.

*(2) Importance of an issue.* You can estimate how important an issue seemed by noting how much time was spent discussing it and how many people expressed an opinion.

*(3) Frequency distribution.* You can classify responses to a question and count the number of people who fit a certain response; for example, three of the group members said they had discussed the desired number of children with their husband, four said they did not, and one did not comment.

*(4) Global evaluations.* Several independent assistants can listen to the tape or read the record and rate the group on several evaluative dimensions, such as involvement versus indifference, positive versus negative views, knowledgeable versus naive, homogeneous versus heterogeneous views, personal decision versus family decision. They make their ratings on five-point bipolar Likert scales:

negative    1    2    3    4    5    positive

*(5) Interobserver reliability.* You can ask another person to listen to the tape or read the record of the discussion. The percentage of answers classified similarly by two such observers indicates the degree of reliability.

*(6) Comparisons across groups.* Lists and frequencies can be compared, for example, to find out if husbands and wives raise the same concerns about contraception.

## SYSTEMATIC NONPARTICIPANT OBSERVATION

**Systematic observation** in a natural setting involves planned, methodical, objective observation of events in their sequence and in their natural context. In contrast to the participant observer, the nonparticipant one does not attempt to experience the activities being observed and does not develop relationships with the people being observed. Another difference is that many people will be observed in comparable contexts so that rates can be calculated and statistical analyses performed.

The observations are recorded in more or less detail, depending on the specificity of the research question. In an exploratory study, the observer might want to write down everything observed so as not to miss potentially important behaviors, conversations, and consequences. If prior information leads you to suspect the importance of certain variables, the record may be selective. Thus at one extreme is the fully descriptive recording of observations, including the physical space, the actors, the general activity, the objects, and the specific actions of people. At the other extreme is selective observations of how frequently specific actions are performed by specific people in specific places. An example of the latter is how often mothers wash their hands with soap while doing household chores, or how often children use the latrine or the bushes to urinate/defecate during school hours. Descriptions of this method are given by Aboud and Alemu (1995), Graeff et al. (1993), Rasmuson et al. (1988), and Weick (1968).

Purpose

What kind of information is usefully obtained through systematic observation? This method is useful when you want to measure a specific event, such as hand washing, beer drinking, nurse-mother interaction, group problem solving. The researcher has usually selected beforehand the physical settings and the actors of interest. The method is also useful for describing events that people do not articulate well because they carry out the process habitually without much thought, because they do not often put it into words, or because they cannot remember all the details. As an alternative to self-report, it is a more accurate record of complex behaviors and is uncontaminated by the respondent's memory and other biases.

Strengths

One advantage of nonparticipant observation is that health behaviors and other observable events can be described in great detail because the observer has no duties other than to observe and record. It maintains the natural sequence of events as well as the contextual antecedents and consequences of the behavior. The record is less subject to observer biases when it is created concurrently and when there is no emotional involvement in the activity. Nonprofessionals can be trained to observe and record reliably. The record is also less subject to participant biases such as memory loss, self-deception, and social desirability. Interobserver reliability can be evaluated during training by having two observers record the same events. Reliability across time and generalization across samples can be examined if contexts are comparable. The data are more amenable to statistical analysis, for example, by coding each unit of observation according to a set of finite categories and analyzing the frequency counts for each category. This means that communities can be compared and statistical relations between events can be inferred. In summary, the strengths are as follows:

- The process provides detailed information.
- Natural sequence and setting are used.
- The process minimizes some observer biases.
- Nonprofessionals can be trained.
- The process minimizes some participant biases.
- Reliability and generalization of data are possible.
- The process is amenable to quantification and statistics.

Limitations

One disadvantage is that the observer must be unobtrusive enough not to interfere with the ongoing activity. People may not be used to strangers recording their actions and may feel uncomfortable at first. However, if the observer is present for a long time, people will usually ignore him or her and carry on as usual; familiar community members should always be trained to do the observing. Because the nonparticipant observer does not question people about their actions or their understanding of events, only the observable events themselves are clues to their meaning. Private events cannot usually be studied this way. The limitations therefore are as follows:

- There may be observer influences.
- There may be omission of subjective meaning of events.
- The process is limited to public events.

Participants

Participants are identified beforehand according to certain criteria. You may decide to observe all interactions between nurses and women attending a family planning clinic during a 2-week period or all women who collect water at five different sites. The criteria here are location and gender. Another option is to randomly or systematically sample from a village to observe for 1 hour mother-child interactions or mothers' hand washing. You may observe mothers make an oral rehydration solution and compare those who did and did not participate in health education. The criteria here are households of mothers with children under 5 years. You determine the number of participants according to sampling procedures to eliminate errors in statistical inferences. Unlike the participants in focus groups, you do not select these ones for their homogeneity, or for the new insights they can provide, but according to criteria and numbers specified beforehand.

Procedure

The procedure consists of an observer taking up an unobtrusive position in the setting and recording events. As an observer, you need to position yourself away from the activity so as not to be seen by participants. However, you need to be able to see and hear the event and its context. You need sufficient training to record events reliably before starting.

Depending on the research question, an observer will record more or less of what is observed. You will decide on this beforehand so that the observer does not need to make such judgments in the field. If you are trying to discover new insights or new explanations, you would want a narrative record. A narrative record includes details of events as they unfold in their natural sequence. Contextual events that precede and follow are also recorded. The time of day (hour: minute) may be written next to the event to indicate its duration and the interval between events. A framework for organizing the data may be partially in place before data collection, but a complete list of codes and categories is developed after (Aboud & Alemu, 1995).

Sometimes the record includes information about a limited number of specific events. Specific events or behaviors are listed on the record, having previously been explicitly defined; as an observer, you check them off whenever they occur and note their duration and the consequence. For example, observers at a health clinic recorded the following health worker behaviors: greets mother, asks mother about her child, asks mother open-ended question, praises mother, asks mother closed-ended question, demonstrates mixing ORS, and has mother demonstrate mixing ORS (Graeff et al., 1993).

Describing the Data

The narrative record requires application of a framework after the data collection to summarize the data. Observations are usually summarized in a way that allows for quantification. For example, the domain is broken down into a finite set of categories, each well defined, that exhaustively cover that domain. Each observation unit is then coded in terms of one category. Frequencies for each category can then be statistically analyzed. For example, the number of mothers greeted by a health worker and the number of mothers shown how to mix ORS are important data; these numbers can be converted to rates if divided by the total number of mothers attending the clinic. Complex categories describing sequences of events can also be used (e.g., health worker poses question, mother responds, health worker acknowledges response with speech or gesture).

When frequencies for certain events, such as breast-feeding episodes, are available, they can be cross-tabulated by demographic variables such as age and sex of child, age and education of mother, and child malnutrition. These frequencies can be examined for statistical association (Richards & Richards, 1994).

## Student Activity:
## Practice your skills at observing

This activity allows you to observe a group problem-solving discussion. You will practice your skills at observing others as they attempt to develop a KAP questionnaire. KAP questionnaires are commonly used in surveys to assess people's *knowledge, attitudes, and practices* in a specific health domain, such as AIDS or child feeding. Divide the class into groups of six: Four will develop the KAP items, and two will independently observe and record everything the group says and does while completing their task.

*KAP task.* Develop a KAP questionnaire on a topic of interest, such as high-risk HIV behavior or diet. Create four or five items to measure each of the following: practice, attitude, and knowledge. Indicate how you would score each answer. You have 20 minutes.

*Systematic observation.* Two observers will position themselves apart from the group but close enough to see and hear everything that transpires. Never talk. Listen and record the group's activities, using the following column headings (time specification may not be necessary here). Your record might look like this:

| Time | Speaker | To Whom | Words or Actions |
|------|---------|---------|------------------|
|      | Marie   | group   | Let's start with the knowledge items. |
|      | Indira  | Marie   | Practice comes first so respondents won't be influenced by what they know. |
|      | Alex    | group   | Here's a possible item: How often . . . |

1. At the end, compare the records of the two observers to see if they match. How accurate and complete were they according to the group? Why did they omit certain events (too busy, thought the comment unimportant)?

2. The group as a whole can work out a framework for coding the group's discussion. To understand the discussion as a problem-solving activity, you might want to use codes such as stating a new item, reworking an item, repeating an item, agreeing or disagreeing,

> stating an obstacle, stating a solution, asking a question, saying what to do, making an off-task comment. Calculate the frequency for each code. Were certain codes more frequent? Do you need additional codes to characterize frequently occurring comments or actions?
>
> 3. Regroup the class. Make a list of the codes and next to each write the frequency for each group. Are some codes more frequent for groups that completed more of the task? There may be more than one way to complete this task successfully.
>
> 4. Develop a list of key behaviors that observers can use in a checklist format for subsequent group discussions.

## PARTICIPANT OBSERVATION

The researcher in this case participates in the daily life or ongoing activities of the people being studied. **Participant observation** involves an in-depth case study of group life from the perspective of someone who has a prolonged, intense involvement in that life, and is based on naturalistic observations and information intentionally solicited. The researcher is the one who becomes involved and who interacts socially with the observed people as they go about their normal activities. Consequently, the quality of the data depends entirely on one researcher. Descriptions of this method are provided by Adler and Adler (1994), Bogdewic (1992), and Rasmuson et al. (1988).

Purpose

Participant observation is used to collect information about the meaning people in a cultural group attach to events in their daily lives. This is the method of choice among anthropologists who want to understand not only what people do but also what it means to them. Asking people why they do what they do is not adequate because people have reasons, assumptions, expectations, and values that are taken for granted and rarely expressed. The researcher tries to collect this kind of information through careful observation and questioning. For example, laypeople often think about illness symptoms and their causes differently from the health professionals they visit. To coordinate efforts, each needs to understand how the other thinks. Particularly when interventions are planned by people from a different culture, participant observations can provide information on the community's values, beliefs, and practices—information that should alter the way the intervention is presented and implemented so that it will be accepted.

Strengths

The advantage of participant observation is particularly salient when the activity of interest is usually hidden from strangers, such as circumcision or wedding rituals. To observe the activity, one must be a participant. A second advantage is that the actions are described within their natural context and sequence of events. This helps to determine natural antecedents and consequences of events. Sometimes ethnographic information about the larger context (e.g., agricultural and ecological conditions, household and political structure) are necessary to compare the case with others. A third advantage is that the meanings of events and the reasons for behaviors can be made explicit by a careful, insightful observer when these meanings and reasons may be obscure to the participants themselves. This will help to design a sensitive intervention that will be meaningful to the community. In summary, the strengths include the following:

- Private events may be observed.
- Events are observed in their natural context.
- Sequence and connection of events are preserved.
- Obscure assumptions and reasons are made explicit.

Limitations

One disadvantage is that the method of recording is time consuming, often taking more than a year to complete a case study of one group. Its credibility depends on the expertise of the researcher, who is more than a mere observer and so must be extensively trained at the university level. The observer's theoretical biases can potentially distort what is observed and how it is described; personal biases may arise from the researcher's emotional involvement in the group under study. An observer who is aware of biases and takes pains to eliminate them can achieve greater objectivity. However, there is no opportunity to assess this without a second observer to provide reliability data. Another disadvantage is that sequences of events do not address the consistency of a connection between two events. Many events precede a health problem but only some of these will be connected to the problem. Without the opportunity for statistical tests, even noncausal associations cannot be tested. Finally, participant observation studies focus on single cases with no attempt to generalize or compare with other cases. Thus the limitations include the following:

- The process is time consuming.
- It requires a highly trained professional.
- Biases emerge from theory and involvement.
- There is no interobserver reliability.
- There is no statistical test of consistent sequences.
- There is no comparison with other cases.

Participants

The participants are a group or subgroup in a community, such as mothers of young children. They are treated as a homogeneous group with a similar culture and therefore a similar set of values, beliefs, and practices. However, individual and family differences may surface; they are referred to anonymously.

Procedure

During a period of time, the researcher observes what is happening, listens to what people talk about, and asks questions to clarify the meaning of events. The meaning of events is derived from the context, from the sequence and connection of events, from people's reactions to events, from the words they use to communicate to each other, and from their explanations given to the researcher. Observations are extensive and descriptive at the beginning; as patterns emerge, the observer becomes more selective in what he or she observes, often asking key informants to clarify inferences.

Becoming accepted as a trusted, unobtrusive participant is one of the most sensitive issues for a participant observer; it is necessary for the observer to gain access to private matters and yet not alter the activity with his or her presence. Trust is the key to privileged information. To become trusted, you will have to be honest, unassuming, nonjudgmental, and accepting of whatever role you are allowed to play within the community. To be unobtrusive, you will have to minimize public displays of recording. Observations continue until no new relevant information emerges.

Data Collection

The participant researcher's record of events takes the form of a daily diary or work schedule, jottings of key words during an event, and expanded field notes of details and personal impressions written at the end of the day. The record includes information on *who* was present, *what* was happening, *when and where* it occurred, *why* it happened (what precipitated it), and *how* it occurred with respect to rules and context. The expanded field notes constitute the core of the data as they include themes, hypotheses, insights, and explanations of events. Information about the physical, economic, and political context also form part of the description and explanation.

Data Analysis

Field notes are used to describe, clarify, and explain the meaning of health-related events from the group's perspective.

---

### *Student Activity:*
### *Become aware of our observer biases.*

Each student will choose a group for which you are already an "insider," such as family, dormitory mates, club, or group of friends. Speak to this group and tell them that you want to record what happens during some naturally occurring event when you are all together, such as mealtime. Address their concerns before beginning to record. The focus of your project is eating practices but you also want to understand the full meaning of "a meal," how people relate to each other while they are eating, and how they relate to the food. On the first occasion, you might be unselective in your observations and write down everything that was said and done. On the second occasion, you can be selective. Try not to be too obvious about your note taking, and write expanded notes immediately after the meal. From this, extract 10 or so conclusions you drew about the meaning of a meal for this group.

1. To find out how accurate you are at observing and inferring what actually goes on during mealtime, I suggest two options:

(a) select an insightful member of your group to act as a "knowledgeable informant" and compare that informant's recall of events with your own notes or
(b) tape-record the mealtime and let another student listen to the recording, then show your list of conclusions to this person and ask how much he or she agrees with each, on a three-point scale (agree, partially agree, disagree).

2. When the class regroups, discuss the difficulties of being a participant observer. Here are some biases that you might have discovered; they are common but unintentional:

- Important events are overlooked. We often forget things that we don't understand or that disconfirm our expectations.
- We think things were done or said that in fact were not.
- We confuse who said what and in what order. If similar things were said on the same topic by different people, it is easy to confuse their statements. Sequences are important, however, because they tell who provoked whom.
- We often think we play a larger role in what happens than we actually do. For example, we think people agree with us more than they do.
- We make inferences about the causes of people's behavior based on whatever information is salient. If someone says, "This food is disgusting," and another person stops eating, we think the former's negative comment influenced the latter's action, when self-report might tell us otherwise.

## KEY INFORMANT INTERVIEWS

**Key informant interviews** involve unstructured questioning of informed individuals to gain a deeper understanding of how community members think about an event. If a close bond develops between the

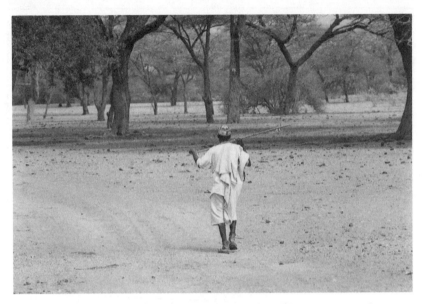

*A key informant is a well-integrated, respected member of the community who can articulate the opinions and concerns of the community.*

interviewer and the informant, the latter will direct the dialogue on the topic of interest. Used in this way, it provides qualitative data. However, if a large number of key informants are sampled from many communities, and they are asked a set of structured questions, their answers can be quantified. Descriptions of both these styles are given by Fontana and Frey (1994), Gilchrist (1992), and Wig et al. (1980).

Purpose

Key informant interviews often accompany other methods because the key informant can provide a lot of information about the community on short order. You may want to know how mothers classify child illnesses or foods; key informants can provide the commonly used terms and mothers' organization of them. You may want to know how mothers treat children with diarrhea so as to develop a structured survey questionnaire; key informants can describe all the methods routes mothers take. Key informants can tell you about sexual behaviors that foster the spread of HIV and how to contact vulnerable people.

### Strengths

As with focus groups, key informants can provide a great deal of information about events, people, and common ways of thinking and acting. If they are well informed and articulate, they may provide new insights and explanations that are useful to a researcher from outside the group. They can be interviewed in less time than other sources, which is important if you want to move quickly to the intervention phase. They can provide information on sensitive matters, such as mental illness and sexual behavior, that others may not want to discuss. Thus the strengths are as follows:

- Key informants provide information about the social and psychological ways of people.
- Their use requires less time and money.
- Sensitive material can be uncovered.

### Limitations

The major limitation is that their views are not tested for representativeness. If informants describe events differently, is it because they are biased or are they describing different subsamples of the population? Informants' value may be limited to homogeneous subgroups and communities that share a culture and a view of reality. The unstructured technique requires a highly trained interviewer. Limitations therefore include the following:

- Reliability or validity cannot be assessed.
- Information may not be representative unless a sampling technique is used.
- Use is limited to homogeneous communities.

### Participants

A key informant is someone from the community who has the following characteristics:

- *Wide contacts* with people in the community and therefore in a position to inform the researcher about community events, that is, thoroughly involved and active in the community

- Good *communication skills*, articulate, willing to talk without reservation and to volunteer information without direct questions
- *Reflective* and therefore able to expand, modify, and clarify the researcher's interpretations of events
- *Trustworthy*

There are different ways of selecting key informants. One is to ask people in the community who is best informed about events in the community and whom they trust to describe their community accurately. This amounts to a popularity contest. Another method is the snowball method. People who are good key informants are asked to name others who fit the criteria.

A more structured sampling technique involves selecting one key informant for every 1,000 people.

Procedure

Here is how a relatively unstructured interview might be conducted. You first ask the key informant some open-ended, broad questions, leaving the informant to direct his or her answer. You may then pose some specific questions, again letting the informant provide as much detail as possible. You may offer specific interpretations to obtain the informant's confirmation or disconfirmation. The interview stops when no new information is being provided. You may return to seek clarification from the informant after collecting more information from other sources. This unstructured format requires a highly trained interviewer who knows how to listen patiently and attentively, how to follow the direction of the informant and probe with questions when necessary, and how to foster a trusting relationship.

Some key informant interviews are more structured, with specific questions asked in a specific order. For example, the WHO's key informant interview on attitudes toward mental illness (Wig et al., 1980) follows a specific set of questions. You first ask some specific questions to determine the informant's range of contacts, power of perception, and recall: "How many blind people living in [name community] do you know by name? How many people who cannot walk or can walk only with crutches living in [name community] do you know by name?" You ask what kinds of healers work in the area, how many healers there are, and what type of patients they treat. Continuing with the topic of healers, you ask what kind of help most people would first seek for 10 different problems, such as fever, convulsions, sleeplessness, and excitement. Finally, you read seven vignettes; each describes the behaviors of someone with a common mental health problem. You ask the informants if he or she knows anyone with such a problem, and then ask whether such a person would have trouble being accepted by their family, by a marriage partner, and by an employer.

Data Collection and Analysis

The data consist of statements made by the key informant that are then organized to answer specific questions, such as what the taxonomies of child illnesses are, what terms are used to refer to types of food, and what the common sexual practices are. Answers to the structured set of questions can be coded and summarized as means or frequency distributions. They can be statistically compared with other communities.

> ## Student Activity:
> ### Pick the brains of a key informant.
>
> Socioeconomic status is one important determinant of health. Some countries have a scale developed by sociologists for classifying a family's socioeconomic status. In industrialized countries, it is usually based on some combination of occupation, education, and income. However, most countries do not have such a scale. You can use key informants to help you create an SES hierarchy to be used in a subsequent health survey. You can do this activity in groups, where one student is selected to be interviewer and the others write down the key informants' comments. Or each student may want to interview a key informant. Select a key informant who comes from a rural village in a developing country. Try both the unstructured and the structured interview formats with different informants from the same village.
>
> *Unstructured Interview*
>
> "I want to get your ideas on something we call socioeconomic status and how people in your community differ in their status.

By 'status,' I mean how important or powerful or influential the person is in the eyes of other people. In most communities, certain people have more influence, other people have some influence, and others have very little influence. Would you say that such status exists in your community? How does it work there?" Write down the important criteria for identifying status and the names of people at different status levels. Continue to probe with questions such as the following: "Who has a lot of influence? Who has very little influence? Why?" The probes should always build on what the informant already said.

*Structured Interview*

Use the three introductory sentences from the unstructured interview: "I want to get your ideas . . . others very little influence." Continue with specific questions about community members who occupy different status positions and the criteria for identifying status. Write names on a ladder from top to bottom as the informant says them, adding and moving names as more names are offered.

1. Who would you say has high status?_____
   Can you name 5 or more?" _____
2. Who has low status? _____
3. Who has middle status? _____
   Are some of these higher than others? _____
4. In some communities, people have high status because of their education, or the amount of land they own, or because they belong to a certain tribe. There are many different reasons that some people have high status and others have low status. What gives a person high or low status in your community?
   Criteria _____

Now let us see how this works with the people you named earlier.

> (Taking each criterion one at a time, make a note next to the names of people who meet that criterion. People at the top of the ladder should have at least one of the criteria, and people at the bottom none. Ask the informant about discrepancies, "Person X is third from the top but seems to have none of these things that give status. Why is that?")

## STRUCTURED SELF-REPORT MEASURES

**Structured self-report measures** include a standard set of questions about a person's health behavior, attitudes, beliefs, or whatever, the answers to which can be quantified and summed to create a composite score. The questions can deal with any topic that a respondent can sincerely think and talk about. For example, questions in a KAP survey concern a person's knowledge, attitude, and practices (behavior); the questions in a verbal autopsy concern symptoms apparent prior to a person's death; the questions in a health locus of control scale concern a variety of forces that influence one's health; the questions in a healthy environment scale concern perceptions of contamination of local water and soil. Multiple questions or items are used to include all possible relevant components. The respondents' answers are classified and given a number to represent some magnitude, such as more or less knowledge, more or less perceived personal control, and more or less healthy behavior (van de Vijver & Leung, 1997).

Purpose

Structured self-report measures are useful when you want to make inferences about a specific population. For example, using correct sampling procedures, you can estimate the percentage of people who practice a certain health behavior, or how positively men view the idea of their wives using contraception. This will be useful information when deciding on the magnitude of a problem. You can also compare the scores for two or more groups, such as husbands and wives on their attitudes toward contraception. Because the same measure is used, the scores for different groups are comparable. This may help you to decide which group is a priority. The scores can also help to evaluate the success of a program if, for example, after a child health program, more people know how to accurately report the symptoms of acute respiratory infection and more people report seeking the services of their community health worker for child illnesses.

Strengths

One advantage of a structured self-report measure is that respondents' answers are comparable and can be grouped into rates or means to provide summary information. Knowing the variation among answers within a sample is one of the most important advantages of this method. The reliability and validity of the measure can be evaluated. The findings are generalizable to the population sampled, and the procedure can be replicated with other samples to determine if the findings generalize to them or do not generalize. Statistical tests can be performed to examine a number of important health questions: (a) whether two variables are associated (e.g., the yearly frequency of diarrhea in a family and use of contaminated water sources); (b) whether two groups differ on some important dimension (e.g., the number of new HIV infections among prostitutes who received and did not receive help setting up a supportive network); (c) which of a number of possible factors are most strongly associated with a health outcome (e.g., a child's malnutrition may be more strongly associated with the mother's education, diet, and frequency of child illness than with the family's income or religion). Finally, the questions do not tax a respondent's memory and answers do not depend on how articulate a respondent is. In summary, the strengths are as follows:

- Summary statistics are available for individuals and groups.
- Statistics will represent the variation in a group.
- The measure's reliability and validity can be reported.
- The data are replicable and generalizable to other samples.
- Statistics will examine what is associated with health.

Limitations

One major limitation is that people often import a measure developed and standardized in a very different culture (the **emic-etic di-**

**lemma**). Consequently, the items and response categories may be incomplete or irrelevant to the population of interest. This is clearly a limitation of the researcher, who has not bothered to check the relevance. It is possible to use a measure that is tailored to the population yet comparable with others (Lonner & Berry, 1986).

A second limitation is that the context is omitted from such inquiries (Guba & Lincoln, 1994). People using this method often do not describe the complete physical and social environment of the population, as one would do in a case study. Yet some aspects of the environment might directly influence people's health and behavior, and this should be tested.

Critics also argue that the desire to minimize the effects of uncontrolled contextual variables leads researchers to strip the testing situation of its natural context (Guba & Lincoln, 1994). Consequently, the researcher is measuring something quite different from the respondents' daily activities and attitudes. This is a serious limitation with two parts. One concerns the generalization of anything, reports or behavior, measured out of context. The second concerns whether self-report in a quiet setting reflects behavior in context. The question of generalization from one context to another needs to be empirically tested. Does a mother who properly mixes ORS in the clinic do so at home when her child has diarrhea? Do a husband and wife, who calmly and rationally discuss contraception with a midwife, also do this at home? There are many examples of actions that do not change in a specified range of different contexts and many examples of actions that do. The question of the validity of self-report has also been tested. A number of biases conspire to reduce the accuracy of self-report: limitations of memory, lack of insight into one's thoughts and actions, and desire to look good. A well-developed test asks for information that is within ordinary persons' memory capacity and uses vignettes to jog their memory; it avoids questions requiring insights about the causes of one's actions and provides an "I don't know" response option; and it phrases questions in a nonleading way. The validity of self-report can be evaluated by noting its consistency with a relevant behavior. In summary, limitations include the following:

- Imported, unmodified measures may be irrelevant, incomplete.
- There is little information on the broader context.

- Behavior is out of its natural context.
- Self-report may not be accurate.

Participants

Participants are selected on the basis of their demographic characteristics, such as living in a certain region, or their health status. Random or systematic sampling procedures provide the investigator with a representative sample whose results can be generalized. When the interview is long and demanding, you may select fewer participants who represent only a subgroup but then replicate the study with other groups to generalize.

Procedure

A large part of your effort will go into finding, modifying, or developing a measure to suit your purposes. Obviously, it saves time and effort if you can find an existing measure that suits your needs. Some have been used extensively in developing countries. Others have been used only in industrialized countries and so will require some modification. Using an existing measure has the advantage of allowing for comparability. However, if a measure does not exist, you must develop your own.

You first outline the relevant content and then seek items to cover the content. Items should have specific wording so that they will be interpreted similarly by all respondents. However, the items may be open-ended (e.g., What is a germ?) or closed-ended (e.g., Can a healthy person have HIV? Yes, No, or Don't Know). Items are usually pretested for clarity, interpretation, and completeness. Then you seek a response format that allows respondents to answer truthfully. You score the person's responses, usually so that you give a higher score consistently for answers in one direction, such as for low-risk sexual behavior. Then you sum scores for individual items to yield a composite score.

Local, high school-educated people are usually trained to do interviews in the local language. They are trained to administer the questions in the same way to everyone, and to show acceptance and attention to all answers. If the questionnaire is initially written in another language, it must be translated and back-translated.

## Data Collection

Interviewers seek permission from each respondent to ask them questions, and then conduct the interview, usually at the person's home. If respondents are not highly literate, the interviewer reads each question and records the answer on the questionnaire form. Anonymity and confidentiality are usually guaranteed. If the questions concern a private matter, such as sexual behavior, respondents can record their answers privately, in the form of tallies and Xs, and put the completed answer sheet in an unmarked envelope.

## Data Analysis

Usually the researcher starts by calculating frequencies for dichotomous yes-no response formats or means for continuous ones such as scores on a 10-item test on practice. Reliability and validity of the measures are then evaluated. The associations between an index of health and a psychosocial variable are examined with rates, ratios, confidence intervals, chi-squares, and correlation. Also $t$-tests and $F$-tests are commonly used to examine differences between groups (see van de Vijver & Leung, 1997, for detailed descriptions). For example, scores on a test of how mothers feed a child with diarrhea may be compared using a $t$-test in which one group includes those who have lost a child and a second group that includes those who have not lost a child to illness.

## Existing Measures

The World Health Organization has developed and validated measures for mental health in adults and children. The **Self-Reporting Questionnaire** (see Harding et al., 1983) has 24 items that are easy to administer and score and that require a simple yes-no answer on the part of the respondent. Here are some examples:

| | | |
|---|---|---|
| Do you often have headaches? | Yes | No |
| Is your appetite poor? | Yes | No |
| Are you easily frightened? | Yes | No |
| Do you cry more than usual? | Yes | No |

The **Health Locus of Control** instrument measures generalized expectancies that self (I; internal), powerful others (P), or chance (C) determine one's health and illness (DeVellis et al., 1993; Wallston, Wallston, & DeVellis, 1978). It includes 18 items such as the following:

If I take the right actions, I can stay healthy.   (I)   Agree   Disagree
My family has a lot to do with my becoming   (P)   Agree   Disagree
  sick or staying healthy.

Ethiopians added a fourth dimension of Powerful Spirits with items such as these:

Amulets protect people against illness.
My ancestral woukabi are responsible for my health or illness.

Scores on the four scales intercorrelate differently in different cultures.

The **McGill Pain Questionnaire** measures the subjective perception of tissue injury or extreme temperature, pressure, and so on (Melzack, 1975, 1987). The short form assesses the severity of 11 sensory experiences of pain, such as burning and shooting, and 4 emotional experiences of pain, such as being fearful. Each descriptor is rated as None, Mild, Moderate, or Severe to indicate whether and how the descriptor applies to the pain experienced. The Present Pain Intensity is also rated on a six-point scale from No Pain (0) to Excruciating (5). Ethiopians added other sensory descriptors such as itchy, crawling, and chilly that were commonly used by their patients. They also used the body drawing from the long form to help patients locate internal and external pain and its radiation.

The **Social Readjustment Rating Scale of Major Life Events** measures the psychological impact of acute stressors experienced in the past year (Holmes & Rahe, 1967; Sarason, Johnson, & Siegel, 1978). Common stressors are listed, and respondents indicate whether or not they have experienced one or more in the past year and how negative the impact was. To the usual list of acute stressors such as death of a spouse, personal injury, or illness, Ethiopians added some chronic stressors such as shortage of food and water, crowded home, and waiting long hours for services.

The **Ways of Coping Questionnaire** measures cognitive and behavioral efforts to manage specific external and/or internal demands that are appraised as taxing or exceeding the resources of the person (Folkman & Lazarus, 1988). There are 66 items tapping eight coping strategies such as Social Support Seeking, Planful Problem Solving, Escape-Avoidance, and Distancing. The respondent rates each example of a coping strategy on a four-point frequency scale. Scores for each strategy can be obtained by summing the ratings.

The **Verbal Autopsy** is a technique for identifying the cause of death by asking structured questions of an adult who cared for the deceased before death (Kamali, Wagner, et al., 1996; Pacqué-Margolis, Pacqué, Dukuly, Boateng, & Taylor, 1990). This is often necessary in rural areas where people die at home and the cause of death is not registered. The questions are about definitive signs and symptoms for each cause of death, and they use local words. The sequence of questions for pneumonia begins, Was his breathing all right before he died? If not, the next question is asked: Was his breathing hurting? For AIDS, the signs and symptoms included fever, loss of weight, diarrhea, vomiting, cough, and skin rash. Trained laypeople conduct the interviews and clinicians use the information to identify likely cause of death. The AIDS verbal autopsy was accurate in that it matched closely the person's HIV status three years prior to death (unknown, of course, to the clinician conducting the interview).

**Self-efficacy** refers to confidence one has that one can perform the required health behavior (Bandura, 1982). People with high self-efficacy are more likely to initiate these behaviors and persist despite obstacles. There are many self-efficacy scales; each is developed for a specific behavior, such as eating proper food. I will describe a self-efficacy scale for teachers who have a new responsibility to teach health to elementary school children (Everett & Telljohann, 1996). Teachers respond to the 16 items using a 5-point Likert scale in which 1 = Strongly Disagree and 5 = Strongly Agree. The numbered responses are then summed for a composite efficacy score. Some items are as follows: I believe I can do a good job teaching students about disease control/prevention. I believe I can evaluate changes in health attitudes. I am able to stimulate students enough that they ask thoughtful health questions.

Developing a New Measure

When developing a new measure such as a **KAP questionnaire,** it is best to learn from others who have worked through the process, even if the topic is different. Developing a poor measure for your "unique" setting is no better than using a good measure developed elsewhere. The following issues must be considered:

How will it be administered? Interview is best for people with little education, but self-administration is possible for highly literate people.

What is the best question format? Open-ended questions requiring short answers might be desirable when assessing knowledge, for example, How can a person get AIDS? Closed-ended questions that require only a Yes-No-Don't Know answer or Agree-Disagree answer place less burden on the respondent's verbal and memory skills, for example, Can a person get AIDS from kissing? It may be best to have some open-ended followed by some closed-ended questions.

What is the best response format and how does one score the responses? The open-ended question requires a verbal response that must be written down verbatim and then scored, perhaps one point for each correct idea. For example, responses to the question on how a person gets AIDS might receive one point for each correct mode of transmission for a maximum of three. (How many do you expect from a layperson?) The closed-ended question should allow for three possible responses: Yes, No, and I don't know. "I don't know" and the incorrect answer are both scored zero; the correct answer is given one point.

Finally, how many items should there be? To enhance the reliability of the measure, it should have many items, perhaps 10 or more. Scores on the items can then be summed. On a KAP questionnaire, you would obtain three separate scores—one for knowledge, one for attitude, and one for practice (but administer the subscales in the reverse order, with items on practice always first). Generating items is a good exercise for a group of people. Afterward, show the items to several colleagues to get their opinion on the clarity of the wording and items to be added. Pilot testing should be used to identify irrelevant items, omitted items, poorly understood items, reliability, and validity.

Here are some KAP items we developed concerning mothers' care of infants over 4 months, where P means practice, A means attitude, and K means knowledge:

P1. What did you feed your baby immediately after delivery?
(breast milk = 1, butter, water & sugar, cow milk = 0)

P2. What do you feed your baby now?
(breast milk + solids = 2, only breast milk = 1, all else = 0)

A. Which of the following are good for your baby and which are bad?

| | |
|---|---|
| immunization shots | Good = 1 |
| amulet around the neck | Bad = 1 |
| sunshine | Good = 1 |
| uvulectomy | Bad = 1 |

K1. What is a germ? (little = 1, causes disease = 1, for max 2)

K2. What is ORS?
(for diarrhea child = 1, prevents dehydration = 1, for max 2)

K3. Does eating carrots prevent blindness? Yes = 1

---

### Student Activity:
### Modify an existing measure
### for your population.

Look at some of the items used by Holmes and Rahe (1967) in their self-report measure of stress called the Social Readjustment Rating Scale. After items were collected, judges rated them as to the amount of readjustment they thought was required by different events, using a standard score of 50 for the amount of adjustment required by marriage. The life change units corresponding to each event are the median rating given by these judges. Respondents in the study sample listen to each event being read to them and indicate whether that event had occurred to them sometime in the past year. The respondent's score is the sum of life change units for the events they experienced.

Sarason and colleagues decided to use the same items but to ask their respondents how stressful each experienced event was on a scale from +3 to –3, where 0 means no impact, +3 means extremely positive, and –3 means extremely negative. This modification allows for cultural and individual differences in the distress resulting from an event.

1. Student groups will meet to examine the Holmes and Rahe scale and modify it for either an urban or a rural population in their country. They can alter the list of events and/or the response format. They will also indicate how to calculate a respondent's score.

2. Afterward, students regroup and discuss modifications made to events and to the response format. Students discuss the advantages and disadvantages of modifying an existing measure compared with developing one's own from scratch.

| Events | Life Change Unit |
|---|---|
| Death of spouse | 100 |
| Divorce | 73 |
| Marital separation | 65 |
| Jail term | 63 |
| Death of close family member | 63 |
| Personal injury or illness | 53 |
| Marriage | 50 |
| Fired at work | 49 |
| Illness of family member | 44 |
| New family member | 39 |
| Change to different line of work | 36 |

## STUDENT ACTIVITY

Select a health problem on which the class wants to collect information. Divide the class into five groups so that each group takes responsibility for one of the five methods. As a class, students will first decide what variables need to be measured, although they may want to add some later after the first round of data has been collected and examined. Working in their separate groups, students will identify variables that are well suited to their particular method and then develop a way of measuring them. When students later regroup, they can decide what to do about variables that were left unmeasured by any group as well as how to sequence the data collection.

# 3

# *FAMILY PLANNING AND CONTRACEPTIVE USE*

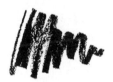

Family planning covers issues that range from the intimate to the global. On one level, planning whether or not to have a child is a private decision made by individuals and couples. At the other extreme are demographers who calculate what the world population will be 25 and 50 years from now depending on how many babies we each produce. Although the desire to limit one's family size predated demographic predictions, the numbers projected for countries such as China and India, with almost half the world's population, were worrisome enough to mobilize national and international activity. India began its family planning activities in the 1950s and 1960s and brought down the number of babies per woman from 6 to 4 in three decades. China began its family planning activities much later, in 1979, and reduced its fertility from 5.5 to 2 babies per woman in the same three decades. Supporting this effort are those helping to develop a variety of contraceptive methods, those who inform couples about their options, and those who provide the service. Family planning is driven not only by numbers; it is considered essential for health and development. As such, it can be seen as a prevention program, similar in scope to child immunization but much more sensitive and controversial (Lee, 1994).

Why is it so sensitive and controversial? It is a sensitive issue largely because it bears on marital relations and sexuality, considered for a long time to be the prerogative of the couple or perhaps the extended family. It is sensitive also because having children is one of those magical events central to religion and nature; people therefore hold strongly to their beliefs about the value of children and the needs they satisfy. Family planning generates a lot of controversy, especially at the U.N. Population Conferences held every 10 years, because certain groups are vociferously opposed to anyone using contraception, others feel that economic and social development is the best contraceptive, and yet others feel it is being imposed unfairly on women. No social revolution is gentle on everyone, and the contraceptive revolution has its battles and its victims. One lesson we have learned is that the face of contraception must become more personal. While technical advances improve contraceptive methods, and planners work out new programs and fertility goals, it is the family planning workers on whom we depend to provide an understanding rather than a coercive face to potential users.

Family planning data seekers have many sources of information. The World Fertility Survey and the Contraceptive Prevalence Survey collected data from many countries during the period from 1975 to 1985, and the demographic and health surveys continue to be conducted and published in the journal *Studies in Family Planning*. These surveys collect information on population growth and total fertility rate (the number of children expected to be born to each woman for the duration of her childbearing years). They then try to match these up with the number of men and women who report using contraception. On the large scale, contraception does seem to work: For every 15% increase in the number of people using contraception, each woman will have on average one less child. The threshold for replacing our country's population is 2.1 children per woman. China and many industrialized countries are therefore reducing not only their fertility but also their populations.

The reasons that certain countries and U.N. agencies have decided to put so much effort into family planning will be discussed first. These will then be compared with the reasons that couples have children. Finally, survey data will be used to show how many people are using contraception in different parts of the world as well as how recent family planning programs have succeeded or failed in promoting safe, personalized methods of contraception.

## THE CASE IN FAVOR OF FAMILY PLANNING

### Unwanted Fertility

The most convincing case for family planning rests on the argument that 26% of births in developing countries each year are unwanted (Bongaarts, 1990). How was this figure arrived at? Bongaarts considered how mothers in 48 different surveys answered the following question: Before your latest pregnancy, what were your thoughts about having children—did you want to have another child, want to wait, or want to have no more children? Choosing the first option indicates wanted fertility; choosing to wait or have no more indicates that the latest pregnancy and birth were unwanted. Of course, this does not mean the baby would be unwanted and unloved. It makes the point that a very large number of women would like to have prevented their pregnancies and yet did not. This is a striking indicator that the need for birth control is not being met. It is particularly high in Latin American countries such as Colombia, Peru, and Mexico, where approximately 40% of births were unwanted. Bangladesh and Pakistan were close to the average with 26%. In the high-fertility countries of sub-Saharan Africa, only 5% to 15% of births were unwanted. These parents want to prevent births but do not have the opportunity to obtain contraception. Meeting this need, and the need of the many more women who will soon be entering this stage of family life, justifies the effort to promote family planning.

### Population Growth and Resource Depletion

Population control is another major reason to promote family planning and contraception use. As I write, the world's population stands at 5.96 billion people. At the beginning of the 1990s, the population of developing countries numbered 4 billion, 80% of the world's population. It is projected to reach the 5 billion mark by the year 2000 and to continue rapid growth for several more decades (Bongaarts, Mauldin,

**TABLE 3.1** Population, Fertility, and Contraception Statistics

| Region | Population (millions) (1994) | Annual Growth Rate 1980-1994 | Total Fertility Rate 1960 | Total Fertility Rate 1980 | Total Fertility Rate 1994 | Contraceptive Prevalence 1994 % | GNP Per Capita Growth Rate 1980-1993 % | Enrollment Primary School % |
|---|---|---|---|---|---|---|---|---|
| Sub-Saharan Africa | 548 | 2.9 | 6.6 | 6.6 | 6.2 | 13 | −0.3 | 51 |
| Middle East & NorthAfrica | 363 | 2.9 | 7.0 | 5.9 | 4.4 | 44 | 0.6 | 86 |
| South Asia | 1,233 | 2.2 | 6.1 | 5.1 | 4.0 | 40 | 2.9 | ? |
| East Asia & Pacific | 1,764 | 1.6 | 5.6 | 3.3 | 2.3 | 74 | 6.8 | 96 |
| Latin America & Caribbean | 466 | 2.0 | 6.0 | 4.1 | 3.0 | 59 | −0.1 | 82 |
| Countries in transition | 414 | 0.6 | 2.8 | 2.3 | 1.9 | ? | −0.6 | ? |
| Developing countries | 4373 | 2.1 | 6.0 | 4.4 | 3.5 | 55 | 2.9 | 84 |
| Least developed countries | 256 | 2.6 | 6.6 | 6.5 | 5.7 | 17 | 0.7 | 52 |
| Industrialized countries | 823 | 0.6 | 2.8 | 1.8 | 1.7 | 72 | 2.2 | 98 |

SOURCE: *The State of the World's Children* (UNICEF, 1996).

& Phillips, 1990). In many countries, per capita economic growth has not kept pace with population growth (compare columns 2 and 7 in Table 3.1). This places an undue burden on the economic resources of countries that are struggling to improve their standard of living. Dense populations lead not only to depletion of natural resources such as arable land, forests, and water but to overstretched services in the areas of education and health.

Population growth is due largely to fertility, the other components being deaths and in- and out-migrations. The **total fertility rate** is the number of children that would be born per woman during her childbearing years if she were having children at the current rate for that country. It is the figure most often used by family planners as an index of whether couples are controlling births. The fertility rate in develop-

*Family Planning and Contraceptive Use*  71

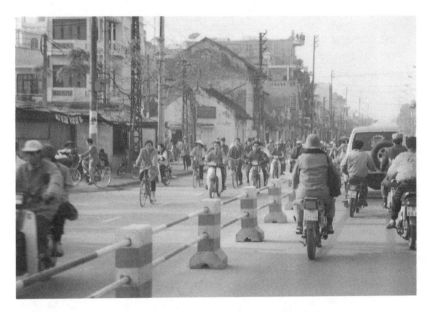

*Vietnam has a population of 75 million, with a fertility rate of 3.7.*

ing countries was 3.5 for the period 1990-1995, down from 4.4 in 1980-1985 and 6.0 in 1965-1970 (UNICEF, 1996). Four regions of the world were responsible for most of the decline, in large measure due to the increasing use of contraception. The largest decline was in East Asia, which now records 2.3 births per woman, similar to the 1.7 births found in developed countries. Latin America, South Asia, and the Middle East have figures of 3.0, 4.0, and 4.4, respectively. However, sub-Saharan Africa has the highest fertility rate at 6.2, showing little change since 1960-1965 (although Kenya dropped from 8 to 6.1 births in this period). The decline in fertility is almost entirely due to the use of contraception, as illustrated by Table 3.1.

The decline in fertility from 1960 to 1995 is also associated with socioeconomic development. A number of indices of socioeconomic development are used: per capita gross national product, infant mortality rates, educational enrollment, and per capita ownership of televisions, radios, and cars (Bongaarts et al., 1990; Mauldin & Ross, 1991). The relationship could be said to work in both directions. A high level of socioeconomic development facilitates a drop in fertility by increasing the demand for birth control and by providing resources to strengthen family planning programs. Also, a drop in fertility facilitates a high level of socioeconomic development, as mothers have more time for employment and make greater efforts to keep their children healthy and educated.

This argument for family planning places emphasis on those countries with large populations and below-60% contraception use, such as Ethiopia, Bangladesh, India, Nigeria, Pakistan, and Zaire. Some of these countries already have a moderately strong program in place; others are only beginning to implement plans. At the same time, efforts should be made to provide opportunities for socioeconomic development so that large numbers of children are no longer seen as necessary for the family to survive economically.

Healthy Mothers and Children

Maternal and child health are also important reasons for promotion of family planning. Many women in developing countries suffer during pregnancy, delivery, and long after because their general nutrition is poor, health services are inadequate, and child care is exhausting. The number of women who die in pregnancy and childbirth is only the tip of the iceberg. Peter Adamson (1996) argues that for every woman who dies, 30 become infected, anemic, or injured. In total, close to 600,000 women die each year, and 15 million a year will be disabled. He estimates that one quarter of the adult women in developing countries are currently affected by injury sustained as a result of bearing children. These injuries go untreated and are suffered in silence because of the "censorship and embarrassment that still surround the issues of sex, blood, and birth in most societies of the world" (Adamson, 1996, p. 3).

**Maternal mortality,** or the number of women who die in pregnancy and childbirth, is usually expressed as the number of deaths from pregnancy-related causes per 100,000 live births (which is a proxy for the number of pregnancies). The maternal mortality rate in the least developed countries is 603 compared with 7 in industrialized countries (UNICEF, 1996). For sub-Saharan Africa, it is 597; South Asia, 482; the Middle East, 200; Latin America, 178; and East Asia, 165. Adamson's figures are higher because they are based on other information, such as

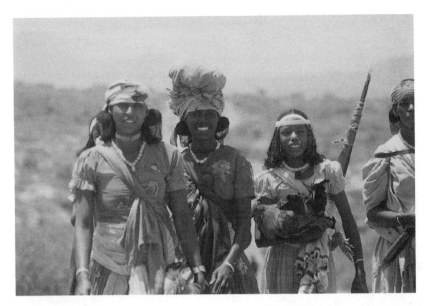

Women in sub-Saharan Africa are likely to use family planning to space rather than limit births, although in Ethiopia, Nigeria, and Zaire, the number who use contraception is low.

surveys and delivery sites, which compensate for the common reluctance to report that a deceased woman was pregnant. His estimates place the maternal mortality rate of sub-Saharan Africa at 980. A total of 21 countries have rates of 1,000 and above (AbouZahr, Wardlaw, Stanton, & Hill, 1996).

Preventing pregnancy and preventing complications that result in death and injury are the two major ways of preventing maternal mortality and morbidity (Freedman & Maine, 1993). Many people believe that if the aim is to reduce maternal mortality, then antenatal and postnatal care should be improved to reduce the risk of complications and death from complications. Adamson, for example, urges that even small district hospitals upgrade their equipment and staff to provide modern obstetric care, such as cesarian sections and other emergency procedures for the 15% of women who need the service. However, most recognize that this strategy alone has not been very successful in reducing mortality due to complications.

Certain groups of mothers are at greater risk of death. This includes women under 20 and over 30, and women who have already delivered three children. Considering the twin goals of reducing fertility rates and maternal mortality rates, several family planning strategies have been proposed for targeting certain groups of women (Trussell & Pebley, 1984; Winikoff & Sullivan, 1987). The most feasible strategy is to target women under 20 and over 39 with parity greater than 5. This would reduce fertility rates by 25% and maternal mortality by 10%. Because it is unlikely that contraception would be acceptable to newly married women under 20, the only feasible strategy for this age group would be to restrict early marriages. Another strategy would target women under 15 and over 30 with parity greater than 5. This would reduce fertility rates by 18% and maternal mortality by 47%. Although the risks of death are higher in pregnant women under 20 and over 40 years, most maternal deaths occur to women between 20 and 34 years because pregnancy is more frequent in this age group. For these reasons, the goal in high-fertility countries has been to promote the spacing of births for women in the 15 to 34 age group and the ending of childbearing for women who are older.

Induced abortions number approximately 55 million per year. Half of these are legal, performed mainly in the developed countries, China, and India (Ping & Smith, 1995). The other half are illegal. When hygienically performed, abortion carries a low risk of death—lower than childbirth. When poorly performed, it often results in severe complications and death. Approximately 200,000, or 40%, of maternal deaths are due to illegal abortions. These figures are most certainly underestimations of the real numbers of women who die from abortion because families are reluctant to report maternal deaths from abortion. However, it is known that abortion is the most common means of fertility control in many countries. Some experts believe that to reduce unwanted pregnancies and maternal mortality, access to safe abortion must be provided in addition to contraceptive methods (Coeytaux, Leonard, & Bloomer, 1993; Simmons, 1986).

The health of children is also enhanced when their parents use family planning. For example, children are more likely to die if their mother is under 20 and over 35 and if they have a late birth order (i.e., at the end of a long line of siblings). This is another reason to stop having children after four or five. Allowing 2 or 3 years to elapse between births, called "birth spacing," may have even greater benefits in ensuring that children survive the first few years. Infant mortality would decline by 24% if children were spaced at least 2 years apart (Trussell & Pebley, 1984). What underlies the statistic is the fact that children with many siblings, spaced close together, compete for limited resources such as breast milk, food, and mother's attention. Children of older mothers who are biologically worn out are more likely to be born with low birth weight (less than 2,500 gm) and to be less successful at breast-feeding. Contraception therefore reduces infant and child mortality if used to space births and if used to end childbearing in older women with many children. A novel counterproposal is to give all young girls 7 or more years of education; this would lower infant mortality rates by 41% and child mortality rates by 60%, all other things being equal (Trussell & Pebley, 1984).

## HOW COUPLES WEIGH THE COSTS AND BENEFITS OF CHILDREN

National population trends and maternal and child mortality are not explicitly involved in couples' reasons for having and not having children. An international study found that parents in agricultural societies were most likely to say that children were economically valuable (Hoffman, 1988); each child contributed resources to the family, not only in terms of labor but also in terms of useful social contacts. If more is better, there is no reason to plan, except perhaps to space births. One hopes that God and nature are favorable. Other parents, in Korea, Taiwan, and Singapore, mentioned that children were valuable in adding a new, stimulating, and enjoyable dimension to one's life. A third reason for having children was the nurturance and love one could experience and express toward children. Despite their different reasons, couples feel a great deal of disappointment when they are unable to have children. In some cultures, the wife's marital and social status is jeopardized as well. Infertility is a surprisingly common problem in many central African countries, where on average 10% of the couples are unable to have children, often as a result of infection (Khanna, VanLook, & Griffin, 1992). Although there are many available orphans to adopt, if childless couples adopt a child, it will usually be one from within the family.

Major societal changes in the number of desired children often result from changes in two particular values that alter the perceived costs of children. Education and economic advancement for individual family members is one value. Fertility declines when parents consider the resources available for each member of the family (Mustafa & Mumford, 1984) rather than for the family as a whole. With fewer children, each person benefits. If children are sent to school, they cost the family more and contribute less in the short term, although their future value increases tremendously. It also means that the woman's labor in home management and child care is reduced, leaving her free to engage in other productive work. Health is another consideration. Women recognize that their health deteriorates after having children as a result of the strains of pregnancy and childbirth and caring for children. This is the case when women have poor nutrition and access to health care. When the marriage bond is close, both spouses may consider the mother's health to be important; however, when continuation of the family line is more important, the mother's health may be less important (Mason & Taj, 1987).

**Maternal depletion** refers to the fact that the health of women declines with the birth of each child. I imagine that for most girls, the first year of marriage is a very trying transition, with the introduction to sex and childbearing. I used to wonder about survey questions asking teenage girls if they were "sexually active." What does *active* mean to a protected girl or one who has been circumcised? Marital or premarital intercourse couldn't possibly be a very actively sought after or exciting experience for a teenage girl in those circumstances. In addition to new household responsibilities, the newly married wife now has a husband and his family to think about. Women and children defer to men and to elders in most things, including eating. Consequently, many young mothers are somewhat malnourished to start with and become further depleted by each growing fetus. In South Asia and sub-Saharan Africa, more than 60% of pregnant women use the services of a traditional midwife or family member to deliver their baby, either out of choice or because the clinic is too far away or closed for the night. Traditional midwives do not have the skills or equipment to handle long labor or a small birth canal, and often do not work under sanitary conditions with clean razors to cut the umbilical cord. The new mother may get infected, bleed excessively, or sustain tears that need time to heal. In some societies, new mothers are allowed to rest with their newborn for 40 days and abstain from sex; in others, the mother walks home with her baby after a few hours and is back to her usual duties. Once again, she may not eat enough to produce breast milk and nourish herself. Given this sequence of events, even a healthy young wife can become weak, tired, and thin. Knowing this, how can anyone possibly think that mothers react with calm fatalism to the death of a child and simply go on having more in the expectation that several will die? Fatalism and expectation are mental states that people talk themselves into after experiencing the death of a loved one. They are ways of coping with an emotionally wrenching experience and not their normal ways of thinking about children.

One useful framework for describing these reasons uses a cost-benefit analysis, which compares the perceived costs of having more children with the perceived satisfactions and benefits derived from having them (Mason & Taj, 1987). The assumption is that the balance will determine whether the person desires a large or a small family and whether the person wants more children than he or she currently has. If the costs outweigh the benefits, then the person should want a small family and want to stop having more children. Such a person should be interested in using contraception.

However, it assumes that people make decisions using a rational process, in the same way as a business manager would tally costs and benefits before introducing a new product. We know that people do not use such a rational process; their decisions are often based on a single cost or benefit that is most important at the time. Furthermore, with many couples, no discussion or decision takes place. It is estimated that 50% of pregnancies are unplanned, and many of these are unwanted (Khanna et al., 1992). For example, in one Yoruba village in Nigeria, 64% of the husbands and wives said no discussion took place, and 70% said no decision was made to have or not have children (Mott & Mott, 1985). Many people believe that God's will and not their own determines whether and when they conceive (e.g., Warren, Hiyari, Wingo, Abdel-Aziz, & Morris, 1990). In other cases, the options are never considered because both husband and wife accept the norm of their community to set no limits on births.

Mason and Taj (1987) compiled the results from many surveys conducted in developing countries that looked at both wives' and husbands' desire for more children. Wives did not differ substantially from their husbands, contrary to the prevailing belief that men want more children than women do. The authors point out that people tend to marry within their social group and as a result have similar socializing experiences and similar values about family roles and family size. This is particularly true when the community homogeneously shares the belief that the main function of marriage is to reproduce (e.g., Ntozi & Kabera, 1991). Young couples fear social ostracism, ridicule, and parental disapproval if they do not produce the expected number of children. Without education, people are unlikely to be exposed to values that question the prevailing norm. Focus group discussions in Ethiopia revealed that the people most likely to recognize the costs of childbearing and the desirability of limiting births were the elder women. Not only had they personally experienced these costs, but they now had the social status to oppose the prevailing value in public (with all but their own daughters, where the grandmotherly "instinct" was stronger). People sometimes think that women have been "conditioned" or forced to submit to social norms of childbearing. The reality is that most men and women approve of the practices they learn socially, if only because they do not think about alternatives, unless with fear or pity.

## THE PREVALENCE OF CONTRACEPTION USE

Approximately 60% or more of couples between 15 and 49 years of age use contraception to space or end childbearing. As Table 3.1 indicates, the rate is 72% in industrialized countries, where the fertility rate is lower than the 2.1 children per woman required to replace the population. In developing countries, 55% of the couples use contraception, largely due to the high rates of use in China (83% in 1996). In the 36 least developed countries, only 17% use contraception. These figures are based on demographic and health surveys conducted in countries and published regularly in the journal *Studies in Family Planning* (Mauldin & Segal, 1988; UNICEF, 1996).

The contraceptives most commonly used in the world today are sterilization (tubectomy, tubal ligation, and vasectomy), 36%; the pill, 15%; intrauterine devices, 19%; and condoms, 10%. In industrialized countries, pills, condoms, and sterilization are equally common. In developing countries, 45% of women and men have had a tubectomy or vasectomy to limit family size, and 24% of women have an intrauterine device (IUD). These methods of contraception are most available and therefore most popular in the two most populous regions of the world. Sterilization is the method "of choice" for most women, for a variety of reasons: It is the only one offered by health workers, or it requires only one decisive action, or it is accompanied by an incentive. When clinicians use the term *tubectomy*, they mean a surgical operation that is irreversible; when they use the term *tubal ligation*, they mean a tying procedure that may be reversible. Under sanitary conditions, sterilization is safe and does not affect one's health or sexual interest (see Box 3.1).

In East Asia and the Pacific, 74% of couples use contraception, in particular sterilization and intrauterine devices (IUD). In South Asia, the rate of contraception use is 40%; sterilization is the most common and IUDs the second most common form. In Latin America, 59% use contraception, the most common forms being sterilization and the pill. Within this region, higher rates are reported for Costa Rica (75%), Brazil (66%), and Colombia (66%), and lower rates for Guatemala (23%) and Haiti (18%). Rates for sub-Saharan Africa are low at 13% and the most common methods are the pill (50%) and traditional methods (30%). Although condoms would be useful in Africa as a means to control births and prevent sexually transmitted diseases such as AIDS, few men use them except for sexual relations outside marriage. It therefore has been difficult to promote their acceptance as a way of spacing births within the family.

Abortion is a common means of preventing births in China, where it is government policy to stop families from having a third child. As a result of widespread resistance and noncompliance with the one-child family policy, rural women gained the right to have a second child if their first was a girl and if they waited four years before becoming pregnant again. However, if a woman becomes pregnant a third time, she may be pressured to have an abortion and penalized if she does not. This depends to a certain extent on the flexibility of provincial officials, who must keep to preset limits on the number of births allowed in their region. Abortions in the first trimester are usually carried out through vacuum aspiration, while abortions in later stages of pregnancy may

### BOX 3.1.
### STERILIZATION IS MORE THAN A STATISTIC IN INDIA

Sterilization is the most popular form of birth control worldwide. In developing countries, one in four couples limits birth through sterilization. Nowhere is it more common than in India, which led the way in early family planning programs, and China, which more recently implemented the one-child policy. John Caldwell and colleagues (1988) feel that statistics about the prevalence of sterilization mask intriguing family dynamics that lead to a decision to have the operation. He and his team of local and foreign researchers observed and interviewed people living in agricultural villages in southern India. About one in three of the population practiced modern contraception—fully 86% of whom used sterilization. Traditionally, there were several means by which families spaced their children, namely, postpartum sexual abstinence for 2 years and breast-feeding. Other than these, people did not use traditional methods such as withdrawal or rhythm. However, in a little more than 20 years, India's fertility rate and infant mortality rate fell dramatically. This is attributed to a strong government decision to promote sterilization during the 1960s and 1970s when Indira Gandhi was prime minister. The pressure was on from all directions in society to persuade people with three or more children to have a tubectomy or vasectomy. There were incentives (loans, livestock, free medicine, housing, and cash) and disincentives (loss of employment or housing) and a visit every 2 months from a health worker who extolled the virtues of limiting the number of children. Usually the young couple were living with the husband's family, as they traditionally do in India until the next son marries. Consequently, the decision to have a tubectomy was usually made by the young wife, with the agreement of her husband and mother-in-law. Now, however, mothers-in-law are less intrusive in the marital affairs of their sons.

The question has been raised about whether people were coerced to have the operation. Several years later, some remain bitter about having had the operation, feeling that they were left little room to choose. Others recall that they were not happy about the way the policy was implemented but are very happy to have fewer children. Two positive consequences were that living children were better cared for by a mother who had been sterilized, and family planning became a topic of public and marital discussion.

> The negative consequences were poor health. Some women complained about weakness, breathlessness, pain all over, loss of appetite, menstrual problems such as severe bleeding, and discharge due to infection. Bhatia and Cleland (1995) attempted to find out whether these symptoms were due to the tubectomy. They interviewed women from the district in south India where Caldwell had been. Women with these symptoms were more likely to have had delivery complications with their last child and to have delivered in a nonhospital setting, whether or not they recently had a tubectomy. Thus the most likely source of problems was the childbirth prior to the tubectomy. Anemia, common infections, and the tubectomy operation itself were also sources of problems for some women. The women's symptoms were real enough, but they were often caused by delivery conditions, nutrition, sanitation, and hygiene. Household sanitation and personal hygiene sound basic and simple. I assure you that in a rural setting it is an uphill battle against the elements of nature and social life.

use saline solution or herbal preparations to remove the fetus. Abortions are also carried out on unmarried women who become pregnant and on those who may transmit genetic defects. The common preference for sons among couples also results in their choosing to abort female fetuses. The ratio of aborted births to live births in China is approximately the same as the ratio in developed countries, namely, 50%. However, the women who have abortions in China are more likely to be married women with two children, whereas women in developed countries who have abortions are more likely to be teenage girls with no children. The number of abortions in China is declining as women become more accepting of the IUD and other methods of contraception (Ping, 1995; Ping & Smith, 1995; Rigdon, 1996).

Traditional methods of birth control are estimated to be used by 14.6% of the population worldwide and are particularly prevalent in Africa. These include the common practices of abstinence, withdrawal, and rhythm, along with prolonged breast-feeding. Breast-feeding continues for 2 years or more in many African countries but is not very effective after the child begins to eat solid foods. The effectiveness of the other methods, of course, depends on the exercise of self-discipline.

Researchers recorded the descriptions of other traditional methods used by rural Ugandans. One involves the use of the umbilical cord of the last-born child, which is worn around the mother's waist until she wants to conceive again. Another involves the mother wearing her son-in-law's clothes when she is menstruating; this is thought to stop her menstrual cycle. Many methods involve the use of herbs, which are drunk in a tea or worn in a belt around the waist (Ntozi & Kabera, 1991). Given what we know about the reproductive process, these methods are unlikely to be effective. The methods chosen suggest to a certain extent whether contraception is desired to space births or to stop producing once the desired family size is reached. Most of the traditional methods are used to space births, and it is often said that this is the prime goal in most African women. In contrast, the prevalence of sterilization in Asia suggests that the goal of these women is to stop bearing children.

New forms of contraception are currently being developed to make the procedures less invasive and less dependent on a highly trained health professional. These include a contraceptive ring inserted into the woman's vagina that releases hormones, a reversible vaccine, injectable vaccines, patches placed on the skin, new IUDs, and female condoms. New developments in male contraceptives are moving at a slower pace, but tests on a male hormone injection have shown promise. The goal is to find a number of viable options from which couples can select the one that suits their needs.

The KAP Gap [Knowledge + Attitude = Practice] - Fallicy

Knowledge of both traditional and modern methods of contraception is generally high in most surveys. Often more than 90% of the samples, and a minimum of 50%, know of at least one modern method (e.g., Mustafa & Mumford, 1984; Tucker, 1986). Similarly, many people approve of contraception, with the exception of objections for religious reasons. The KAP equation assumes that *knowledge + attitude = practice*. However, the low use of contraception in many countries suggests that knowledge and attitudes do not predict use. The discrepancy between knowledge, attitudes, and practice is referred to as the "KAP gap." Knowledge about contraception and positive attitudes are necessary, but they are certainly not sufficient.

One obvious reason is that husbands and/or wives want more children. The figure quoted previously indicated that 75% of couples in developing countries, and more in sub-Saharan Africa, want to have more children. They might be interested in using contraception to space births but not to stop having children.

An often-cited reason is poor access to family planning services. Despite efforts to expand these services, 40% of women in South Asia, Southeast Asia, and Latin America do not have access, which usually means that they live farther than 10 km from such services. In sub-Saharan Africa, 90% do not have access. Even with access, there are considerations of the cost of time, transportation, waiting at the clinic, numerous return visits, lack of privacy, and disrespectful treatment by health professionals (Schuler, McIntosh, Goldstein, & Pande, 1985). Efforts made to remedy the extent and nature of family planning services in a region will be discussed later.

Another reason is that women might fear the invasive nature of modern contraception. Some believe that pills will have a permanent effect on their reproductive organs and prevent them from having children in the future. They think they work by burning up one's vital fluids and drying the uterus, and that pills will lead to early menopause and old age. Mothers fear the pill will heat up their breast milk, giving the nursing child rashes and diarrhea, and dry it up so the child will be thin and sickly. Others fear pain, weakness, weight loss, infection, changes in the menstrual cycle, and effects on their sexuality (Eschen & Whittaker, 1993; Nichter, 1989). Without knowing the seriousness of these side effects, women may become concerned about the reproductive and sexual functions of their bodies as well as their roles of wife, mother, and daughter in the family system (see Box 3.2).

For these and other reasons, women who are less educated are less likely to use modern contraception. In contrast, women with higher incomes, women who are more educated, and women who are employed outside the home consider family planning to be an important goal in their lives. Most studies find that these women are more likely to use modern contraception. Not only do they want to limit their family size for economic reasons, they are more likely to understand the side effects on their bodies, to be treated courteously by health professionals, and to be able to cope with the costs (Ntozi & Kabera, 1991; Tucker, 1986).

## BOX 3.2.
## FOLK BELIEFS ABOUT
## MODERN CONTRACEPTION

Mark Nichter (1989) talked to women in Sri Lanka to find out what they thought about modern contraception methods, such as the pill, condoms, intrauterine device, and sterilization. Most of the women had not used any of these techniques, but they had heard about them. And what they heard was bad news. Pills are said to have a heating effect, burning up one's vitality; they also dry up one's uterus, which leads to early menopause and old age. This is how pills are supposed to prevent pregnancy, they said, but the result is that one is permanently unable to have children. Furthermore, pills cause weight loss, nausea, vomiting, general weakness, dizziness, burning sensations in one's abdomen, and pain in many sites. Condoms are said to produce heat and burning due to the rubber and the friction (it's like wearing rubber shoes). IUDs are said to produce heat and profuse bleeding, which are needed to eliminate the fetus. In addition, many women thought the loop would get pushed up into their stomach or perhaps their head during active intercourse. It is amazing that the same complaints are mentioned by women around the world who have never themselves used the contraception method.

Nichter concludes that we are too quick to judge the information as groundless rumors. Others call these ideas "false beliefs" (Torrey, 1967). Nichter prefers to call them culture-based common sense. *Common sense* is a good term for these ideas, in that it means sound practical judgments about everyday matters. Common sense is psychologically sound but not necessarily scientifically sound. And although these ideas may come from a culture, they may also come from a universal need to make cause-effect sense of something as important as sexuality and reproduction. The study of how and why people create ideas about the causes and effects of things that happen to them has a long history in the psychology of social cognition. We know that people feel the need to search, in particular, for causes of negative and unexpected events. We also know that people identify causes by looking for something that happened close in time or space to the negative or unexpected event. Consider these beliefs:

- You will get a cold if you stay in a cold or drafty place.

> - If a woman has a deformed baby, it's because she stared or laughed at another's deformed baby when she was pregnant.
> - If a girl menstruates before her marriage, she must be a nonvirgin.
> - If a man urinates in the light of the moon at night, he will get a sexually transmitted disease.
>
> These beliefs make sense considering that the negative event and its folk cause often occur together. But we are rarely systematic in our search for causes. Do we ever ask ourselves: How many times have I been in a cold or drafty place when I did not catch a cold? How many times have I caught a cold when I was not previously in a cold or drafty place? If lean girls typically menstruate at 15 years, and marry at 12 years, then they will be virgins.

## WHAT MAKES A FAMILY PLANNING PROGRAM EFFECTIVE?

Numerous programs have been tried in developing countries to increase the use of contraceptives. Their goal is to speak directly to the 25% of women who do not want to have more children, and to target teenage and older women and those who have more than five children. In particular, they feel effort should be concentrated in six countries with large populations and low contraception use, namely, Ethiopia, Bangladesh, India, Nigeria, Pakistan, and Zaire (Mauldin & Ross, 1991).

Some of these programs are the Menstrual Regulation program in Bangladesh; PROFAMILIA and MEXFAM in Colombia and Mexico, respectively, which target men, women, and adolescents; the 40-day postpartum consultation visit in Tunisia; postabortion services in Turkey and India; and contraceptive services at clinics for AIDS and other sexually transmitted diseases (Eschen & Whittaker, 1993). In Bangladesh, for example, the Women's Health Coalition is a privately funded nongovernmental organization controlled by women to offer a variety of services in maternal and child health. They have six clinics in rural and urban sites. The drawing card is its menstrual regulation service. This refers to an aspiration evacuation of the uterus to end pregnancy early in women who might otherwise have a risky abortion. It is usually performed manually in Bangladesh using a syringe and a hollow flexible plastic tube. The success of the contraceptive program rests on the timing of the message—when the woman is most likely to be concerned about unwanted pregnancy. The long-term objective is to reduce the need for menstrual regulation services by counseling women in the selection of preventive contraception. Approximately 25% of clients' time at the clinic is spent with a counselor discussing their individual needs and finding out about methods of contraception. In the course of 1 year, 73% of the women left the clinic with a contraceptive device (Kay & Kabir, 1988).

However, when choosing to develop and implement a program, it is important to know which programs are most effective and most cost-effective. After 20 years of experience, it is possible to examine and compare different programs. The index most often used for evaluating a program is the increase in the number of people using contraception in comparison with a control group who lacks the program. Measures of the strength of the program itself have also been used to evaluate the process. Lapham and Mauldin (1985) provide 30 items that can be placed in the following four broad categories: policies of the country, service activities, evaluation, and methods made available. Mauldin and Ross (1991) evaluated 98 countries in terms of the strength of their programs and found that availability and services were the two most important determinants of contraception use and fertility decline. East Asian countries were most likely to have strong programs; South Asia and Latin America, to have moderately strong programs; and Africa and the Middle East, to have weak programs. Services are particularly important. Four noteworthy aspects of service will be discussed in more detail. They include

1. incentives and costs,
2. media communication,
3. community-based distribution, and
4. worker-client exchanges.

Incentives and Costs

Costs, payments, and incentives are another feature of family planning programs (Elder & Estey, 1992; Ross & Isaacs, 1988). If production and distribution were solely a commercial enterprise, there would be a cost to the consumer for contraception. This is usually the case with condoms, and there is clear evidence that the higher the cost, the fewer the condoms sold (Harvey, 1994). However, in many developing countries, family planning was initiated by nongovernmental organizations and then taken over by national governments. These governments then decided whether or not to provide free services or to charge for services. On the one hand, there is the desire to make contraception affordable to all who need it, and, on the other, the need for organizations and governments to recover some costs of the program.

Some governments provide payments to acceptors, especially those who choose sterilization; payments to providers and recruiters on a case-by-case basis; and incentives to communities and families who limit births. For example, regions in India, Sri Lanka, Taiwan, and Thailand provided cash, retirement bonuses, education funds, livestock, and symbolic medals to couples who accepted sterilization or otherwise refrained from having more children. One incentive scheme promoted birth spacing by rewarding women with the gift of a piglet when they spaced their next pregnancy. Women who accepted contraception use were given a piglet to fatten for 8 months; if they refrained from getting pregnant during this period, they could get an additional pig. During the 3-year period of this program, no woman who accepted a pig ever got pregnant (Elder & Estey, 1992). Some governments impose penalties on those who exceed the regulated number of births. Singapore, for example, gave housing, schooling, and employment opportunities to families with one or two children, and removed these benefits on the birth of a third child. China imposes penalties on women who have a third unauthorized child and on provincial governments who exceed their birth quota for the year.

Ethical considerations become relevant when the payments and penalties are coercive enough to restrict an individual's or couple's right to decide freely and responsibly the number of children they can care for. To a certain extent, governments also have this right, and so must responsibly decide the population size that can be maintained by the economy of the country without endangering future generations and natural resources. Thus both social and individual freedoms must be respected in the decision to impose benefits and penalties. The criticism against a purely voluntary system is that it works too slowly in countries that need fast action, where having children is more a matter of chance than a freely made decision and where there is otherwise no motivation to become informed about contraceptive options. Usually the magnitude of the payment affects whether it is seen to enhance or restrict freedom of choice. Payments that cover the cost of the sterilization operation and long-term payments that provide old-age security in lieu of children are seen as enhancing a poor person's option to choose contraception as well as providing an incentive. Because many people in the international community are uncomfortable and suspicious about cash-for-contraception schemes, follow-up surveys have been conducted to ask people if they are satisfied or regretful; 90% express sincere satisfaction and do not mention money as the reason for ending their fertility (Cleland & Mauldin, 1990).

Payments to providers and communities are thought to lead to too much social pressure being placed on couples by people who have ulterior motives for wanting them to accept contraception. Penalties not only restrict individual choice but impose a burden on the children of the family, who are innocent of wrongdoing. As for charging a fee from the client, some suggest a two-tiered system taking "from each according to his or her means." That is, couples who are able to afford contraception pay for it, while those who are not get services free. This allows for some cost recovery by agencies and increased affordability for poorer couples.

Message Through the Media

Use of the mass media to increase awareness and acceptance of family planning has been tried in several countries with some success. A visual message is not sufficient to arouse interest, unless it borders on the outrageous (such as one recently seen on the back of a bus advertising condoms with a picture of a green zucchini being touched by a yellow feather). In Nigeria, where urban dwellers are likely to have televisions, variety shows and soap opera dramas provide a convenient context to popularize contraceptive use (Piotrow et al., 1990). The typical soap opera, for example, has the right mix of family problems and reconciliations, which unfold with great hilarity as well as grief. Most viewers identify with the characters. In three Nigerian cities, a number of family planning episodes were inserted into already established TV programs. They were humorous, dramatic, and entertaining. The media developers were careful to find out beforehand, from men and women, what kind of message would be culturally acceptable and address viewers' concerns. Scenes were previewed and evaluated by potential viewers. The number of new contraception acceptors increased fivefold in the city where the campaign lasted 3 years and threefold in the city where it was run for 1 year. Many new acceptors said they had watched the programs. But an equal number heard about family planning from friends, relatives, and health professionals who were indirectly affected by the media campaign. In summary, television programming with role models that appeal to a targeted audience can have a significant effect on contraceptive use, not only on those who watch the program but indirectly by gaining an attractive reputation that is spread by word of mouth through interpersonal channels. Radio and magazine promotions have also been used to promote vasectomy in Brazil and Guatemala with positive but less striking results (Foreit, de Castro, & Franco, 1989; Piotrow & Kincaid, 1988). Radio messages often lead to an increase in knowledge about contraception but have little effect on attitudes or acceptance for personal use.

Community-Based Distribution

Making contraceptives such as pills, injectables, and condoms available in rural communities eliminates the need for people to travel repeatedly to get materials or checkups. This is particularly crucial in Bangladesh and India, where women do not travel far from home, and in Africa, where clinics are located far from most of the population. Bangladesh in particular has been the site of efforts to make family planning available in one's own home (Bernhart & Kamal, 1994; Phillips, Hossain, Simmons, & Koenig, 1993; Simmons, Baqee, Koenig, & Phillips, 1988; Simmons, Koblinsky, & Phillips, 1986).

In Bangladesh, the demand for contraception traditionally has been low. Therefore, it has been important to foster demand by carrying the message to people in their homes. During the past decade, community-based distribution, or outreach, programs of NGOs and the International Centre for Diarrheal Disease Research in Dhaka have been reviewed. Home visits by a woman field-worker are labor intensive but satisfy the wife's need for privacy and for social support from her husband. In this culture, field-workers must be women; they are recruited from the community, have an eighth-grade education, and are trained for 4-6 weeks. They are given a certain population to visit on a monthly basis and are supposed to make a forceful case for using contraception. In addition, they discuss the needs and interests of the couple, contraindications to using a particular method, and possible side effects. If the couple wants pills or an injectable, they can be distributed there. If the couple wants sterilization or an IUD, the field-worker will arrange for travel and an appointment at the nearest clinic. Not only did the workers succeed in meeting the need for contraception in distant places, they crystallized the desire in people who were uncertain and awakened an interest in others.

The program in Guatemala had 552 urban and rural distributors (Bertrand, Pineda, Santiso, & Hearn, 1980). Although 30% had not received any formal course in family planning, this did not seem to affect their success as measured in terms of the number of couple-months of contraceptive protection sold during a 12-month period (pills, condoms, and foam). Many of the distributors sold the products in their homes or in a shop along with other products. They also actively promoted family planning by organizing group meetings and visiting homes. The average number of couple-months of protection sold per distributor was 35 in the urban area and 11 in the rural areas. Most of their clients were regular users, although a significant number were new acceptors. A similar program used traders in a Nigerian city market to distribute contraceptives (Lapido, McNamara, Weiss, & Otolorin, 1990). During the period from 1986 to 1989, contraception sales increased from 32% to 48%, with an average of 5.3 per month for each trader. Although the market may not be an ideal place to introduce contraception to new users, it is a site very accessible to regular users of the pill and irregular users of condoms.

One of the benefits of home visits, other than convenience and privacy, is the social and psychological support of a spouse. Husbands are very influential in a woman's decision to accept contraception. Programs aimed at couples help the wife and husband communicate about their mutual and separate concerns and make a decision that will be more sustainable than if made separately. One such program was carried out in a semiurban district in Ethiopia (Terefe & Larson, 1993). Health assistants from the local health stations made one or two home visits to discuss contraception and to address personal questions about its benefits and side effects. Married women between 15 and 49 years were randomly assigned to be visited alone by the health assistant or to have their husbands present for the visit. Although more than 60% of the husbands were in favor of family planning, none of the couples were using contraception at the time of the visit and the rate of contraception use in the community was 2%. After two months, 15% of women visited alone became users, whereas 25% of those visited as a couple had begun birth control. Twelve months later, birth control was maintained by 5.6% of the alone group and 16.4% of the couple group. More interesting was the finding of a delayed acceptance by 11.6% of the alone group and 16.4% of the couple group, since the 2-month visit. The message was presumably remembered and considered more attractive after the couple had time to discuss its relevance to their own goals.

Worker-Client Exchanges

Family planning workers, whether they are professionals in a clinic or midwives in a village, have the tough job of persuading couples to use contraception. Many in the past saw themselves as teachers whose role was to instruct, coerce, and reprimand. Bullying and shaming people into using contraception cannot work in the long term. Some combination of forthright disclosure, confident commitment, and empathic listening is needed, given the ambivalence of most women toward contraception. Workers become credible and persuasive by being both an expert and a person with whom the woman can identify. This is why some programs try to have their contraceptive users act as enthusiastic facilitators among their friends and neighbors.

Poor, illiterate women are often not given the time, information, and respect they deserve. The thought of coming back every few months for a resupply, and getting abuse, would dissuade anyone. A clear demonstration of the communication problem was provided when researchers sent couples posing as interested clients to different clinics. The lower-class couple were themselves not very knowledgeable about family planning and asked few questions. They were treated as inferior, given less information that was often inaccurate, and dismissed sooner than the middle-class couple (Schuler et al., 1985). This is the kind of bias that drives a large gap between rural illiterate people and health professionals, a gap that is counterproductive to promoting family planning.

To learn good communication skills, workers are studying the GATHER framework:

G = Greet client in friendly and helpful way.
A = Ask client about family planning needs.
T = Tell client about available methods.
H = Help client decide which he or she wants.
E = Explain how to use chosen method.
R = Return visits should be explained.

Simulated clients are then used to evaluate the quality of the worker-client interaction. Clients from the rural areas are hard to recruit for this kind of simulation. They are too afraid to go into a clinic and afraid they might be pressed into doing something they will regret. Nonetheless, this is one way to assess the interpersonal skills of workers (Huntington & Schuler, 1993).

GATHER is a worker-driven agenda for communicating about family planning needs. In some cultures and settings, the successful interaction would have to be less driven by the worker and more controlled by the client. Although health workers are expected by their clients to be in control and to give advice, there are ways to make the communication a dialogue. One is to stop after each letter of the GATHER framework and listen to the client. Active listening is an art that some come by naturally and others must practice. An active listener encourages expression and shows interest in what is said without talking. It is a mistake to think we have to fill silence with talking and "empty" mental spaces with knowledge.

## STUDENT ACTIVITIES

1. Do a local survey of "false" or folk beliefs concerning modern contraception or any other health issue. Include any of the ones you have read about here and add others that are suitable for your sample. Here are some extras that you might find interesting to include:

a. People get colds from being cold.
b. People will eat what is good for them when they are hungry.

2. As a result of lobbying from various anti-abortion groups, who fear that family planning aid money is being spent on providing abortions, national policy makers of a certain country are trying to determine if this is indeed the case. They must also consider the pros and cons of various policy options such as withholding funding, continuing funding, or setting strict, enforceable conditions. Imagine that you have been hired as a consultant to provide relevant information and figures so that a decision can be reached on funding family planning programs. You must be unbiased and complete in providing information, but then take a position. Choose a region or a country as a focus for your information-gathering efforts. Consider these arguments: Those in favor of funding family planning programs say that the money is being used to promote nonabortion contraceptives and that eliminating funding for these programs will only increase abortions as women seek to control births. Those who oppose funding family planning say that the money is being spent on providing abortion services and that setting conditions on the use of funds isn't effective because "the assistance frees up other money that can then be used for abortion" (Vobejda, 1996, p. 16).

# 4

# THE AIDS/HIV PANDEMIC

*Michaela Hynie*

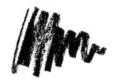

In 1981, the medical community announced the discovery of a hitherto unknown illness, acquired immunodeficiency syndrome (AIDS). In the mid-1980s, it was determined that AIDS is a late-stage infection by a retrovirus, the human immunodeficiency virus (HIV). The extensive spread of HIV, the virus that causes AIDS, is assumed to have begun in the late 1970s and early 1980s among men and women with multiple sex partners in East and Central Africa and among homosexual and bisexual men in specific urban centers in the Americas, Western Europe, Australia, and New Zealand. The epidemic has since spread throughout the developing and industrialized world. As of December 1996, it has been estimated that 26.8 million adults and 2.6 million children have been infected with HIV since the onset of the epidemic. Of these 29.4 million, 6.7 million adults and 1.7 million children have developed AIDS and, of these, 5.0 million adults and 1.4 million children have died of it. In 1996 alone, the last year for which we have figures, there were an estimated 2.7 million new HIV infections among adults and 400,000 new HIV infections among children. In 1996, 1.5 million deaths were estimated to be attributable to HIV/AIDS: 1.1 million among adults and 350,000 among children (UNAIDS, 1996b).

If you have trouble imagining these numbers, translate them into a community of similar size. For example, the population of Tanzania is roughly equal to the number of people who have been infected with HIV. So is that of Canada. If you imagine all Canadians under the age of 21, that gives you a rough estimate of the number of people in the world who have suffered from AIDS. The number of deaths due to AIDS and HIV is equivalent to Canadians under 16 years. If your population age structure is more like Tanzania, then imagine that all Tanzanians under the age of 8 contracted AIDS, and the smaller number of those under 6 died of it, and you will have a frightening picture of the human cost of this disease.

AIDS is characterized by a severely weakened immune system; people living with AIDS ultimately succumb to life-threatening opportunistic infections such as pneumocystis carinii pneumonia and cancers such as Kaposi's sarcoma and lymphoma of the brain. In developing countries, AIDS is typically associated with diseases of the digestive system and is characterized by severe weight loss. Approximately 60% of adults infected with HIV will develop AIDS within 12 to 13 years from the time of infection. Except for the development of self-limiting, flulike symptoms in the weeks following infection, many infected persons are asymptomatic between initial infection and the development of AIDS. Others will develop HIV-related illness before they have the symptoms of AIDS. Survival times after AIDS onset are short although they have increased from 1 year to about 3 years in industrialized countries as a result of improved health care. In developing countries, however, the progression from infection to symptomatic illness may be more rapid in than in industrialized countries and survival after AIDS onset continues to be less than 1 year. At this point in time, there is no known cure for AIDS and there is no vaccine to prevent HIV infection. Moreover, a vaccine is not expected to be available at any time in the near future. (Facts and figures from this paragraph are found in Coates et al., 1996, and UNAIDS, 1996a.)

## BOX 4.1.
## TYPES AND SUBTYPES OF HIV

There are two different types of virus that causes AIDS, HIV-1, and HIV-2. HIV-1 is the more common of the two types and is the one that is typically reported in HIV prevalence rates. Although HIV-2 also leads to AIDS, it appears to be less easily transmitted than HIV-1 and to have a longer incubation period. HIV-2 is transmitted through heterosexual intercourse and blood transfusions, and infection rates appear to be equal between men and women. Although vertical transmission from mother to child of HIV-2 has been reported, it seems to occur less frequently than for HIV-1. HIV-2 is more prevalent than HIV-1 in West Africa, where the AIDS incidence is lower than in Central and East Africa. Outside of West Africa, high rates of HIV-2 infection have also been reported in Cameroon and Angola. In the Ivory Coast, epidemic levels of both types of virus, HIV-1 and HIV-2, have been observed.

There are also a number of subtypes of the HIV-1 virus. In the last 4 years, 10 genetically distinct subtypes have been identified. The major group (group M) contains subtypes A to J. A second group of subtypes, group O (Outliers), contains a set of highly heterogeneous viruses. The different subtypes are found at highly varying rates around the world. Subtype B is found most commonly in the Americas, Japan, Australia, the Caribbean, and Europe. Subtypes A and D are found primarily in sub-Saharan Africa. Subtype C is typically found in South Africa and India whereas subtype E is found in Central African Republic. The other subtypes are of very low prevalence and highly localized.

Certain subtypes may be predominantly associated with specific modes of transmission. For example, it has been suggested, but not confirmed, that subtype B is associated with blood transmission and is therefore transmitted primarily through contact between men who have sex with men and injection drug use. Subtypes D and E are assumed to be transmitted via the mucosal route and are therefore associated with heterosexual transmission. Moreover, certain subtypes may be more infectious than others. Specifically, subtype E may be spread more easily than subtype B.

In the future, additional genetic subtypes will likely be discovered and the known subtypes will continue to spread. It is unclear whether these genetic variations make a difference in terms of responses to antiviral therapy or

> prevention by vaccine. In terms of the behavioral prevention of HIV infection, however, the type of HIV makes no difference. Sterilizing injection equipment, using condoms, and adopting safer sex behaviors continue to be the most effective methods of preventing HIV infection for all known HIV types and subtypes (Miyazaki, 1995; UNAIDS, 1995).

## MODES OF HIV TRANSMISSION

There are three primary modes of transmission of HIV. Although the risk of transmission through one act of unprotected heterosexual intercourse with an HIV-infected partner is small—estimates range from .0004% to 1%—unprotected sexual intercourse is the main route of HIV infection. Worldwide, between 75% and 85% of HIV infections in adults have been transmitted through unprotected (i.e., without a condom) anal, oral, or vaginal intercourse. Heterosexual intercourse accounts for approximately 70% of HIV infections and man-to-man intercourse accounts for a further 5% to 10%. There are no documented cases of the transmission of HIV between two female sexual partners. A number of factors have been associated with an increased risk of sexual HIV transmission during vaginal and anal intercourse, including duration of the sexual relationship, frequency of sexual contact, gender of the infected partner, lack of male circumcision, the presence of genital ulcerations due to chancroid, syphilis, or herpes sores, the presence of other nonulcerative sexually transmitted diseases (STDs) such as gonorrhea, chlamydia, and trichomoniasis, and sex during menses (Carlin & Boag, 1995; Haverkos & Quinn, 1995; Kimball, Berkley, Ngugi, & Gayle, 1995).

HIV transmission also occurs through blood and blood products, primarily through the use of infected needles, syringes, or other skin-piercing instruments or through blood transfusion. The virus can also be transmitted through donated organs and semen. Transfusions of blood or blood products account for 3% to 5% of adult HIV infections whereas the sharing of infected injection equipment between injection drug users accounts for 5% to 10% of adult infections and is the dominant mode of transmission in several countries. The proportion of adults infected through injection drug use (IDU) appears to be increas-

> **BOX 4.2.**
> **MORE PRECISE AND SENSITIVE TERMINOLOGY**
>
> In the past few years, we have realized that our former use of terms and labels for people who are at risk for HIV was not accurate and not sensitive to them as persons. Here are some of the changes.
>
> *Groups engaging in risky behavior* is the phrase that replaces *risk groups*. Although the term *risk groups* is frequently used in this and other health-related texts, the people in these groups are likely to receive HIV only if and when they engage in certain behaviors. To focus on the behaviors, rather than the people, we have now adopted a more precise term.
>
> *Injection drug users* replaces the term *intravenous drug users*. The new term includes people who inject subcutaneously and intramuscularly as well as those who inject intravenously because all three forms of injection put people at risk for HIV infection.
>
> *Men who have sex with men (MSM)* is used in addition to the term *homosexuals*. Men who have sex with men may also be heterosexual or bisexual in their orientation. It is the sexual act rather than the sexual orientation that increases the chances of infection.
>
> *Sex workers (SW)* replaces the term *commercial sex workers* in some contexts because many sex workers receive remuneration in kind rather than money for the sexual services they provide.

ing (UNAIDS, 1996a). Formerly, we used *IDU* to refer to intravenous drug use; in the past few years, this and other terms have been changed as a result of our attempt to be more precise and socially sensitive to people whose behavior puts them at risk for HIV (see Box 4.2 on precise and sensitive terminology).

Finally, HIV transmission can occur from a mother to her child during pregnancy, delivery, or breast-feeding. This is called vertical, perinatal, or mother-to-child transmission. More than 90% of HIV infections among children are the result of vertical transmission and approximately 25% to 35% of children who are born to mothers infected with HIV become infected themselves. It is estimated that up to 15% of vertical transmissions may occur through breast-feeding alone (Mertens & Low-Beer, 1996; UNAIDS, 1996a).

## MEASURING THE MAGNITUDE OF AIDS AND HIV

AIDS was first identified by the presence of uncommon and unusual diseases, such as Kaposi's sarcoma and candidiasis of the esophagus, trachea, bronchi, or lungs. The U.S. Centers for Disease Control and Prevention (CDC) generated guidelines for diagnosing AIDS in the mid-1980s that were based on clinical case observations of the presence of these unusual diseases. These guidelines were then adopted by the World Health Organization (WHO) for use in other industrialized countries. However, the CDC guidelines are not suitable for developing countries because of the lack of facilities for diagnosing most indicator diseases. Thus several other definitions for diagnosing AIDS have been proposed for use specifically in Africa and in Central and South America (Buehler, De Cock, & Brunet, 1993; Piot et al., 1992).

However, diagnosis of AIDS on the basis of AIDS symptoms alone is problematic. The clinical definitions have been found to miss more than 50% of AIDS cases in some settings, most notably in Africa. Thus, without a sensitive case definition of AIDS, based on observed features rather than laboratory tests, most cases still go unrecognized in Africa (Jager, Heisterkamp, & Brookmeyer, 1993). The most accurate figures are therefore based on estimates, using selected sentinel sites where laboratory tests are available, for example, and extrapolating from them to the population.

More reliable diagnoses are possible using laboratory tests to detect the presence of HIV. The presence of HIV is typically determined through the use of ELISA tests (enzyme-linked immunoabsorbent assays), which test for HIV antibodies in the blood. Another test, the Western blot, can be used as a confirmatory test after positive results are obtained with the ELISA. The Western blot test detects HIV proteins directly and is more reliable than the Elisa, which can produce false positives at rates near 30%. The ELISA antibody tests are now widely available in developing countries and are increasingly used in combination with clinical case definitions to identify cases of AIDS and HIV infection (Cohen, 1996; Piot et al., 1992).

The epidemic can be monitored using either prevalence rates or incidence rates. Prevalence rates are obtained by estimating the number of persons living with HIV/AIDS in one specific region at a specific time and then dividing by the total population of that region. Prevalence rates essentially represent the total number of people who have been infected in the past, minus the number of infected people who have died. In contrast, incidence rates represent the number of new HIV infections, or new AIDS cases, during a specific time period such as a year. Incidence rates have the advantage of permitting tracking of trends in HIV infection, AIDS onset, and AIDS deaths from year to year (Bongaarts, 1996).

The magnitude of the AIDS epidemic was initially monitored by relying on reporting of AIDS cases to the WHO. However, because of the high rates of underreporting, the WHO now monitors the epidemic by estimating the rates of HIV infections, AIDS cases, and AIDS deaths. Global and regional HIV prevalence estimates are calculated from data collected from published and unpublished serological surveys and studies and regional and national reports. Estimates for pediatric AIDS and HIV infections are typically based on estimates of the number of HIV-infected women and their fertility patterns and on the rate of transmission from an infected woman to her infant (approximately 25% but it varies from 20% to 50% depending on the country).

Past trends and future predictions can then be estimated from these data through various mathematical models. Future predictions are typically achieved with one of three basic procedures: statistical extrapolation, back-calculation, and dynamic models. Statistical extrapolation is used for short-term predictions of future rates and is based on past incidence rates only. Back-calculation predicts future AIDS patterns by examining past incidence rates plus knowledge about the disease progression, such as incubation times and effects of interventions. Dynamic models use the same information as back-calculation models but also use information about modes of transmission and transmission probabilities. Because dynamic models require more specific information than back-calculation models, the use of these models is more restricted (Bongaarts, 1996; Chin, 1990; Jager et al., 1993).

Estimates of prevalence and incidence in the general population are based on surveys of blood serum collected from people who are in contact with health services, such as pregnant women in antenatal clinics and blood donors, both considered to be groups at lower risk of HIV. However, serosurveys are also carried out by sampling directly

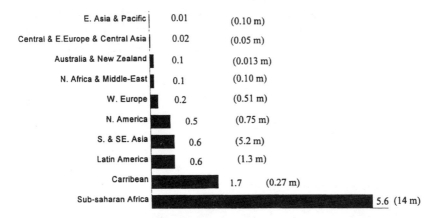

**Figure 4.1.** Estimated Percentages (and Numbers) of Persons Living With HIV/AIDS* by Region at the End of 1996
SOURCE: Based on data obtained from the UNAIDS web site (November 1996): www.us.unaids.org.
NOTE: The global total is 22.6 million. The current rates and numbers may be different; contact UNAIDS on the Internet for the latest figures.
*Percentage of persons living with HIV/AIDS equals the number of persons with HIV/AIDS in one specific region at one specific time divided by the total population of the region.

from the general population (e.g., Wilkins et al., 1991). Other populations surveyed for seroprevalence are those that are considered to be at high risk for infection, namely, patients in STD clinics, sex workers, migrant workers, truck drivers, and female bar workers (Anderson, May, Ng, & Rowley, 1992).

## INTERNATIONAL PREVALENCE RATES AND PATTERNS

Prevalence rates of infection vary widely between regions and between different populations within the same region as a function of sexual practices and patterns of STD infection. Regions differ not only in their rates of infection but also in the primary means by which HIV infection is transmitted (see Figure 4.1).

Statistics from the end of 1996 suggest that prevalence is highest in sub-Saharan Africa (5.6%), where it is estimated that there are 14 million adults and children living with HIV/AIDS. Slightly more than 50% of the 13.3 million infected adults are women, and heterosexual transmission is the dominant mode of HIV transmission. The rapid spread of the epidemic in sub-Saharan Africa has been attributed to social factors, such as the migratory labor system that separates men from their home communities for long periods of time (Goldin, 1994), greater sexual activity at a younger age, and higher levels of transmission efficiency due to the presence of facilitating factors such as STDs (Kimball et al., 1995). Some 700,000 children have been infected, accounting for more than 85% of all cases of children infected through vertical transmission (UNAIDS, 1996a).

There is considerable variability in HIV prevalence rates both within and between countries. Among certain groups of people such as sex workers (SWs), the rates of infection can be as high as 80% as in Nairobi, 55% in Abidjan, and 55% in Djibouti. The general adult population can show rates varying from 0.1% in Sudan to 18% in Botswana. Seven countries—Kenya, Malawi, Rwanda, Tanzania, Uganda, Zambia, and Zimbabwe—found that more than 10% of women attending urban antenatal clinics were HIV positive. Rates tend to be higher in urban areas where transportation and commerce converge, although the epidemic is gradually spreading to small towns and rural areas.

The prevalence rate is second highest in the Caribbean (1.7%), where it is estimated that 270,000 persons are infected with HIV. The earliest group with risky behavior in this region was homosexual and bisexual men, but there was a rapid increase in heterosexual transmission in the mid-1980s (Kimball et al., 1995). More than 40% of currently infected individuals are women, and heterosexual intercourse is now the primary means of infection. Possible reasons for the rapid shift to heterosexual transmission include high levels of endemic STDs and the relative frequency of bisexual behavior compared with exclusively homosexual behavior. The epidemic has varied widely in this region, with some countries such as Cuba showing 0.02% infection and others such as Haiti and Barbados with 4%.

There are approximately 1.3 million adults and children with HIV infection in Latin America, where the prevalence rate is currently 0.6%. Brazil and Mexico together account for more than 70% of the region's infections; active urban centers on the east coast are the main locations. The primary mode of transmission is through men who have sex with men. However, since the late 1980s, there has been an increase in heterosexual transmission and IDU transmission. At this point in the epidemic, women make up 20% of the population living with HIV/AIDS but the rates of heterosexual transmission are rapidly increasing. It is hypothesized that the dramatic increase in HIV transmission to women in this region has been facilitated by traditional sex roles and possibly high rates of cervical pathology (Kimball et al., 1995; Parker, 1996).

South and Southeast Asia also have a prevalence rate of 0.6%, which represents approximately 5.2 million people currently living with HIV/AIDS—4.7 million of them adults. The epidemic began in this region in the late 1980s but its progression has been explosive. Unlike other regions where the yearly incidence rate is declining, the rate of new infections here has climbed from .15 per 1,000 adults in 1990 to .55 in 1995 (Bongaarts, 1996). There are significant variations between countries in this region, with Thailand and India showing the highest prevalence and the largest number of infected people. The epidemic in India is increasing at an alarmingly rapid rate. For example, 50% of the sex workers tested in Bombay were infected, along with 36% of the patients attending STD clinics and 2.5% of pregnant women attending antenatal clinics (UNAIDS, 1996b). In Thailand, HIV prevalence increased in sex workers from 3% in 1989 to 29% in 1993. The dominant mode of transmission is through heterosexual intercourse, although it began with IDU in Thailand and continues to be primarily centered on IDU in Myanmar (Dwyer, 1996). Currently, more than 30% of those infected in these countries are women.

The prevalence rate in North America is 0.5%, with 750,000 currently living with HIV/AIDS. The epidemic was first documented among homosexual men in the United States, and men-to-men sexual intercourse continues to be the dominant mode of transmission, followed by IDU transmission. However, heterosexual infection has been increasing during the last decade, especially in urban populations with high rates of IDU, crack use, and STDs. Approximately 20% of persons living with HIV/AIDS in North America are women.

Western Europe has a prevalence rate of only 0.2%, or 510,000 persons. The pattern of transmission is similar to that of North America, where men-to-men intercourse is the dominant mode of transmission, followed by IDU and heterosexual intercourse, and where 20% of those currently infected are women. However, there is considerable variation among European countries with respect to HIV transmission patterns.

For example, IDU is the dominant mode of transmission in Italy and Spain despite the predominance of men-to-men transmission in Europe overall.

Only 13,000 persons are currently infected with HIV in Australasia, representing a prevalence rate of 0.1%. In Australia and New Zealand, infection rates have plateaued and may even be decreasing. The primary mode of transmission is men-to-men intercourse, with IDU and heterosexual intercourse accounting for a smaller proportion of infections. As in other industrialized countries, approximately 20% of those infected are women. The epidemic was acted on quickly in these countries through cooperation between the government and NGOs, and the epidemic appears to have been contained (Dwyer, 1996).

Rates in North Africa and the Middle East are only .1%. This translates into 100,000 persons infected of whom 20% are women. Transmission is primarily through IDU, followed by heterosexual intercourse. However, the data coming from Northern Africa are relatively incomplete so the actual status of the epidemic in this region is difficult to assess.

In Central and Eastern Europe and Central Asia (the former Soviet Union), the epidemic is only beginning to take hold. The prevalence rate is only 0.015%, with 50,000 persons estimated to be living with HIV/AIDS. Currently, the dominant mode of transmission is through IDU, followed by men-to-men sexual transmission, but these patterns differ by specific region. Approximately 20% of those infected are women.

Finally, prevalence rates are still very low in East Asia and the Pacific (0.001%), where it is estimated that there are 100,000 persons living with HIV/AIDS. It is further estimated that 20% of these individuals are women. Transmission is equally prevalent via IDU and heterosexual transmission. Men-to-men transmission is less common but still a significant source of infection.

The different patterns of the epidemic's spread can be summarized using the three-pattern classification system devised by the World Health Organization (Kimball et al., 1995; Piot et al., 1992). We now recognize that the **pandemic** has escaped a simple system, because each country and region seems to have its own pattern and dynamics. So, consider the system to be a simple way of summarizing what is now a very complicated reality.

*Pattern I* countries demonstrated an extensive spread of HIV/AIDS that began in the late 1970s or early 1980s. Men who have sex with men and injection drug users have been the most affected people, but heterosexual transmission is currently increasing. Most industrialized countries fall into this category.

*Pattern II* countries also showed an extensive spread of HIV/AIDS that began in the mid-to-late 1970s or early 1980s, but heterosexual transmission has dominated throughout the epidemic. Sub-Saharan Africa is classified as having a Pattern II epidemic.

Some countries have been classified as *Pattern I/II*. These regions initially resembled Pattern I countries in that the epidemic began in the late 1970s or early 1980s and initially affected men who have sex with men and injection drug users. During the mid-to-late 1980s, however, these countries began to resemble Pattern II regions, where heterosexual transmission was the primary mode of transmission. Latin American countries and the Caribbean are classified as Pattern I/II.

*Pattern III* countries are defined as those where the introduction or extensive spread of HIV/AIDS did not occur until the mid-to-late 1980s. In some of these countries, HIV prevalence remains low, whereas others are showing rapid and extensive spread. This category includes countries in South and Southeast Asia as well as Eastern Europe. The early response of some countries, such as Thailand, has led to systematic surveillance and prevention measures that promise to slow rates of infection.

## PREVENTION STRATEGIES: WHOM AND WHAT TO TARGET

Preventing HIV infection through behavioral change is currently the most effective way to control its spread. Where the pattern of transmission is through sexual intercourse, three behaviors are promoted: abstinence, fewer sexual partners, and condom use. Simply put, the ABC message of safe sex is A = abstinence, B = be true to your lover, C = condoms. Past successes and failures of various programs have helped to clarify the issues, and it is now clear that many individual and cultural factors need to be considered (Mann, 1991). These include the roles of men and women, social norms for sexual behavior, attitudes toward condom use, sensitivity to frank discussion of sex, and difficulty in reaching groups who engage in risky behavior because of social exclusion.

The question of whom to target has generally been resolved in favor of directing efforts at groups of people who practice risky behavior. In countries with relatively small health budgets, it is more cost effective to promote the ABC message with groups who show increasing rates of infection, such as sex workers, STD patients, and young males at school or in the military. Testing individuals, counseling those who are infected, and notifying their partners is not feasible in developing countries. Rather, the message is directed at all members of the group. In many cases, these groups are hard to reach because they are stigmatized by the larger society. Nonetheless, this strategy has been tried with homosexual men in industrialized countries and sex workers in developing countries, with some success. The down side of this strategy is that members of these groups become even more victimized as a result of being linked with the disease. Moreover, the message may be shunned by other sexually active adults who do not want to identify with the stigmatized group (e.g., E. Green, Zokwe, & Dupree, 1995). In countries where the virus has established itself in the general population, as in Uganda, targeting only specific groups will not be adequate to contain the epidemic (Kimball et al., 1995).

The question of what to target has changed over the years. Aggleton (1996) distinguishes between early programs aimed at changing knowledge, attitudes, and sexual practices of individuals, and later programs that have a broader social scope. Information obtained from KAP (knowledge, attitude, practice) surveys revealed how people viewed the disease and what risky behaviors were common in a region. However, the expectation that practices would change following instruction was naive. At a minimum, people have to feel personally at risk before they will change (Janz & Becker, 1984), and they have to have some control over their protection.

Currently, prevention efforts take into account how social and cultural norms influence sexual behavior and why certain groups lack control over their exposure to infection. For example, in every culture there are "unspoken rules" concerning how free or constrained men and women are in choosing sexual partners. These norms are not easily broken unless there is a concerted and coordinated change at the community level. In most countries, women—married and unmarried—lack the power to refuse sexual intercourse and to insist their partner wear a condom (e.g., Heise & Elias, 1995). Information gleaned from KAP surveys as well as anthropological accounts of social norms and gender roles provide some background to the interventions that follow.

Knowledge, Attitudes, Practices

In Africa, where the incidence of AIDS is high and AIDS has been in existence since the early 1980s, virtually all participants in all recent surveys report having heard about AIDS. Box 4.3 shows the kinds of questions people might be asked as part of a KAP survey. Most people also know that AIDS is transmitted sexually as well as from a mother to her child (Irwin et al., 1991; Lagarde et al., 1996; McGrath et al., 1993). However, in parts of the world where the epidemic is in its earlier stages, knowledge of AIDS is less extensive. In Latin America, knowledge of the existence and sexual transmission of AIDS is relatively high, but one study undertaken in Managua, Nicaragua, found that fewer than 5% of the respondents knew that AIDS could be transmitted during pregnancy (Pauw et al., 1996). In India, where the epidemic is more recent, up to 40% of sex workers in some areas are unaware that AIDS is spread sexually (Asthana & Oostvogels, 1996; Bhave et al., 1995).

Perceptions of personal risk vary widely across surveys. Even in high-prevalence areas, often only a small minority of people report feeling personally vulnerable to the infection. However, surveys in Uganda and Senegal found that 65% to 80% of people in these regions were afraid that they would get AIDS (Lagarde et al., 1996; McGrath et al., 1993). These wide differences in reported perceptions of personal risk are remarkable and may reflect the presence of media messages as well as the number of AIDS patients among one's personal contacts.

It is generally assumed that if people perceive themselves to be at risk, then they will take steps to change their behavior. At the very least, this requires knowing the behaviors that place one at risk and the appropriate means of reducing risk. The ABC message sounds simple, but other inaccurate beliefs about AIDS often prevail. For example, several studies have found that many people believe that AIDS is

## BOX 4.3.
## KNOWLEDGE, ATTITUDES, PRACTICES

Here is an example of the types of questions that might be asked in a KAP survey concerning HIV and AIDS. The letters to the left of each question represent the feature (knowledge, attitudes, practices) that is being addressed.

K 1. Have you ever heard about AIDS? Yes ___ No ___

K 2. How does one get AIDS? _____

K 3. Can you get AIDS through . . .

|  | Yes | No | Don't Know |
|---|---|---|---|
| . . . sexual intercourse? | ___ | ___ | ___ |
| . . . mosquito bites? | ___ | ___ | ___ |
| . . . injections? | ___ | ___ | ___ |
| . . . mother to fetus? | ___ | ___ | ___ |
| . . . touching? | ___ | ___ | ___ |
| A 4. Is AIDS curable? | ___ | ___ | ___ |
| A 5. Do you feel at risk for AIDS? | ___ | ___ | ___ |

(or, What are the chances you might get AIDS?)

K 6. How do you prevent AIDS? _____

K 7. Do you know what a condom is? Yes ___ No ___

P 8. Have you ever used a condom during intercourse? Yes ___ No ___

P 9. Have you had sexual intercourse with someone other than your regular partner in the previous 12 months? Yes ___ No ___

P 10. Have you changed your behavior or way of life since having learned or heard about AIDS? Yes ___ No ___

If yes, how? _____

SOURCE: Adapted from Lagarde, Pison, and Enel, (1996).

curable or at least not fatal (Caprara et al., 1993; Ford et al., 1996; E. Green et al., 1995; Irwin et al., 1991; Orubuloye, Caldwell, & Caldwell, 1993).

More important, there are several misconceptions about how HIV transmission can be avoided. One misconception that appears to be present worldwide is that one can tell by looking at a person whether or not they are infected. The notion of asymptomatic infection is difficult to understand and, as a result, people assume a healthy looking person must be healthy (Bhave et al., 1995; Ford et al., 1996). Two associated beliefs are that HIV infection is connected to cleanliness and to physical strength. Thus many believe that cleaning oneself after intercourse and maintaining good personal hygiene will prevent AIDS (Asthana & Oostvogels, 1996; Ford et al., 1996). Furthermore, because illness and infection are associated with weakness, people believe that being strong and in good health will protect them or that some people have a natural immunity to the disease (Asthana & Oostvogels, 1996; Irwin et al., 1991).

In addition, there are myths that AIDS is transmitted through casual contact, such as handshakes, sharing food, kissing, coming into contact with an infected person's clothing or their sweat, or through breathing the same air as an infected person. These myths interfere with proper care of patients. Many also believe that AIDS can be transmitted by mosquitoes (Asthana & Oostvogels, 1996; Caprara et al., 1993; Ford et al., 1996; Golden & Anderson, 1992; Irwin et al., 1991; Lagarde et al., 1996).

When asked about changes they have made to their behavior in the wake of AIDS, many respondents state that they have made no changes (Caprara et al., 1993). In some cases, this is because they do not perceive themselves to be at risk, so the motivation to change their behavior is lacking (e.g., Pauw et al., 1996). A more frequent reason people give for not changing their behavior is that they currently have only one sexual partner (McGrath et al., 1993). However, monogamy is an effective means of preventing HIV infection only if it is practiced by both partners. Numerous studies have shown that both men and women are aware of this, and that women, in particular, fear the possibility of infection as a result of their partner's sexual activity, despite the fact that they themselves are monogamous (Heise & Elias, 1995; McGrath et al., 1993; Parker, 1996).

Those people who have changed their behavior typically claim to limit the number of sexual partners they have and occasionally to limit their interactions with prostitutes. Others report being more selective in their sexual partners (Ford et al., 1996; Lagarde et al., 1996; McGrath et al., 1993; Pauw et al., 1996). One unfortunate outcome of this new selectivity is that older men are now seeking younger women, whom they perceive as unlikely to be infected (Ulin, 1992).

Although condom use is one of the most effective means of preventing infection, knowledge of condoms is extremely limited in many countries and rates of condom use are very low (Kimball et al., 1995). Williams (1992) reports that knowledge about condoms among women in Africa ranges from as low as 8.2% in Mali to 87.3% in Botswana. Rates of ever having used a condom are even lower, ranging from 0.2% of women in Burundi and Senegal to a high of 12.8% in Zimbabwe. As a result, condom use is rarely reported as a behavioral response to AIDS (Ford et al., 1996; Lagarde et al., 1996; Orubuloye et al., 1993; Pauw et al., 1996; Schopper, Doussantousse & Orav, 1993).

Although use of condoms is low, it may be increasing. A cross-sectional survey conducted in Malawi with pregnant women found that condom knowledge had increased from 16% in 1989 to 90% in 1993 (Taha et al., 1996). During the same period, intermittent condom use increased from 6% to 15%, but consistent condom use did not change significantly, remaining below 0.3% at both time points. Thus an increased knowledge of condoms did not appear to be associated with increased use. On the other hands, UNAIDS (1996a) reports successful social marketing of condoms in Vietnam and Ethiopia in the past few years, which has presumably led to increases in their use in these two countries.

The failure to cite condom use as a means of preventing infection reflects not only a lack of knowledge about condoms but also doubt that condoms will be effective in preventing transmission. In fact, several studies have uncovered negative attitudes about condoms and condom use. These attitudes are fueled by a lack of familiarity with condoms, the generally poor quality of condoms that have been available in developing countries, and the association between condoms and casual or commercial sex (Bhave et al., 1995; E. Green et al., 1995; Heise & Elias, 1995; Irwin et al., 1991; Orubuloye et al., 1993).

The following beliefs about condoms are common: Condoms tear, condoms reduce sensation and pleasure during intercourse for both men and women, and condoms can come off during intercourse and work their way into the woman's womb or stomach, thereby causing illness, sterility, or even death. Some cultures believe that semen contains properties that are beneficial to women and that the use of condoms denies women these health benefits. Moreover, in cultures where fertility is highly valued, the fact that condoms prevent pregnancy as well as disease is viewed as a serious shortcoming (Heise & Elias, 1995; Irwin et al., 1991; Orubuloye et al., 1993; Ulin, 1992).

In sum, despite relatively high levels of awareness of both the illness and its connection to sexual activity, misconceptions about the nature of the infection and its modes of transmission are rampant. There is considerable variability in people's perceptions of personal risk and in whether or not they have changed their behavior in response to the threat of AIDS. The majority of those who have changed their behavior report limiting their sexual activity but very few have opted to use condoms to prevent transmission. Social marketing techniques may be more successful at changing this practice than traditional health education techniques.

Social Norms for Sexual Relations

People who are part of a culture and a community learn from others how to conduct themselves. The implicit and explicit rules of a culture and a community are referred to as "norms." There are norms for how people relate to one another in their marriage, in their social and sexual relations, and in daily interactions. Of relevance to HIV infection and prevention are the norms concerning genital care, sexual abstention, sexual networking, and gender roles.

Among the African sexual practices that foster transmission of HIV infection, the one that seems to have received the most attention is that of "dry sex," which refers to procedures undertaken to dry or tighten the vagina prior to intercourse to increase sexual pleasure. This practice occurs in Malawi, Nigeria, South Africa, Zaire, Zambia, and Zimbabwe. Numerous means are used to reduce vaginal secretions including the insertion into the vagina of leaves, powders, stones, or pharmaceutical products; wiping the inside of the vagina with a cloth or tissue; and drinking a special porridge. A study in central Zaire found that one third of the married women had used a drying substance at least once (J. Brown, Ayowa, & Brown, 1993). Although it seems likely that damage to the vagina and/or penis through dry sex practices would facilitate

HIV infection, evidence supporting this association is inconsistent (Sandala et al., 1995).

Another African practice that has been suggested as a possible facilitator of HIV infection is female circumcision. Because the operation is often performed with unsterilized instruments and frequently leads to infection and hemorrhaging, it seems likely to increase the risk of HIV infection. Long-term effects include recurrent urinary tract infections, chronic pelvic infections leading to infertility, problems in pregnancy and childbirth, and increased likelihood of female genital trauma during intercourse. As a result, it seems likely that female circumcision would facilitate HIV infection. However, female circumcision is not common in the areas with the highest rates of transmission, and currently there is no evidence that this practice is associated with increased HIV transmission (Armstrong, 1991; Kimball et al., 1995; Lancaster, 1996). However, for other reasons, the WHO is actively discouraging this practice.

The practice of male circumcision has been consistently associated with reduced HIV transmission. It has been argued that lack of male circumcision facilitates HIV infection both indirectly, by increasing susceptibility to other STDs, which in turn facilitates HIV infection, and by potentiating HIV infection itself. Some cultures have abandoned their traditional practice of male circumcision, and it has been suggested that they should be encouraged to retain this practice and that perhaps male circumcision should be promoted throughout Africa (Haverkos & Quinn, 1995).

Patterns of sexual abstention have been of some interest both as a means of preventing HIV infection and as a factor that increases risk of infection. Abstention is a natural means of avoiding sexual activity in sub-Saharan Africa, where there are often complex rules regarding prohibition of intercourse and where women are expected and encouraged to enforce these rules. This includes abstaining when pregnant, when menstruating, for several months postpartum, and while breastfeeding. Some have suggested that familiarity with sexual abstention could facilitate the promotion of sexual control in situations where couples differ in serostatus. In particular, it has been suggested that women might feel empowered to refuse sexual intercourse under these circumstances. However, prolonged sexual refusal may threaten the wife's status and lead to the husband either abandoning his wife or seeking sexual activity with another woman or an additional wife. Moreover, polygamous societies tend to tolerate multiple partners for men even outside of the formal marital system, thereby increasing HIV risk (Heise & Elias, 1995; McGrath et al., 1993; Orubuloye et al., 1993).

*Sexual networking* refers to patterns of multiple sexual relationships that do not fit the fully commercial character of prostitution in that they often involve companionship and domestic services along with sex and cash. It is common among men in many African and Latin American cultures; it is also a way for women in urban East and Central Africa, who remain unmarried or have lost a husband due to death or divorce, to seek economic support through a sexual liaison (Heise & Elias, 1995; Hudson, 1996; McGrath et al., 1993; Standing, 1992). Women may engage in a number of steady relationships in which men contribute either money or resources to the women's households to help them survive. As economic conditions become more troubled, these sexual networks become increasingly common and more central to women's financial support.

Sexual networks are also supported by traditionally polygamous cultures where men, either officially or unofficially, have several female partners, as well as by migrant work practices (McGrath et al., 1993; Orubuloye et al., 1993; Standing, 1992). For example, it is not uncommon for men who work in the city to have a "town wife" and a wife back home who takes care of the land. For men, there is an association between sexual relationships and domestic needs that makes it natural to take another wife, either formally or informally, in one's second residence.

Sexual networks are a concern with respect to the HIV/AIDS epidemic because they spread infection more efficiently, particularly when people have numerous regular or casual partners. If each individual in a sexual network is associated with one or two individuals in other sexual networks, then the introduction of even one infected person can spread the infection throughout the networks to a large number of people. This is the case with long-distance truck drivers who, because of their widespread contacts, have the potential to spread the infection from urban to rural areas (Hudson, 1996).

The plight of women in this epidemic has been of considerable concern in recent years. Preventing infection in women is important not only for their own sake but also because of vertical transmission to their children (see Box 4.4 on children). To protect themselves, women need

> **BOX 4.4.**
> **CHILDREN AND AIDS/HIV**
>
> The number of children infected with HIV has been increasing and will continue to grow as the number of women of childbearing age with HIV increases. Children who become infected with HIV progress to disease and death much more rapidly than do adults. This is partly due to the vulnerability of infants' immune systems, but infected children's morbidity and mortality is further accelerated by the lack of accurate diagnosis, clinical care, and pharmacological support. It is estimated that 25% of all HIV-infected newborns will die within their first year of life and that 80% will die before age 5.
>
> Children are also victims of the HIV/AIDS pandemic through the deaths of their parents. A study carried out in the Dominican Republic, Kenya, Rwanda, Thailand, Uganda, the United States, and Zambia estimated that the number of children under the age of 14 orphaned by AIDS had already surpassed 1 million in these seven countries alone. It is estimated that the number of children orphaned by AIDS could reach 2 million by the year 2000. Orphaned children face not only bereavement from the loss of one or both parents but also reduced resources and stigmatization. Children who lose both parents can be a difficult burden for grandparents or aunts and uncles, who undertake the care of their orphaned relatives but lack the resources to care for these children. Children orphaned by AIDS are frequently ostracized by their community as a result of their parents' illness, regardless of whether or not they themselves are infected with HIV. The care of children orphaned by AIDS is rapidly becoming a serious social problem throughout the developing world (Kamali, Seeley, et al., 1996; Preble, 1990; Preble & Foumbi, 1991; UNAIDS, 1996b).

to be able to control both their own sexual activity and that of their partners. However, for many women, neither of these goals is easily attainable. Rape and sexual assault are examples of extreme lack of control but are more common than reported. In the United States, prevalence rates of rape are estimated to be 18 per 1,000 adult women. In 1988 in South Africa, the prevalence rate was estimated to be 34 per 1,000. The majority of victims are assaulted by men they know (Heise, 1993; Heise & Elias, 1995). Even within a marriage, women do not generally have control over their sexual activity.

Women also lack control over the sexual activity of their partner, yet that is the main source of infection for them. Many women feel unable to challenge their husband's or partner's infidelity because doing so places their relationship, economic security, and physical safety at risk. Furthermore, norms that strictly limit women's sexual activity are often juxtaposed with ones that tolerate or even encourage sexual infidelity among men (Heise & Elias, 1995; Kirby, 1996; McGrath et al., 1993; Orubuloye et al., 1993; Parker, 1996; Wilkins et al., 1991).

To protect themselves from HIV infection, women must rely on men not only in limiting extramarital sexual liaisons but also with respect to condom use. However, in most places, condom use is a male prerogative (Heise & Elias, 1995; Ulin, 1992). For example, Irwin and her colleagues (Irwin et al., 1991) report that in their sample from Zaire, an overwhelming majority of both men and women believed that the decision to use condoms belonged to the man alone. In Kinshasa, Zaire, one third of the women who attempted to convince their husbands to use condoms succeeded (Schoepf, 1993). Often women who ask their partner to use a condom are accused of infidelity or are believed to be accusing their partner of infidelity. In either case, the partner often reacts with anger and derision (Heise & Elias, 1995; Parker, 1996).

Women who are sex workers have to overcome not only traditional sex roles in their attempts to sustain safer sex practices but also social class expectations that dictate that they should yield to their "socially superior" customers. Moreover, poverty often makes them fear losing customers and unable to refuse greater sums offered to them in exchange for having unprotected intercourse (Schoepf, 1993). For example, in a study of sex workers in Bombay, India, 98% reported that they would be afraid of losing clients if they insisted on condom use (Bhave et al., 1995). However, sex workers may actually have more success in negotiating condom use than other women because negotiation is already part of the sexual exchange (Ulin, 1992) and because they are not dependent on any one man and therefore can refuse further contact. This suggestion is supported by the successes that have been achieved with interventions among sex workers in numerous countries (Asthana & Oostvogels, 1996; Bhave et al., 1995; Ford et al., 1996; Visrutaratna, Lindan, Sirhorachai, & Mandel, 1995).

The impact of social and cultural norms on sexual behaviors has led planners to realize that effective interventions ultimately need to address social norms. Some of the needed changes, such as changing the economic relations in Africa, are beyond the realm of public health interventions. However, public health campaigns can acknowledge and address some of these issues by engaging in communitywide interventions, by encouraging men and couples to change their behavior, and by including components of empowerment in their intervention efforts.

## INTERVENTIONS TO PREVENT HIV INFECTION

The examples described here focus on prevention of the heterosexual spread of AIDS because it is the dominant mode of transmission in the world. Interventions with the general population and with groups having risky behavior will be reviewed. Keep in mind that frank discussion about sex is generally avoided in many societies (Dwyer, 1996). Nonetheless, mass media and focused community programs have tried to reach selected groups and the general population to increase knowledge, encourage "zero grazing," and promote condom use (Gillies, 1994; Krause, 1996).

### School and Community Education

School-based interventions can educate an entire generation of individuals and can be introduced before students become sexually active. However, traditional approaches to sex and contraceptive education have met with limited success (Kirby, 1985, 1996). An AIDS prevention program designed for high school students in the Philippines is a good example of a traditional school-based education program (Aplasca et al., 1995). Health education and value education teachers were trained to deliver a 12-lesson AIDS education curriculum covering human sexuality and sexually transmitted diseases, AIDS and the immune system, development of self-esteem, decision-making skills, and refusal skills. Condom use was discussed with respect to HIV prevention, but the focus of the program was to encourage the delay of sexual initiation. Results were reported for AIDS-related knowledge and attitudes at baseline and at 8 weeks following the end of the education session. Students in the intervention schools displayed significantly greater improvement in knowledge of AIDS biology, transmission, and prevention, and expressed more compassion for people with AIDS. However, students in the intervention group did not differ from nonintervention students in the preventive behavior they intended to use. Thus, although the education program was successful in increasing knowledge, it did not seem to influence intentions to engage in safer behaviors.

The latter finding is typical for education programs. Study after study has found that providing accurate information alone is not sufficient to change behavior (Kirby, 1985, 1996). However, education programs may have more success if they use interactive methods. The CONNAISSIDA project conducted in Kinshasa, Zaire (Schoepf, 1993), relied on small group dynamics and exercises such as role-plays, case studies, and simulation games to instruct and motivate women in a low-income community. The four-session intervention was conducted with a small group of sex workers and with members of a local church's Mothers Club. Three months following the intervention, all but 1 of the 15 sex workers reported using condoms regularly; but five months later, many had stopped using condoms on a regular basis, in large part as a result of dissuasion efforts by their clients. All 60 of the mothers had approached their husbands about using condoms; however, only one third were successful.

The results of this intervention suggest that a dynamic, interactive educational program can motivate individuals to change their behavior and provide them with the confidence and skills to do so. This parallels findings from industrialized countries, where comprehensive small group interventions have been found to be highly successful (Janz et al., 1996). Although the Kinshasa intervention was initially successful, the sex workers were unable to maintain behavior change, in part because of men's resistance, and many mothers were unable to overcome their husbands' refusals to change their behavior. This underscores the need to include men in community interventions.

Couple Education and Counseling

The importance of including men in HIV interventions is highlighted by the success of a counseling program conducted in Kigali, Rwanda (Allen et al., 1992). A large number of women were selected from outpatients attending maternal and child health clinics. The women viewed a 35-minute educational video in small groups of 10 to 15 and then participated in group discussions led by a physician and a social worker. Free condoms and spermicides were distributed, with attention given to condoms as the preferred method. Women then received their HIV test results and HIV counseling. Women were requested to return every 6 months for medical questionnaires and HIV testing. Those who took condoms or spermicides were asked to record all sexual contacts with and without their chosen method, return every 3 months for assessment of compliance, and obtain more contraceptives as needed. Some 26% of their male partners also volunteered to view the AIDS video and receive an HIV test. One year after enrollment, women who were HIV positive were more likely to be using condoms than those who were HIV negative (35% versus 16%). Moreover, women whose partners had been tested were three to four times as likely to be using condoms as spermicides, regardless of serostatus. The strongest predictors of condom use in the group as a whole were a positive HIV test in the woman and counseling of her partner. Importantly, at the 24-month follow-up, rates of new infection decreased very little among women who were tested alone but decreased by more than 50% if their partner was also tested.

Individual testing and counseling is cost and labor intensive and is typically not conducted in Africa. Counseling is available in Asia and Latin America, but government policies about disclosure of HIV status and partner notification make people reluctant to attend the programs (Kimball et al., 1995). Moreover, there is considerable debate over what constitutes appropriate counseling (Aggleton, 1996; Kimball et al., 1995). Content of the counseling in the Kigali intervention and lack of appropriate control groups make it unclear which part of the intervention was more effective, the video or the counseling. The important point of this intervention, however, is that counseling couples rather than women alone enhanced condom use.

Community Healers

One means of changing behavior in a community is the use of respected community leaders. A novel educational intervention was devised in South Africa that included traditional healers (E. Green et al., 1995). Traditional medicine continues to play a large role in developing countries, and traditional healers are highly respected members of their communities. They are likely to come into contact with individuals who are suffering from AIDS or STD, and they are likely to wield considerable influence over their clients and communities.

Green and his colleagues trained an initial group of 30 traditional healers in HIV/AIDS and STD prevention in a 6-day training workshop. These workshops included, among other topics, AIDS epidemiology, traditional healers' STD-related beliefs and practices, counseling issues for at-risk populations, care and support of HIV/AIDS patients, and educating other healers about HIV/AIDS. Seven months later, a second workshop was held for the original group of healers. By this time, the original group had trained an additional 630 traditional healers (the second generation). The authors also estimated that the healers probably counseled up to 229,320 clients during this time.

A group of 70 second-generation healers were sampled from several regions and assessed with respect to their knowledge and attitudes regarding AIDS/HIV. All 70 healers in the second-generation sample had heard of HIV and 51 gave a fully correct definition; 60 gave fully correct answers regarding symptoms of AIDS, 65 correctly reported on transmission, and 50 gave correct answers regarding prevention. Of the 70 healers, 68 reported that they had counseled their patients to engage in safer sex and all 70 reported that they had also advised friends, family, or people in their community about AIDS or STDs. In addition, 69 reported having advised patients to use condoms and 56 reported having shown patients how to correctly put on a condom using a model. Thus healers can be fairly useful in spreading education and preventive messages to their communities and to other healers. This method of promoting safer behavior shows considerable promise.

Community Interventions

Another way of achieving behavior change is through community-wide interventions. A community education program was implemented in two communities in Managua, Nicaragua (Pauw et al., 1996), and results were compared against two similar communities that did not receive any intervention. The education intervention involved a house-to-house campaign, school activities, and events in public meeting places, all of which emphasized HIV transmission and prevention and the role of condoms in preventing sexual transmission. During the house visits, correct condom use was discussed and demonstrated. In addition, HIV prevention leaflets, stickers, posters, calendars, and T-shirts were distributed along with free condoms in the intervention neighborhoods. One year later, levels of knowledge increased in both the intervention and the control samples but the increase was only marginally greater in the intervention areas. Attitudes toward condoms, condom use, and sexual practices all changed in desired directions in both intervention and nonintervention communities, but once again the magnitude of the change was only marginally greater in the intervention samples. Condom use continued to be low, with less than 20% of women and less than 40% of men ever using a condom.

The results of this study are somewhat disappointing. The community intervention was quite thorough and did achieve some changes, but given the changes in the control neighborhoods, it is not clear that the improvements were actually due to the intervention itself. It is possible, however, that obtaining change with a large-scale community project like this one requires prolonged intervention. Communitywide interventions from North America have also demonstrated only small and slow changes (U.S. Centers for Disease Control, 1996). It is also possible that longer term interventions, or community interventions paired with more focused interventions, might produce better results.

Targeting Groups Who
Engage in Risky Behavior

Community interventions have been successful with groups such as sex workers and injection drug users who frequently engage in risky behavior (Des Jarlais & Friedman, 1996). An example of a highly successful project is the condom promotion program established in Chiang Mai, Thailand (Visrutaratna et al., 1995). This intervention is particularly notable because it targeted both sex workers and owners of commercial sex establishments and because the investigators managed to obtain the cooperation of every sex establishment owner in the district. Small group training sessions were given in every brothel every 3 months for a year. These sessions were additive so that they reinforced the initial messages and also provided basic information to new workers. Topics addressed information about HIV transmission and AIDS, personal risk, demonstrations of the proper use of a condom, and coaching on how to convince a reluctant client to use a condom. Discussion groups were held after each session to allow workers to identify additional problems. Innovative means were devised to communicate information, and efforts were made to make the sessions fun.

Brothel owners were recruited through the cooperation of the more influential brothel owners in the district. Brothel owners were convinced to promote a "condom only" policy by emphasizing that they would save money by not having to pay for STD services for their workers, and that workers would be able to work longer and more consistently if free of disease. Every brothel owner posted a sign indicating the "condom only" policy and spoke to each client about condom use before the client entered the sex worker's room, explaining that the client must use a condom and asking to see if he had one. If he did not produce a condom, he was offered one.

Evaluation was conducted by young men posing as clients who tried to convince workers to consent to sex without a condom. Before the intervention, 42% of workers succeeded in refusing a client's persuasion to have unprotected intercourse. Two months after the intervention, 92% successfully refused. One year later, 80% successfully refused the persuasive appeal.

This intervention had several important components. First, it used an interactive, small group approach. Second, it capitalized on and encouraged the workers' sense of community. Third, it created a local norm by convincing all brothels in the district to conform to the condom policy. Fourth, the workers were supported in their safer sex behavior by the owners of the establishments, who would intervene on their behalf with difficult clients.

In sum, intervention strategies that provide information alone in a traditional format are unlikely to be effective in changing behavior. Interventions that use dynamic, small group interactions are more successful in that they convey information as well as providing peer support and opportunities to build feelings of self-efficacy and self-esteem. However, condom use requires cooperation between women and men, and thus interventions with women alone will not be successful unless women are given the means to enforce their decision to use condoms. For sex workers, this means support from owners of the establishments and enforcement mechanisms. For married women, this requires support from their spouses. For unmarried women in the general population, it will probably require changes in social norms at the level of their peers. Most of the successful interventions are labor intensive and long term, and thus require resources, support from authorities, and acceptance of new rules of conduct. Ultimately, understanding and influencing sexual behavior require a consideration of and sensitivity to individual, interpersonal, communal, and cultural factors—in short, all of the forces at work in determining complex human behavior.

## STUDENT ACTIVITY

In her article in the *Guardian Weekly* (1997), Phyllida Brown stated that because about 90% of all AIDS research worldwide is funded by the United States, American priorities are setting the global agenda. Yet most people suffering from AIDS live in developing countries. American priorities are to develop a drug cocktail that will treat AIDS, but the costs, which amount to $20,000 for a year's course, are so high as to be prohibitive for any other government to consider. Because of the new faith being placed in treatment drugs, the push to develop a vaccine has receded. Behavioral interventions are the only hope now in developing countries. If you were a consultant to UNAIDS, where would you advise putting research funds—into treatment drugs, vaccines, or behavioral interventions?

# 5

# COMMUNITY PARTICIPATION AND AGENCY INVOLVEMENT

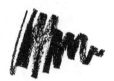

There are many players on the field of health. They include the children and adults who seek and obtain health care; village health committees who plan, for example, where to locate a new clinic; community health workers who conduct primary care activities; health professionals such as nurses and doctors; district and regional health teams who manage the services in their area; ministries of health at the national level; governmental and nongovernmental organizations (NGO), both local and foreign, who perhaps initiate and provide resources for specific activities; and international agencies such as the World Health Organization (WHO) and the United Nations Children's Fund (UNICEF). There is no simple way of discussing how these bodies organize and coordinate themselves to get the job done, even with the aid of an organizational flowchart with boxes and arrows. However, by 1975 people began to realize that health care was not reaching people who need it most, namely, the rural poor who often make up 90% of a nation's population. At a large WHO- and UNICEF-sponsored conference in Alma-Ata in 1978, the source of the problem was identified and a solution proposed. Briefly stated, the problem was said to be due to a huge discrepancy in the worldviews of two teams of players. One team consisted of urban, educated ministry staff and health professionals who designed and conducted services as they saw fit. The other team consisted of rural people who usually lived far from a clinic, had a nonmedical understanding of health and illness, and wanted relief from their pain and illness. Although much had been learned about how to prevent and cure illness inexpensively, the rural poor were not benefitting from the knowledge. The few resources available in developing countries were going to expensive city hospitals.

The solution was primary health care (PHC), which was spelled out in the Declaration of Alma-Ata as "essential health care made universally accessible to individuals and families in the community by means *acceptable* to them, through their *full participation* and at a cost that the community and country can afford."

Furthermore, it was stated that people have a *right and duty to participate* individually and collectively in the planning and implementation of their health care. All attending countries agreed with this declaration, but they found it difficult to implement for obvious reasons: Bureaucracies had long been operating with a top-down approach; financial support for rural health was sometimes less than $1.00 per person per year; health professionals did not have the skills or attitudes to foster community involvement; and community members often did not have the capacity to initiate and implement full participation.

Nine years later, at a meeting in Bamako, Mali, the representatives of sub-Saharan African countries announced specific strategies for community-level participation (see McPake, Hanson, & Mills, 1993):

- Substantial decentralization of health decision making to the district level
- Community-level management of PHC
- User financing under community control
- Provision of basic essential drugs

On the basis of these policy statements, governments set up district health offices with personnel trained in management and health, village health committees (VHC), training centers for community health workers (CHW), and schemes to raise money from users. These were structural adjustments that served to identify a specific role such as the CHW or a team such as the district and village health committees. Through these roles and committees, people could participate.

## WHAT DOES IT MEAN TO PARTICIPATE?

The word *participate* is vague; it means simply to take part or share in something. The term *involvement* is not much better, although it implies being included in the operation, being concerned and interested. Perhaps this is sufficient as a minimal definition of community participation: to take part in some aspect of the health operation because of genuine concern and interest. Beyond this, one can go on to describe and measure the quantity and quality of an individual's or group's participation using specified criteria. One framework for describing participation is that of Cohen and Uphoff (1980). They suggest looking at the kind of involvement (from reaping the benefits to making the decisions), the means to participate, and the people involved. An elaboration of these three dimensions gives a clearer picture of the many ways communities can participate.

Kind of Involvement

Under the traditional top-down approach, people participate mainly by attending clinics and benefitting from the services. They may get more involved if they help to construct or operate a community-based preventive scheme under the direction of health personnel; the schemes are often related to safe water, sanitation, and disease control. The bottom-up approach has something else in mind, namely, that people control health activities in their community in partnership with health professionals, government officials, and perhaps external agencies (see Box 5.1). This includes the following:

- Identifying their health problems (called "felt needs")
- Setting priorities (which problems are most severe)
- Making decisions about how to solve the problems
- Managing community resources (buildings, people, funds)
- Planning and implementing activities that solve the problem
- Monitoring the success of the program

In brief, Rifkin, Muller, and Bichmann (1988) describe **community participation** as a *social* process whereby specific groups with shared needs living in a defined geographic area *actively* pursue identification of their needs, make decisions, and establish mechanisms to meet these needs.

The Means to Participate

Certain vehicles for participating are available. One may be part of an organized group such as the village health committee, a group that helps disabled people, or a self-help group for alcoholics. Many communities also have neighborhood volunteers to find out if anyone is sick in the neighborhood and connect them with a health worker. There is the community health worker who provides health services and promotes people's involvement, and perhaps also a community organizer who promotes and supports groups organized for a specific purpose. Another vehicle would be a general assembly of all residents held once or twice a year to discuss health issues and become informed about past activities and future plans. This would be the place for people to elect their health committee.

People Participating

The idealistic view is that people will be eager to participate because it is a means to increase control over their lives. However, the reality is that even under ideal conditions, not everyone will become involved. There are many reasons people do not participate even after they have been encouraged and the personal benefits are apparent.

- They may be shy about speaking in a group.
- Some people feel they have too little knowledge about health and illness to make a contribution.
- Some people may feel that they cannot control their health because it is controlled by spiritual forces and healers through their special powers.
- Being in control means that one feels responsible for the outcome, to be praised or blamed. This is the down side of participation.
- Finally, some people are too busy; they do not have the time or resources to leave their family and attend a meeting. If such people feel they can trust others to convey their opinions, then their participation is implicit.

> **BOX 5.1.**
> **HEALTH AND/OR EMPOWERMENT**
>
> Whether the needs should be specific to health or more broadly identified as power is a hotly debated topic. In the eyes of many current activists, the former health-oriented framework is suspect because the goal is limited to health and initiated by outsiders. Success is measured in terms of improvement of health and the number of people involved. In the eyes of many pragmatists, the latter empowerment framework is idealistic because the goal is power, control, and self-determination for the least powerful people in a society. Outsiders may be asked to respond to the community's decisions rather than to initiate them. Success is measured in terms of how people perceive social change. Rifkin (1996) outlines the two positions and then attempts to resolve the nasty conflict by siding with Cohen and Uphoff's opinion that both positions are workable and valuable. She goes a step further by suggesting that participation is a learning process, that the outcome is neither controlled nor predictable because it results from the dynamic interaction of all those involved, and that progress should be measured from the people's point of view. I think Rifkin is trying to suggest that arguing over the value of health versus power is unproductive. Whether the goal is short-term progress in health or long-term progress in self-determination, we would all agree that learning, social interaction, and perceived progress are critical variables.

People participate in groups and as individuals. The two contexts require somewhat different skills but both make essential contributions. On the one hand, groups do a better job than individuals at solving problems. The number and quality of their solutions are better. The reasons are perhaps obvious: More information is available from which to create solutions; members evaluate each other's solutions and eliminate the poor ones; and people enjoy the social benefits of a group, which helps sustain their involvement (Cartwright & Zander, 1968). However, getting lost in the group has its drawbacks. For example, group members may make improper decisions because of pressure to agree with the most extreme opinion (called "groupthink"). The larger the group, the less control and the less sense of responsibility any one person feels for the outcome (called "diffusion and confusion of responsibility"). Finally, tightly knit groups often feel the need to protect and enhance their group and so become hostile and competitive toward other groups. Thus identifying too strongly with a group at the expense of maintaining personal values and responsibility can be detrimental to good decision making.

Participation often takes place with professionals, and this has its own pitfalls (see an interesting case from South Africa by K. Kelly & Van Vlaenderen, 1996). Rarely is the community group on equal footing with the professionals in terms of technical knowledge and skills. Health promoters now see their role as facilitators of "power," helping community members acquire the skills, attitudes, knowledge, and technical support they need to control the things that influence their health (Robertson & Minkler, 1994). In this capacity, professionals are like consultants whose resources are selected and used by the community at the community's invitation. This creates a triangle of influence—the individual on the community, the community on the individual, and each with the professional.

## BENEFITS AND COSTS OF PARTICIPATION

Idealistically, there are many benefits to be gained from community participation despite the costs of time, energy, and responsibility. Some of these were seen in the successful rural community development schemes of the 1960s and 1970s (Cohen & Uphoff, 1980; Foster, 1982). With greater community input, resources will be allocated according to the needs of the community. For example, if a village is more than 10 km from a clinic, then personnel from the clinic will go to the village for regular "outreach" activities rather than insisting that mothers walk to the clinic. People may demand that health professionals be more consumer-friendly. Thus the obvious benefit is that community members will feel that the clinic is "theirs" and so will maintain it in good shape and use it more.

A second benefit is that people will become informed about health and so will adopt healthy preventive behaviors; improving health behaviors is more effective and efficient than improving health services. A third benefit is that more resources will be discovered and directed toward health—in particular, community resources such as people with untapped skills, money, and material. People are the greatest resource of a community, and their skills have not been well developed or used to improve health. A fourth benefit is that the individual and group capacities developed for one health project will be sustained and will spill over to other projects, thus having a widespread and long-term effect. This is called the "ripple effect"; a small change sets off other changes, which continue. A nice illustration of the ripple effect comes from a water project. In the process of working together to provide their community with sources of clean water, people developed capacities in organization, leadership, and communication. They were helped by a social agent who had been trained in health and community organizing. They subsequently used these capacities to organize their village for child immunization, with greater success than villages who passively received clean water (Eng, Briscoe, & Cunningham, 1990).

Advocates of community participation hope that the process not only will affect health but will have a broader impact on social equality (the health versus empowerment issue). The goal of long-term participation is that people gradually adopt a more self-reliant or autonomous attitude, thinking and acting for their own and others' welfare and not depending on professionals. This, of course, takes time and depends on the nature and success of their community activities. Some people feel that attitude change is more important than material or health benefits (see Foster, 1982). In one sense this is true: In the course of working on a failed project, people may have developed useful capacities that allow them to be self-reliant and initiate another project. On the other hand, a self-reliant attitude without any short- or long-term benefit is hollow.

Some of the costs for community members have been alluded to already. Community participation takes time and energy as well as the inevitable mental stress associated with taking responsibility for one's decisions and actions, especially when these affect others. Another cost is that the project will take longer and involve more person-hours if more people are involved; those in a hurry will find this frustrating unless they remember that many intangibles are being accomplished in addition to the health outcomes. A final cost is that the legitimate needs of any particular participant may *not* be met. If a group of women in the community want family planning services, but they are a small minority and others are vociferously opposed, then they will likely not have their needs met. Similarly, UNICEF may think that infants need to be immunized against the six killer diseases, but community participants may decide that this is not their priority.

Inevitably, tensions arise between the felt needs of a community and its medical needs as identified by professionals. Communities have sometimes selected priorities that professionals feel run counter to health promotion, such as stocking pharmacies with inessential drugs (e.g., vitamin C) given through injection, making and selling herbal remedies, creating a cooperative store that sells junk food cheaply, and isolating people who are HIV positive. Conflicts such as these point to the need for initial agreement among all participants that decisions will be based on certain criteria. These would include information gathered by community members about the health status of citizens, resources available to tackle the problem, and values of participants concerning their preference for one goal over others. With all this information laid out on the table, positions and disagreements will become clear and easier to resolve.

## WAYS TO RAISE COMMUNITY PARTICIPATION

A number of writers have stated that the rural development projects based on community participation 20 to 30 years ago were not an "unqualified success" (Foster, 1982). By looking at ones that succeeded and ones that failed, we can maximize our chances of success in the health field. Foster points out that community health has certain advantages over the previous rural development schemes. One is that health has a single focus and is a high priority for most people. Professionals involved in health have prestige, whereas those involved in community organizing for unfocused or multiple purposes did not have much status or a career ladder. Finally, curative health services provide speedy and observable results (although preventive services provide long-term benefits that are not so obvious).

Oakley (1989) offers an excellent outline of the conditions that are conducive to participation. They are particularly important for induced participation, where an external agency brings money to spend on health and then tries to mobilize the community to get involved. They should be part of a checklist that governments, donors, and planners use when their goal is to increase community participation in health.

## Identifying the Community

Do you identify the community in terms of geography or in terms of shared values and organization? Health professionals and governments prefer the former; anthropologists and sociologists prefer the latter. The real issue is which criterion suits the project and maximizes success. Geography provides a convenient unit that parallels other administrative units and minimizes the distances people must travel to participate. The criterion of shared values helps ensure that participants will agree on needs and activities. However, even people with similar socioeconomic status have diverse opinions about health needs and strategies. It must be understood from the beginning that not everyone's needs will be met but that certain criteria can be agreed upon for defining priorities.

## Focusing on Health

Communities who feel that their health needs are satisfied and other needs are more urgent are not fertile ground for a community health project. Because external money is often budgeted for a specific activity such as health, and because professionals receive specialized training, redirection is not often possible. Foster (1982) points out that health is a good focus for spontaneous or induced community participation, because it is high priority for most people and its benefits are immediate and visible. Rifkin (1990) offers two reasons that maternal and child health is a good focus for community participation: Health overlaps with many of the tasks and preoccupations of women, and formal and informal networks among women are used to discuss and solve health problems. Thus, even within the health field, it may be important to concentrate efforts on a few priorities, chosen by the community from a menu of options, rather than spreading manpower and money too thinly to have any impact.

Supports Internal to the Community

Oakley points to several supports that need to be in place in the community. One is that some health care infrastructure must exist—some services or activities in which people can get involved. At least some health resources need to be available in the community, in the form of health workers or vaccines, to demonstrate the administration's commitment to support health. Similarly, logistical support is needed to provide a place for meetings, transportation of resources, and communication. Most important is the existence of community organization and honest leadership. The skills required to make group decisions, initiate and coordinate activities, and manage resources can be improved with training, but there must be evidence that organizations, leadership, and group skills have begun to develop in the community. Muller's (1983) comparison of three villages in Peru that differ on this dimension is a striking reminder that a community must be receptive in spirit and in structures (see Box 5.2).

Supports From Outside the Community

If communities are to make decisions and manage resources, they must have a government bureaucracy that allows for such initiatives. The ministry of health, for example, must be flexible enough to allow a community to reallocate some resources. The ministry should have decentralized some of its powers as well as its resources. In some cases, communities raise money to finance their activities. However, the initiative for a new activity often comes from an external agent, such as a nongovernmental organization (NGO). NGOs are not part of a government but are registered in a particular country, receive public and/or private funding, and have a document outlining their purpose and procedures. For a number of reasons, NGOs are useful supporters of community participation: They have experience in health development, they are more flexible and less restricted by bureaucratic rules, they have resources to contribute, and they are prepared to work closely with a few communities. In particular, NGOs have skills in gathering information, running an organization, managing funds, and evaluating outcomes. Community participants may find it useful to adapt and adopt these skills. NGOs are currently under pressure from their fun-

> ## BOX 5.2.
> ## WORKING WHERE YOU ARE WELCOME
>
> Frits Muller used to provide curative services to 40 villages in the Andes of Peru, the center of the former Inca civilization. During these visits, he and his team tried to persuade villagers to select someone as a CHW and send him to be trained in their donor-funded program. Villagers selected 34 CHWs; 25 returned after the 2-week training; and 15 were still active 3 years later. Muller describes three villages that responded very differently to the offer. In the words of Muller, "Occoran rejected it; Pinchimuru collaborated with it; and Pampaccamara—to whom the program was not offered originally—demanded assistance from it." Why? Occoran, with only 36 families, had no institutions, no forum for meeting regularly as a community, and no leader other than the traditional healer. At the insistence of the local school teacher, they reluctantly met and selected a young man—who never returned to the village after being trained. For lack of interest, lack of organization, and lack of leadership, the opportunity was lost. Pinchimuru with 76 families was also poor; the traditional healer was a respected man. However, the Pinchimuru folks met and selected the son of the healer as their CHW. When he returned, they gave him money for supplies, followed his example when he started his own vegetable garden, but weren't involved enough to help him build his own health post or a village well. Pinchimuru had greater sustaining power than Occoran because it had community organizations and leadership already in place from prior campaigns. Families in the third village, Pampaccamara, grew enough crops to sell in nearby towns. They had previously organized to fight for land rights and so had strong organizations with effective leadership. They met regularly as a community and raised money to construct a local school, health post, community center, and post office. They tried unsuccessfully to get the ministry to assign someone to their health post. So, without waiting for an invitation to the CHW course, they selected someone at a general meeting and sent him. He was trained and worked for 4 months at the health post. When the government realized what a wonderful placement that would be for one of their own professionals, they sent a government health worker who essentially outranked the CHW. Demoted and discouraged, the CHW withdrew (Muller, 1983).

ders to maximize community participation in their projects to enhance their sustainability (see the later section on NGOs).

Training Skills and Attitudes

Oakley makes the point that attitudes and skills conducive to community-based health must be acquired at all levels of the system, particularly among health professionals, community leaders, and community health workers. Health professionals receive formal education in clinical skills but little training in communication, management, organization, and epidemiology. They tend to have a negative attitude toward community participation because the community's plans may conflict with the medical decisions and medical activities for which they were trained. They are often less than enthusiastic about working in rural communities because they come from cities and prefer to work in urban sites where the equipment is more sophisticated and the schools for their children are more progressive. Without training in community skills and attitudes, professionals can become a counterproductive force, lobbying to maintain money and decision-making power in the urban centers. A survey carried out in Rwanda (Freyens, Mbakuliyemo, & Martin, 1993) found that 83% of health workers in peripheral clinics responded negatively to the question, "Do you think it would be a good thing if the community took the initiative in health promotion activities?" Their reason was that people lacked ability and resources. When asked to suggest acceptable activities for the community, they proposed limiting activities to identifying problems, paying for drugs, managing the ambulance, choosing community health workers, and maintaining the health center. Community leaders and health workers therefore need training in participatory skills, such as how to communicate, organize, delegate, and consult.

My own experience in Ethiopia was with Community Health Departments that provided training in epidemiology, management, and participatory skills, partly through course work and partly through extensive experience in nearby rural villages. Hands-on experience in a village meant visiting each family to collect information on everyone's health, discussing problems and resources with leaders and organizations concerned with health and other sectors (agriculture and education), identifying priority problems, conducting activities, and so on. The experiences were not always pleasant—wet clothes in the rainy season, uncomfortable accommodations, electricity shortages, language differences—and urban students sometimes felt "rural" culture shock. Consequently, students learned a wide range of adaptive and participatory skills, but the attitudes they acquired would best be described as mixed: They saw the benefits of community-based health and supported its promotion; they felt empathy for rural folk and respected their strengths; and they were not eager to spend their lives in a rural village. As professionals, they were too well trained to remain in a rural setting for longer than 10 years before being promoted to a more senior position. However, the rural training paid off in the end because, in their senior positions, they determined policy and allocated resources that facilitated community-based health.

Setting Up the Means
for People to Participate

Oakley describes the sequence of actions to be taken in setting up a Community Health Committee. The district or regional health manager, or an external agent, approaches village leaders to explain the purpose of the health project. Either through selection or election, people from different subgroups in the community are approached to serve as committee members. They collect information about community health problems and resources and select one problem to work on. With the help of the formal health system or an NGO, they set objectives and activities, delegate responsibilities to people, and monitor the process. Thus the committee is one vehicle for participation.

The health committee can also open other means for people to participate, for example, by arranging for the selection of people to be community health workers, trained traditional midwives, and volunteer neighborhood workers. These people, in turn, arrange the means for community members to participate in groups or individually. For example, adults and school children may participate in informal education sessions aimed at building capacities in health knowledge and skills. Sometimes the community is asked to conduct a rapid participatory appraisal of the needs of their community through focus group discussions and mapping. In some communities, there is a formal mechanism for people to convene at a public assembly at which they elect committee members, discuss the budget, and propose new needs.

## TWO INTERNATIONAL PARTICIPATION SCHEMES

### Community Health Workers

Until recently, more than 70% of people living in developing countries lacked access to health services, meaning that they lived more than 10 km from a clinic. This is because a large chunk of health ministry budgets went to financing hospitals with the accompanying expensive equipment and highly paid staff. One of the goals of the Alma-Ata Declaration was universal access to health services. The proposed solution was the **community health worker (CHW)**, also known as the barefoot doctor in China. CHWs were to be community members who had completed at least primary school and who, with some training, could perform basic preventive and curative services in their communities. The community was expected to build a health post for the CHW and to reimburse him or her for the time spent on community health. Because most communities already had a midwife (or traditional birth attendant) who helped deliver babies, the decision was made to retrain these women with modern techniques that reduced the risk of infection and continue using their services. The CHW along with the trained traditional birth attendant (TTBA) and the village health committee were to form a nucleus of informed and active community members who would mobilize and manage resources for health.

Different countries have had different experiences with CHWs, but all have experienced some successes and some failures (Galvez-Tan, 1983, and Hilton, 1983, are only two of many reader-friendly accounts in the book *Practising Health for All*). Many journal articles have been devoted to evaluating the functioning of CHWs 5 or 10 years after they were trained. In Ethiopia, studies found that more than 50% of the 11,915 CHWs and 11,743 TTBAs trained were no longer functioning. They had returned to being farmers or had disappeared. This was very disappointing. Many problems could be identified: CHWs were often selected by the village leaders and were not representative of or acceptable to the community; CHWs complained they often did not have a health post or report forms because the village health committee did not fulfill its obligations; CHWs were not respected by their communities because they did not have drugs to offer; and they were not financially supported by their community. These were common problems experienced by workers in many countries throughout Africa, Asia, and Latin America (e.g., Johnson et al., 1989; Robinson & Larsen, 1990; Sauerborn, 1989; Walt, Perera, & Heggenhougen, 1989).

I am familiar with one innovative but simple attempt to make the scheme work better (Ayele, Desta, & Larson, 1993). Functioning and nonfunctioning CHWs from a rural district in Ethiopia were located. Given that authorities above the CHW were the source of most problems previously described, the intervention focused on enhancing support from community leaders and health professionals. Only CHWs who were performing at least one of their functions were included in the intervention (see Box 5.3). On average, the 102 CHWs included in the study were 30-year-old farmers, had completed fifth grade, and served a community of 2,500. Only one third had an active health committee to provide support.

Fekadu Ayele was a district health manager and so he visited the communities to mobilize community support. Meetings with the community and its leaders were used to inform them of their responsibilities toward the CHW, the CHW's job description, and the need for an active health committee. Half the CHWs received two other inputs: a 5-day refresher course to improve their knowledge and skills, and monthly supervisory visits from the nearest health assistant, who should have been supervising but rarely did. When functions performed by the CHWs were assessed and compared with the baseline, the refresher-supervised group showed an increase by the second month, which they maintained at the 6-month follow-up. The CHWs who only received help with community support showed no change during the 6 months. The former group increased the number of activities they performed per month from 13 to 19, whereas the latter remained at around 12 activities per month. Measures were also taken of community support, such as supervision by community leaders, remuneration, and having a health post built. Few of the CHWs managed to get more money or a health post, but the refresher-supervised group were more likely to get support from their community leaders. It does not seem to be sufficient

> **BOX 5.3.**
> **THE BUSY LIFE OF A**
> **COMMUNITY HEALTH WORKER**
>
> The job description of a community health worker includes the following activities:
>
> 1. Immunization of children under 1 year
> 2. Maternal health including prenatal checkups and family planning advice
> 3. Child health including growth monitoring and diarrhea management
> 4. School health
> 5. Home visits
> 6. Health education to groups and families
> 7. Environmental health including waste disposal, safe water, malarial sites
> 8. Curative services
> 9. Outreach services for families living outside the village
> 10. Referrals to clinics with a nurse or doctor
> 11. Epidemic control
> 12. Registration of births and deaths
> 13. Submitting reports to higher levels

to visit the community on one or two occasions to mobilize support for the CHW. Rather, the problem needs to be tackled from both ends. Mobilizing the community is one part; the other part is enhancing the capacities and status connections of the CHW so that he or she gains credibility in the eyes of the community.

Once again, the major problem with CHWs, as with all health services, is that they are not used by enough people. However, accessibility is not an issue here: CHWs live and work in the community; what they lack is credibility. Community members think CHWs have little to offer. Preventive services to a large extent depend on the persuasive powers of the CHW and therefore his credibility. We have to have faith that health behavior will prevent an illness because we do not see a concrete outcome, which is the absence of an illness, and the outcome does not come quickly. For example, if the CHW suggests that people fill malarial swamps and construct a safe water well, the outcome will be fewer cases of malaria and diarrhea, resulting in fewer deaths in the following year—an outcome that will be apparent to someone who keeps statistics but perhaps not to anyone else. In contrast, the immediate and observable consequences of curative treatment and pain relief are obvious. For the CHW to gain the credibility needed to work on preventive projects, he or she may need to promote curative services and sell drugs and contraceptives. Although, in the end, the CHW will need to earn respect by having caring interpersonal skills and by improving the health of the community, he or she may require a boost from local and external authority figures.

The Bamako Initiative

In 1987, African ministers of health met in Bamako, Mali, under the sponsorship of the WHO and UNICEF, to propose solutions to the problem of financing health services. Because of their crushing debt and trade imbalance, many governments are unable to properly finance essential drugs and health worker salaries. The Bamako Initiative relies on the solution of user financing under community control. An evaluation of this initiative, as applied in five countries, has been made (McPake et al., 1993). The authors point out that the initiative was supposed to enhance community participation, possibly in deciding how to raise, manage, and use funds for community health services. It appears to have been successful to a large extent in mobilizing community resources and in some cases community control over these funds for community needs. But it has not changed the tendency for local elites and males to dominate the leadership and decision-making structures.

The method of raising fees was quite different in the five countries. In two countries, Kenya and Nigeria, user financing was instituted at the village level by the community health worker, who could raise money by charging for drugs. By providing funds at the grassroots level, these countries hoped to encourage the development of health posts in small villages to increase the number of people who had access to drugs and services. Other countries, such as Guinea, Burundi, and Uganda, collected prepayments or user fees at existing health centers;

the purpose here was to strengthen institutions that already existed but, because of lack of funds, could barely function.

Through household surveys, focus group discussions, and exit polls of users leaving the clinic, people were asked questions such as what they thought of the quality of service, how they afforded the fees, and how much money was raised for the community. The overall evaluation in terms of acceptability, affordability, and quality was positive. Most people had a safety net of friends and family from whom they could borrow money when it was needed; they said charges for drugs and services were affordable. People were positive regarding the community health worker and the increased availability of drugs. It is not surprising that people's respect for the community health worker increased as a result of him or her having a desirable commodity for sale, and the worker's motivation, in turn, improved. The money raised was put into salaries for community health workers, bonuses for health professionals who have had no pay raises, repair of facilities, and recovery of drug costs. The amount of money actually raised was lower than expected because there were not enough users. Low use is a common problem in many developing countries. Consequently, although community members and users were positive about changes brought about by the initiative, the services are not yet self-financing. There continues to be a problem of people in need not using available curative or preventive services.

## FRAMEWORKS FOR EVALUATING COMMUNITY PARTICIPATION

When the stated objective of a project is to enhance community participation, there are several sets of criteria for evaluating the level of participation achieved. Uphoff's criteria include the levels of participation, who the participants are, and how participation occurs (Cohen & Uphoff, 1980). They were used to evaluate the following project in Nepal. The criteria never seem to be applied in a systematic way by evaluators, perhaps because there is no need to coordinate or combine them. Consequently, the following project in Nepal uses some but not all the criteria (see Box 5.4 for Uphoff's dimensions). Rifkin's subjective

> **BOX 5.4.**
> **NORMAN UPHOFF'S**
> **DIMENSIONS OF PARTICIPATION**
>
> 1. What kind of participation occurs?
>    - in decision making
>    - in implementation by contributing resources, coordination, administration
>    - in reaping the benefits
>    - in evaluating the project
>
> 2. Who participates?
>    - local residents, local leaders, government personnel, foreign personnel, and so on
>    - disaggregated by age, sex, education, ethnicity, income level, and so on
>
> 3. How does participation occur?
>    - local or outside initiative
>    - what are the incentives (voluntary, paid, coerced)
>    - organized groups and/or individuals
>    - regular or irregular, direct or indirect, empowered or unempowered
>    - Descriptive information about context and purpose of participation

indicators reflect the quality of participation (Rifkin et al., 1988). They were used to evaluate the project in the Philippines. Subjective ratings are made by nonparticipants after observing related activities and interviewing community members, local project staff, and external agents. The ratings are made on a 1 to 5 scale for each of five criteria: needs assessment, organization, resource mobilization, management, and leadership (see Box 5.5 for the NORML criteria). The scale numbers refer to narrow (1), restricted (2), fair (3), open (4), wide/excellent (5).

A Case Study of Two Nepalese Towns

Uphoff's criteria for evaluating community participation was applied by Sepehri and Pettigrew (1996) to two village projects in Nepal. The health post in Ghandruk was organized by the Annapurna Conservation Area Project, a local NGO, to be controlled by the community; the health post in Sikles was state run. Both offered preventive and curative services. They were evaluated five years after the NGO project had started in Ghandruk.

*What kind of participation occurred?* In this case, *participation* refers to decision making, financing, and benefitting from use. Ghandruk's health post was initiated by a local NGO but currently supported by a health committee, a community health worker, health volunteers, and two clinic staff. A revolving drug fund was initially established with contributions from the NGO and the community. Sikles had a similar structure and drug fund, but the state rather than the community made major decisions. Ghandruk differed in another respect, namely, the NGO had mobilized people to construct private latrines, a village water supply, and day care; they also organized regular cleanups.

Despite these differences, there was little difference in the two communities' use and awareness of health activities at the village level. The health committee of Ghandruk rarely met because its members were indifferent. Less than 10% of people in the two communities knew such a committee existed. Less than 20% of the people knew that a community health worker existed. None of the midwives was active or known. Health volunteers were more popular; 44% of the Ghandruk people interviewed and 30% of the Sikles people used or knew of their services (the differences is probably not significant). The health volunteers were performing only promotion and education functions; they had never replaced the drugs they sold and no longer did any treatment. The health posts had been used by 30% of the people in each village; 40% had treated themselves and 2% had sought services from a distant hospital. The community-run system, unfortunately, was no better known or used than the state-run system.

*Who participated?* It was clear from interviews that the Ghandruk residents did not participate greatly—in electing key players such as

*Community and Agency Involvement* 143

committee members or health volunteers, in making decisions, or in using the services. They may have contributed manpower to building and maintaining the latrines, water supply, and day care. Decisions were in the hands of relatively well-off men, who seemed to think the job was too puny for them. The external NGO had to remain active to keep community preventive activities going.

*How did people participate?* This refers to qualitative aspects of involvement. The initiative came from outside the Ghandruk community, and in many respects it remained there. People participated individually by using the services of the volunteer and clinic staff; they liked the services received. Otherwise, community organizations that should have been providing ways for people to participate were dysfunctional.

The project at Ghandruk was not more successful than the one at Sikles in fostering participation or use of health services. However, it appears to have been more successful in reducing illness; only 24% of the households contacted had an ill member in the previous 2 weeks compared with 81% in Sikles (and compared with 36% in the same community 7 years prior). This may be attributed to the water and sanitation activities organized by the NGO. Another NGO called CARE undertook to raise community involvement in its water projects in Indonesia with somewhat more success. It too has been evaluated using Uphoff's dimensions (Eng et al., 1990).

A Case Study in the Philippines

Rifkin's framework (see Box 5.5) was applied to a health project run in the Philippines by the Rural Missionaries of the Philippines and funded by Missionary Medical Actions of the Netherlands (Laleman & Annys, 1989). Community health workers (CHWs) existed in several villages but their services were not used and they received no money for their services. They asked for help. The Rural Missionaries decided to use maternal and child health services as an entry point to put the CHWs in contact with community members by offering services that were needed but technologically simple. They attended training sessions and, again, started with enthusiasm, but they were not successful in broadening their work to support other projects demanded by their communities. The major players in this program were the staff from the Rural Missionaries, the CHWs, and the communities. The authors gave the following scores for the five criteria:

Needs assessment: 2
Organization: 2
Resource mobilization: 2
Management: 3.25
Leadership: 3.25

Needs assessment was rated 2 because health professionals made a household survey but never fully analyzed or presented its results to the community. Eyeballing survey responses suggested to staff that CHWs should have extensive training in curative and preventive health. CHWs only "wanted some information on home remedies, the use of herbal medicine and acupressure, and some practical tips on infant feeding." Because they got more training, their needs were not correctly assessed and met, according to the authors. The value of this criterion is arguable. What we are missing at this time is evidence that assessing and satisfying the needs of the CHWs would also satisfy the needs of community members and thus contribute to the success and sustainability of the program.

Organization was rated 2 because maternal and child health was considered too narrow a base for an organization to succeed. Mothers Clubs were organized but they did not broaden their scope to include other activities. Thereafter, only villages with many existing organizations in place were encouraged to recruit and train CHWs. It is an obvious point that communities with well-established organizations have a reservoir of leadership potential and resource mobilization that will generalize to the health sector.

Resource mobilization was rated 2 because mothers were asked to pay for drugs alone. They were not asked to pay more to support the MCH program. It seems the CHWs were satisfied to volunteer their services.

Management was rated 3.25 because the CHWs now are full partners in planning, implementing, and monitoring their program; they sometimes take the initiative to make their own decisions.

Leadership also received a rating of 3.25. Although professionals from the external agency initiated and sustained the project during the first few years, CHWs soon began electing their own leaders. They took training in community organization, leadership, and communication skills and discussed among themselves the qualities required in a leader. The main limitation was that CHWs did not fully represent the poor in that none of them had come from this background.

A Few General Points From
a Case Study in Pointe St. Charles

Because there are few written case studies of health projects to which the frameworks have been applied, I collected data on a local project in Pointe St. Charles to see if I could use the criteria. I went with a skeleton set of questions to be asked of all the key informants, with variable follow-up questions to pursue mechanisms or structures specific to that project.

*Who and how people participated.* Uphoff's criteria were easier to apply objectively in the project I studied. The context was a lower class neighborhood in Montreal where there has always been a high rate of illiteracy and unemployment. A group of medical students 25 years ago spoke to the community about their plan to set up health services; now the project is funded by the government but controlled by the community. The clinic hires 88 full-time workers, one third of whom come from the community. For example, all 9 family care workers, and 20% of the nurses and social workers, come from the community. None of the 9 doctors is local. More than 10,000 of the 13,000 community members had registered at the clinic, although in 1 year only 37% may actually have made an appointment for services. Others will have been contacted and visited at home. Usually only about 100 citizens attend the annual general assembly where members of the board of directors are elected and proposals are voted on and amended. Other assemblies held on specific issues attract up to 600 citizens. Each year board members are elected from the community. Affiliated with the clinic are a group of 15 to 20 community organizations organized by groups such as Young Mothers, Elderly, and Action Watchdog. Thus, in this Montreal community, there was evidence of many vehicles for participation from

> **BOX 5.5.**
> **INTERVIEW QUESTIONS**
> **FOR NORML EVALUATION**
>
> 1. *Needs Assessment*
>    How were health needs identified?
>    Did the community have any role in conducting needs assessment and in analyzing health needs? Was there an opportunity to voice nonhealth needs?
>    If a survey was conducted, who designed and conducted it?
>    Was it used to gather information or to initiate discussion?
>    Was it used to help the community make decisions?
>
> 2. *Organizations*
>    How were organizations focusing on health needs development?
>    What is the relationship of health professions to these organizations?
>    What is community representation on these organizations, and can they identify needs other than health needs?
>
> 3. *Resource Mobilization*
>    What resources has the community contributed?
>    Who decides how resources will be used?
>    Can these resources be directed to whatever programs are needed, or is their use limited?
>
> 4. *Management*
>    To whom are the health workers responsible?
>    What are the decision-making structures?
>    Have the structures remained in the hands of certain groups/individuals, or do they include other groups more representative of the community?

using the clinic services to making decisions, and many people were involved.

*Needs assessment.* This criterion concerns whether professionals make the decision that health services are needed by the community or

> **5. Leadership**
> How was the leadership chosen and how has it changed? Which groups does the leadership represent?
> Is the leadership dictatorial, paternalistic, consultative, charismatic, or inactive?
> Has the leadership made decisions to improve the health of poor citizens?

whether community members assess and identify their needs. I asked, "How did the project get going?" and "Who decides what the community needs and what services are provided?"

My local project received a score of 3 for community participation in needs assessment because external professionals initially decided on the basis of health statistics and physician availability that the community needed low-cost health services. They consulted with community leaders and parent organizations and met the initial expressed need for a children's playground. At this point in time, however, needs are raised by individuals or groups in the community and discussed with citizens who make up the elected board. So now they would rate a score of 5 for needs assessment.

Most health projects will have a problem with this criteria because, if their funds are earmarked for health activities, they cannot fund activities for building a church even if that is a priority for the community. However, if health is viewed as physical, mental, and social well-being, most funders should be satisfied with activities related to education, food production, housing, and water, which are indirectly related to health.

*Organizations.* This refers to the existence of community organizations prior to the program, which were involved in setting up the health program, as opposed to organizations created by outsiders to support health. If organizations existed, they should have had broad involvement from the community and have been able to make their health and nonhealth needs impact on the program.

In the Pointe, a number of community organizations existed before the clinic was formed, and many have subsequently been fostered and supported by the clinic, regardless of their health focus. Clinic members on the board have strong links with other community organizations through their previous and ongoing membership in these organizations. The Community Development Team at the clinic spends most of its time in activities that support community organizations, such as Action Watchdog, recreation centers, antipoverty groups, and schools. The president of the board of directors is a member of the Consortium of Community groups and in this capacity meets regularly with the mayor and representative of other groups. Thus the score for organizations was initially 3 but is now probably 5 in that community organizations existed independently of the health project and were involved in creating community control over the clinic during the second year of its existence.

Many communities will have no health-related organization to work with when the external agency arrives, and so the village health organization must be created. There are a number of potential hazards in this situation. The organization will initially need supervision, training, and funds. At the same time, without undermining the organization, the agency must encourage full community participation in the organization's activities, and discourage domination by the traditional elite. It may be impossible to address all these issues. Rifkin (1990) reports that only one out of four planned and supported health committees in Cameroon succeeded in overcoming these difficulties.

*Resource mobilization.* This criterion refers to how many resources have been committed by the community and how much control the community has in deciding how to use these resources. The resources are usually labor, people, and funds. The goal here is self-reliance.

In the Pointe's local community clinic, most of the funds now come from the government, which pays for health services, and only 33% of the clinic staff come from the community. Thus the score for resource mobilization would be a 2, indicating little resource commitment from the community and restricted control over funds by the community.

The major problem for communities in developing countries is their lack of trained people and funds. People from the community rarely finish school or get the grades to enter a health sciences training program. Funds are difficult to raise, although the Bamako Initiative has had some success with drug sales and user fees.

*Management.* This refers to who makes decisions, delegates tasks, and supervises the planning, implementation, and evaluation of the program. At the local clinic I studied, the external agency initially made decisions and supervised the community health workers. Thus the initial score for the project's management was 1. But at this time, the score would be more like 4 because health workers are supervised by service teams and a coordinator, who are ultimately responsible to the board.

*Leadership.* This refers to whom the leaders represent in the community—the high-status minority or a broader band of citizens. It may also refer to the development of leadership skills, one important aspect of capacity building. At the community clinic in the Pointe, the formal leaders are citizens elected to the board that makes the final decision on most clinic matters. Leaders cannot become entrenched as there is a 4-year limit on their positions as board members. Most have had prior experience in a position of responsibility in another community organization. Still, they are given some training sessions by the coordinator in how to manage a budget, their rights and responsibilities according to the charter and the law, and their contract with the health professionals' union. Many new board members need the help of a supportive coordinator to enhance their decision-making skills and self-confidence. At this time, the leadership criterion would be rated 5 for representing a broad spectrum and being consultative.

The major problem here is the domination of leadership roles by the external agent, by health professionals, or by the traditional elite. Initially, these leaders make the project move ahead quickly and predictably. Charismatic local leaders provide a successful alternative in that they mobilize people to commit time and energy to the project. Very often one reads reports suggesting that personal conflicts, petty grudges, selfish people, poor managers, power-hungry elites, and ignorant leaders were the cause of failure. The substantial amount of research that has been conducted on leadership popularity and effectiveness documents that certain qualities such as lack of knowledge, low self-esteem, and uncontrolled emotions do lead to poor leadership. On the other hand, flexibility, charisma, confidence, communication skills, and problem solving are useful in this type of setting. To a certain extent, different communities may need different kinds of leaders. Also, perhaps charisma, confidence, and inflexibility are needed to get a project off the ground while flexibility, consultation, and problem solving are required to extend and maintain the project.

Four Common Problems

There appear to be a few major problems or conflicts commonly found in this work:

- There may be conflict in the agenda of community members, community elite, and professionals.
- There may be conflict regarding broad needs versus a focus on a few health priorities.
- There may be conflict between long-term empowerment and/or short-term health status.
- A final problem is that research on community participation is not advanced enough to identify which qualities actually contribute to success.

Are all five NORML qualities essential, or are some more important? The answer requires studies that provide NORML ratings for many different cases along with an index of success for each. How does one measure success? Evaluation of the Bamako Initiative included questions on acceptability and quality that were asked of people in household surveys, focus group discussions, and participant settings (McPake et al., 1993). They also used some objective indices of cost recovery and use rates. Likewise, to enhance the credibility of community participation and the NORML qualities, independent measures of community acceptability and use must be examined in relation to them. If acceptability and use questions were asked at baseline, before some special effort was made, and then at regular intervals during the following 10 years, it would serve as a subjective index of success to be correlated with progress in terms of the five qualities.

## NGOs WHO PROMOTE PARTICIPATION

Organizations external to the community are often interested in helping to promote participation. They bring expertise and money with the intention of using these to help the community develop what it needs to manage its own health. The agents then move on. The U.N.

Development Program (UNDP) is one such international organization. A host of nongovernmental organizations (NGOs) are involved in large and small projects.

## How Are Nongovernmental Organizations Involved?

NGOs can work closely with a community to transfer skills and develop organizational structures. They are very interested in promoting community participation and sustainability (see Korten, 1987, and other articles in the supplement). They are beginning to do this through partnerships with local NGOs who are present in the region that they want to support. Developing country NGOs may lack the funds and resources needed to support health but have the expertise to understand and work with the community. By helping to develop the capabilities of a local NGO, especially one with proven stability, international organizations can be assured of sustainability.

Despite the many examples of good aid (Millwood & Gezelius, 1985), there are stories of projects that did not live up to their potential. NGOs have been criticized for a number of shortcomings (Downs, 1993; Streeten, 1987). One is the eternal conflict between the needs of a local community and the demands of donors. For example, donors may demand democratization and gender equality in the project whether or not meeting those criteria will hinder other aspects of development. NGOs have had to become skilled at maintaining proper development priorities while satisfying their donors. Another criticism is that mechanisms for monitoring NGO activities are not always well developed (A. Green & Matthias, 1996). Independent evaluations from the local and foreign country need to be a standard component in all projects.

CARE, or Cooperative for American Relief Everywhere, is a large NGO with affiliates in many countries and a head office in New York. Its 1991-1992 biennium budget was U.S.$1,270 million raised from the public and matched by government grants. It manages more than 200 projects in 41 developing countries, sometimes providing food-for-work to develop an infrastructure but generally assisting long-term development in health, forestry, agriculture, water, and small enterprises (Ruggiero, 1993).

One CARE project took place in West Java Province, Indonesia, in the early 1980s. The goal was to provide safe drinking water to 40% of the rural villages, using holding tanks and a gravity-flow water system. To build and maintain the water systems, CARE developed a partnership with each village. The village provided workers to help with construction and maintenance; CARE provided materials and employed Indonesian field-workers to do most of the construction, community organizing, and education activities. Field-workers stayed in a village for 1 or 2 years, decreasing their involvement as the community took over maintenance. Ruggiero (1993) found from CARE reports that in 5 years, the number of villages with functioning water systems increased from 18% to 62%, surpassing the target of 40% set by CARE. This led to a 37% reduction in diarrhea deaths. A spinoff in increased child immunizations was discussed earlier as one of the indirect benefits of this project (Eng et al., 1990).

In conclusion, a final judgment cannot yet be written on the value of community participation and its chances of success. We do know that it will take many forms in different communities, and that some of these will be better than others. The analysis of case studies must continue for many years because only by induction can we start to see which paths are approaching the goals of health and development. Many people have voiced disappointment and pessimism at the obvious gap between the rhetoric and the reality of participation. Rifkin (1996) attributes the gap to unfounded rhetoric, on the one hand, and misguided attempts to engineer reality, on the other hand. The rhetoric of "empowerment" led us to believe that participation would lead to power and that poor people would be only too willing to seize power when it was offered to them. Community participation was expected to solve all the problems of underuse of modern health services and scarce resources. Few projects can fulfill these monumental goals. Furthermore, at least some people find participation in management and organization to be a "disempowering burden" rather than the reverse (Labonte, 1996). The reality of community participation is rooted in the details of daily life and the willingness of men and women to do the boring as well as the exciting activities. Attempts are bound to be misguided because there is no universal guide to successful community participation. There are several frameworks to help one organize components for consideration in the planning step. Organizing frameworks may be better than fixed blueprints, at this stage, because they allow for flexibility and creativity. When enough different projects have been tried and evaluated, we may know more about the necessary and sufficient conditions for successful community participation.

## STUDENT ACTIVITY

Where do you stand on the issue of empowerment versus target-oriented community participation? Debate the pros and cons of each approach from the perspective of planners in the ministry of health who have funds to improve life in a rural village (in a developing country).

Or you could debate the issue more broadly using the following as your resolution to define the two opposing positions: Resolve that the empowerment framework is superior to the target-oriented framework.

Examine several nongovernmental organizations operating close to you in terms of the centrality of community participation in their agenda. Apply Uphoff's or Rifkin's framework to evaluate their operation. Invite someone working for the organization to come to class and discuss grassroots issues with you—not only the ideology but also the problems of putting it into practice.

# 6

# NUTRITION FOR CHILD GROWTH AND DEVELOPMENT

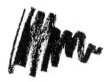

The visible side of malnutrition is the young child whose ribs show through the skin of a diminutive body, and whose large brown eyes stare with helplessness and innocence. For a Westerner, the context of this image is a refugee camp where children wait patiently, bowl in hand, for a meal. Sometimes the children have distended bellies, not because of full stomachs but because of stomach muscles that are too weak to remain taut. A child may also become malnourished after a severe illness. Because of famine, war, displacement, or illness, these children are severely malnourished. They may never get the help they need and may soon die. Or they may come to the attention of emergency aid people or health workers and survive. I recently saw a television flashback to the Ethiopian famine of 1984-1985. An Irish aid worker was sadly pessimistic about the chances that the wasted baby in her arms would survive. The infant was not only starving, she was sick. Fast-forwarding to the present, the journalist introduced that child, now a young adolescent with the poise and quiet modesty typical of girls in her culture. She had survived, although many others had not. After recovering, she had left the camp with her father and gone to more fertile regions. Today she appears to be healthy, happy, and articulate, although she obviously recalled little of her earlier ordeal.

Severe malnutrition, in this form, is usually treatable in a hospital or in the wing of a clinic specially set up for mothers and their babies. Given proper nourishment, even severely malnourished children put on weight and begin to grow again. However, their mental and social health may not recover as quickly and may require more than nutrients.

The less visible side of malnutrition is the many children, particularly in rural areas of developing countries, who eat less than their bodies require. As a result of having less food and less of the right kinds of food from 6 months of age on, they have shorter stature but not necessarily thinner bodies. In fact, they may have a healthy weight for their height. Nevertheless, short height is indicative of inadequate nutrition, generally over a period of months. The problem of malnutrition is also less visible when the child is mildly or moderately malnourished rather than severely malnourished. However, it now appears that even the less obvious forms of malnutrition have an impact on a child's health and development—physical, mental, and social.

Despite the number of international bodies set up to deal with undernutrition, many people in developing countries still suffer from malnutrition. In developing countries, about 35% of children under 5 years are underweight, totaling close to 200 million. Some countries in sub-Saharan Africa do not produce enough food to meet the needs of their growing populations. Although 90% of the population may be involved in agriculture, most are called subsistence farmers because they grow barely enough for their families, with little left to sell. Many other factors are responsible for malnutrition in these and other countries. In particular, the unequal distribution of food within a community and within a family results in a large number of underprivileged women and children receiving fewer calories than they require. Also, infection and parasites prevent the body from fully using what is ingested. The magnitude of the problem as well as the severity of its outcome make malnutrition one of the most pressing issues to be resolved.

## MEASURING MALNUTRITION

*Malnutrition* refers to nutrient intake that is not sufficient to meet the body's needs for growth and activity. The nutrients most likely to be needed and missing are energy, protein, vitamin A (also B and C), iodine, and iron (see Box 6.1 on nutrient sources and deficiency disorders). The body's requirements differ somewhat depending on the person's age, gender, activity level, and recency of illness. For example, people between 20 and 40 years require more than at other ages, but young children also have heavy demands from their growing bodies and brains. Adult men require more calories than women; farmers, fishermen, and women with no household appliances require more than those in sedentary occupations; and children who have recently recovered from a bout of diarrhea need a week of extra food to make up for what they have lost.

One method of measuring malnutrition is to assess habitual food intake. Another is anthropometry, or the measurement of body height and weight. These methods are both commonly used to assess energy and protein nutrition. Two other methods, namely, conducting biochemical tests and observing clinical signs, are more useful for the assessment of micronutrients such as iron, iodine, and vitamins. Iron-deficiency anemia, for example, can be detected by looking at the color of the membrane under the lower eyelid; iodine deficiency, by the size of the goiter; and vitamin A deficiency, by the presence of xerophthalmia, an eye disease. These clinical indicators are not always reliable across examiners, but they may be used to identify a population with potential nutrition problems. Two extreme forms of malnutrition can be reliably identified by their clinical signs. One is **marasmus** in which the signs of calorie malnutrition are indicated by prominent ribs, wrinkled skin, and an extremely wasted appearance. The other is **kwashiorkor** in which the signs of protein deficiency are evidenced by a round "moon" face and edema or swelling of the lower limbs. These are severe forms of energy and protein malnutrition that require immediate medical treatment. However, because mild and moderate energy-protein malnutrition are more common, we will look more closely at their measurement.

## Habitual Dietary Intake

One frequently used assessment involves weighing the food that a person will eat and calculating the amount of calories, protein, carbohydrates, and fats in the foods. Tables are available to translate the weights of most foods into the weights of these nutrients (Food & Agricultural Organization [FAO], 1985). These are then compared with the daily recommended amounts for people of different genders, ages, and levels of activity. For example, 250 ml of milk (3.25% fat) contains 12 gm of carbohydrates, which contribute 48 kcal; 8 gm of protein, which contribute 32 kcal; 9 gm of fat, which contribute 81 kcal; plus minerals, vitamins, and water.

In summary, this is how your body calculates its kcal energy requirements:

| | a *male* of 65 kg or | a *female* of 55 kg |
|---|---|---|
| If you are 20 to 39 years old and | | |
| for 8 hours sleeping | 500 | 450 |
| for 8 hours social/personal activities | 1,000 | 750 |
| for 8 hours of occupational activity | 3,000 | 2,200 |
| add on pregnancy needs | | 350 |
| add on lactating needs | | 550 |

Children's food requirements are based on age but not on body weight as is the case for adults; it would not make sense to have overweight children eat more and underweight children eat less. Children require slightly more than 1,000 kcal daily in their second year and 1,200 kcal daily in their third year. In comparison, rural Kenyan children in one study received on average 848 kcal, Nigerian children 738 kcal, and Egyptian children 1,119 kcal (Bentley et al., 1991; Wachs et al., 1992). Approximately 11% to 13% of caloric intake should be protein. At one time, it was thought that protein deficiency was a major problem, and international agencies developed low-cost protein foods for distribution. However, we now realize that a well-rounded diet is more important, giving priority to energy and then to other nutrients (*energy-nutrient malnutrition* may soon replace the term *protein-energy malnutrition*). If insufficient energy is available, then the body uses protein for its caloric, or energy, value instead of for its growth value. Protein provides the building blocks, but without the energy "cement" to hold it together,

> **BOX 6.1.**
> **NUTRIENTS, THEIR SOURCES,**
> **AND THEIR DEFICIENCIES**
>
> *Energy:* Energy is needed for all internal bodily activity as well as for mental activity, physical work, and play. Energy comes from foods high in sugars, starches, and fats. These include fruits such as bananas, tubers such as potatoes, animal or vegetable oil, grains, and rice. Energy deficiency results in lowered activity, lower body heat, slowed growth, and use of body stores until they deplete, at which time the person looks wasted and marasmic.
>
> *Protein:* The amino acids that make up protein are necessary for bone and other tissue growth. They are found in legumes such as lentils and in meat, fish, and eggs. Protein deficiency results in lack of bone growth and stunting.
>
> *Vitamin A:* Vitamin A, specifically retinol, is found in leafy green vegetables, yellow or orange vegetables and fruits, and fish-liver oil. A deficiency in vitamin A results in difficulty seeing at night (xerophthalmia) and the inability to absorb other nutrients such as iron. It may have other more general effects on resistance to infection.
>
> *Iodine:* Iodine is an element found in the ground that is then ingested through food. Many regions of the world lack iodine, so it is added to a substance such as salt. Iodine deficiency manifests as a goiter, an enlargement of the thyroid gland in a futile attempt to produce thyroxin. Iodine deficiency in a pregnant mother impairs the nervous system development of her unborn child and results in cretinism and reduced mental capacity. Iodine deficiency in children may also retard mental development.

there would be no structure (Cameron & Hofvander, 1983; Walker, 1990).

Measurement of food intake requires constant monitoring of the foods eaten by each member of the family on a given day, which is very time consuming and intrusive. On the other hand, if we want to find out merely whether any foods containing vitamin A or animal protein

> *Iron:* Iron is found in breast milk in sufficient quantities for the first 6 months of life; the iron in cow's milk is less usable by infants. Most of the iron we eat comes from grains, legumes, and some vegetables. A lesser amount is found in animal meat. Iron-deficiency anemia results from a diet low in iron and a loss of iron stored in bone marrow, from blood loss, and from parasites such as hookworm. The consequences are lowered activity and a feeling of tiredness, lowered alertness, and perhaps reduced mental activity. However, too much iron can be toxic.
>
> SOURCE: Based on Cameron and Hofvander (1983), *Manual on Feeding Infants and Young Children.*

are commonly eaten, we take a 24-hour recall of foods eaten without being too concerned about the exact amounts. In many cultures, people do not eat vegetables or fruits, and children may not drink milk after they stop breast-feeding. The absence of certain nutrients, such as vitamins, means that other nutrients, although present in the diet, will not be fully absorbed or useful to the body. Infections and parasites in the digestive tract also prevent full absorption. For these reasons, the measures of food eaten do not entirely represent the nutrients available to the body for its requirements.

Anthropometric Indicators

Weight and height are an easier and perhaps more valid measure of a child's nutritional status. These measures reflect how much food is being absorbed and used for growth, minus how much is lost due to illness. The child's weight and height are compared with the median weight and height of a sample of fairly well-fed children of the same age and gender, taken from the National Center for Health Statistics in the United States. Malnutrition is identified in children who are more than two standard deviations below the median for their weight (underweight) or height (stunted). This is taken to indicate moderate to severe malnutrition. The World Health Organization (1983) advocates the use of these medians and standard deviations as international reference values because they predict mortality and morbidity and because well-fed children in most countries meet these standards. However, some countries have devised their own references values.

Using the Waterlow classification (see Table 6.1), children who are below minus two standard deviations from the median height for their age are considered moderately to severely stunted. Formerly, less than 90% of the median height was the method for calculating stunting, but standard deviations provide a more consistent unit of measurement. **Stunting** is an index of chronic or long-term malnutrition because it implies that insufficient protein for bone growth (and energy) has existed for months or years. **Wasting** is an index of current malnutrition because it usually occurs immediately as a result of lowered energy intake or severe illness. Children who are below minus two standard deviations from (formerly less than 80% of) the median weight for their height are considered moderately to severely wasted. Thus, regardless of how tall they are, they are too thin. **Underweight,** indexed by weight for age in comparison with the reference, combines the other two in that it reveals the lack of growth in both bone tissue, which contributes to height, and fat and muscle tissue; again, minus two standard deviations is the cutoff for moderate to severe. Under nonfamine conditions, most underweight children will be stunted rather than wasted (Keller & Fillmore, 1983). Road to Health graphs have been prepared for use in clinics around the world, on which a child's weight and height can be plotted in comparison with the 100% and 80% levels. A child who drops below the 80% weight line can be clearly identified and given extra attention (Gerein & Ross, 1991).

The circumference of the child's mid-upper arm is also a quick way of assessing nutritional status, although it is less reliable than weight or height. Children between 1 and 5 years of age should measure 16 cm and over; those whose circumference falls below 13.5 cm can be considered moderately to severely malnourished. It is a quick way of identifying regions that need emergency food aid.

## PREVALENCE OF MALNUTRITION

The major index of malnutrition is the weight of children under 5 years of age. A reduction in weight gain usually begins after 6 months, when no solid foods are given to supplement breast milk and when

**TABLE 6.1** Waterlow International Standards for Malnutrition, Given as a Percentage of the Median and in Standard Deviation Units (SD) Below the Median

| Indicator | Mild | Moderate | Severe |
|---|---|---|---|
| Height for age | 90%-94% < 1 SD | 80%-89% < 2 SD | < 80% < 3 SD |
| Weight for height | 80%-89% < 1 SD | 70%-79% < 2 SD | < 70% < 3 SD |
| Weight for age | 80%-89% < 1 SD | 70%-79% < 2 SD | < 70% < 3 SD |

diarrhea depletes energy stores. Across all developing countries, the prevalence of moderate to severe malnutrition based on weight for age is 35% (see Table 6.2). This translates into close to 200 million children under 5 being underweight. For some separate countries, the prevalence is 69% in India, 67% in Bangladesh, 48% in Ethiopia, 40% in Indonesia, 36% in Nigeria, 34% in the Philippines, and 34% in Guatemala (UNICEF, 1996). The rate is generally much higher in rural than in urban areas and in girls than in boys, particularly in South Asian countries. Most of the underweight children are stunted rather than wasted. This implies that they have been receiving less than the required amount of protein and energy for a number of months. Fewer are wasted: 7% in sub-Saharan Africa and 13% in South Asia.

Deficiencies in specific nutrients are now more widespread than previously thought. For example, vitamin A deficiency can lead to blindness, and even mild deficiencies increase the risk for childhood diseases. It is estimated that 5 to 10 million children become deficient enough in vitamin A to develop vision problems. Iodine deficiency resulting from naturally low levels of the element in certain regions affected about 1 billion people in 1990. These figures are based on the prevalence of an enlarged goiter in a region, although there can be serious problems even before a goiter becomes detectable. Across all developing countries, 15% of the schoolchildren from 6 to 11 years had a detectable goiter. Almost half the people in Kenya, Zaire, Ethiopia, Turkey, and Peru, and one quarter of those in India and Nigeria, had or were at risk for iodine deficiency. The rate in most of these countries is declining with the introduction of iodized salt, a low-cost way of provid-

**TABLE 6.2** Prevalence of Moderate to Severe Malnutrition in Developing Countries

| Region | Underweight | Wasting | Stunting |
|---|---|---|---|
| Sub-Saharan Africa | 31% | 7% | 41% |
| Middle East & North Africa | 12% | 5% | 24% |
| South Asia | 64% | 13% | 62% |
| East Asia & Pacific | 23% | 4% | 33% |
| Latin America & Caribbean | 11% | 3% | 21% |
| Developing Countries | 35% | 6% | 42% |

SOURCE: UNICEF (1996).

ing iodine. Iron deficiency leading to anemia is another major problem, affecting close to half the children in sub-Saharan Africa and South Asia. It is particularly prevalent in women living in developing countries, where an estimated 47% between the ages of 15 and 49 are anemic (Merchant & Kurz, 1993; UNICEF, 1996).

Mothers also suffer from protein-energy malnutrition, and this affects not only their own health but that of their children. It is estimated that 45% of the women 15 years and over living in developing countries are stunted from chronic malnutrition (Merchant & Kurz, 1993). A mother with inadequate weight gain during pregnancy is likely to deliver a low birth weight baby; 33% of the babies born in South Asia and 16% of those born in sub-Saharan Africa were under 2,500 gm (Kramer, 1987; UNICEF, 1996). These rates reflect current undernutrition in mothers, although they are necessarily underestimates because a mother with minimal intake will lose body stores of nutrients to her fetus at her expense.

## CAUSES OF MALNUTRITION

Famines due to drought and repeated crop failure have been responsible for many cases of malnutrition over the centuries. In Ethiopia, the well-known famine of 1984-1985 affected 7.8 million people and claimed the lives of 1 million (Kloos & Lindtjorn, 1993). Donor aid came too late for many, and the relief centers became places where infection spread rapidly. Man-made factors, such as excessive state control over production and pricing that had led to reduced food production and chronic malnutrition in the years prior to the famine, exacerbated the problem.

Factors other than famine are largely responsible for chronic malnutrition in many countries. The major ones to be discussed are the inadequate production and distribution of food, the prevalence of disease, and children's eating habits.

Food Production and Distribution

Inadequate food production is common in sub-Saharan Africa if one compares the calorie requirements of the population and the food produced. However, it is also the case for Afghanistan, Bangladesh, Bolivia, Peru, and Haiti. Governments in these countries may be reluctant to import grains to make up the difference because they lack foreign currency. In some regions, people prefer to grow crops, such as tea or coffee, for cash. The income earned from cash cropping may benefit children if high-quality foods are bought. On the other hand, children suffer if their diet depends on family food production. An important part of the solution lies in agricultural development—improved seeds, high-yield grains, tools, fertilizer, and livestock management (Brun, Geissler, & Kennedy, 1991; Shack, Grivetti, & Dewey, 1990).

Disease

The second cause of malnutrition is disease, in particular diarrhea and measles. Infection is both a cause and a consequence of malnutrition. Sick children become malnourished through a number of different routes. The obvious one is that sick people generally do not have a good appetite and so eat less. As we learned in Chapter 1, diarrhea prevents much of what we eat and drink from being absorbed by the intestines (Keusch, 1990; Stephenson, 1994; Waterlow, 1992). Also, mothers often give their children less food and fluid during an episode of diarrhea, in the mistaken belief that this will stop the diarrhea, but it only stops the symptoms. Children rarely regain lost weight after illness because it requires a diet with 30% more energy and 100% more protein than usual; this extra meal a day for at least a week is called "recovery feeding." Many children become so wasted and dehydrated that they die (e.g., Favreau, Yunus, & Zaman, 1991). The wasting and dehydration

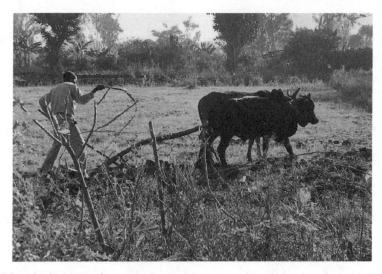

*Although often 90% of a country's population is rural, traditional methods of farming do not supply enough food.*

could be prevented with a solution of salt-sugar-water either in the homemade cereal-based version or the UNICEF sachets of oral rehydration salts.

Malnutrition therefore cannot be fully eliminated unless people have access to, and use, uncontaminated drinking water that is free from parasites, virus, and bacteria. Boiling kills germs, but that is not the solution for most rural people. They need water that has been pumped up from deep underground. Only 60% of rural people in developing countries have access to safe water and only 20% have access to adequate sanitation such as latrines. Immunization against common childhood diseases and use of oral rehydration are also important preventive measures. Currently, only 60% give oral rehydration to their children (UNICEF, 1996).

Eating Habits of Children

Eating habits of children, otherwise known as child feeding practices of mothers, are the third major cause of malnutrition. Even when food is available, children may not be given the needed quantity or quality.

It is not uncommon to find well-nourished adults, with above-threshold body-mass index, in the same household as stunted children (Lindtjorn & Alemu, 1997). Child feeding manuals advocate giving only breast milk for the first 4 to 6 months, supplemented with solid foods after 6 months. Children need food 5 or 6 times a day for the first three years. Breast-feeding is not currently a major problem, although the trend toward modernization puts it in jeopardy. Rather, the major problem is during the weaning stage, from 6 to 24 months of age, when traditional practices and maternal preferences limit the foods a child will be fed.

*Breast-feeding.* Breast-feeding is widespread in developing countries and is the main reason that children under 6 months are rarely malnourished. Breast milk provides not only the essential nutrients for the first months of life but also the mother's antibodies, which protect the child from infection. The early introduction of bottle feeding and solid foods not only increases the risk of diarrhea but reduces the mother's milk supply. Maximum breast milk production requires suckling every 2 to 3 hours with complete emptying; this does not occur if the child receives other liquids or food. One study found that the bottle was given before 6 months of age to most children living in Asia and Latin America, with or without breast milk. In contrast, many African children are exclusively breast-fed for 6 months and in the rural areas may receive breast milk for 2 years (Boerma, Rustein, Sommerfelt, & Bicego, 1991). Many cultures do not have a tradition of drinking animal milk, so when breast-feeding stops, the child will rarely drink cow's milk (Adair et al., 1993).

Modernization sadly brings with it a tendency to think that new commercial products are better than natural or homemade ones. While breast-feeding is increasing in some industrialized countries, it is declining in many developing ones as better educated urban women choose bottle feeding and infant formula. Winikoff and Laukaran (1989) examined the answers they received from 4,469 urban mothers of children under 24 months, interviewed in Bangkok, Bogotá, Nairobi, and Semarang, Indonesia. They concluded that although more than 90% of the women had begun breast-feeding, those in the first three cities did not continue for long. By 2 months of age, 70% of the children in Bangkok and Bogotá and 31% of those in Nairobi received food; more than half received milk in bottles. Remember that children who receive these substitutes are more likely to get infections and less likely to take all the mother's breast milk, so she begins to produce less. The mothers, however, seemed unaware of this chain of events. When asked why they gave their infants bottled milk, the mothers claimed that their milk supply was inadequate or the baby was dissatisfied. Rarely did they intend to stop breast-feeding to return to work. So, without intending to stop breast-feeding, they had given their infants bottled milk, which in turn reduced their own milk production, and this led to the feeling that breast milk was not sufficient. The important question, then, was why they had started bottles in the first place. Many of the women recalled hearing about the benefits of baby formula from advertising and health professionals, despite its prohibition. Hospital practices of separating newborns from their mothers also contributed to early bottle feeding (see also Hull, Thapa, & Wiknjosastro, 1989). Since then, UNICEF (1993) has begun to promote breast-feeding in delivery hospitals, where the source of the problem partly lies. A hospital is designated as "baby-friendly" if it follows 10 steps that encourage breast-feeding and bans formula freebies.

*Feeding children in the weaning stage.* Child feeding practices in the period from 6 to 24 months are most likely to contribute to measurable malnutrition in the second year. The term **weaning foods** refers to the semisolid foods that are given to children, along with breast milk, to provide extra energy and other nutrients. The key variables are timing, amount, and quality (Walker, 1990).

Timing is a problem when supplementary foods are not given at 6 months, the age when breast milk is no longer sufficient. Some mothers delay until the child is 18 or 24 months. For example, 41% of the children in one Ethiopian study received no solids before 12 months, and 47% of underprivileged Punjabi girls received no solid foods before 18 months (Aboud & Alemu, 1995; Cowan & Dhanoa, 1983).

The amount of food given is often less than required. Nigerian children in their second year, for example, were receiving on average 738 kcal, or 60%-70% of their requirements, and Kenyan children 850 kcal, or 80% of their caloric requirements (Bentley et al., 1991; Sigman, Neumann, Baksh, et al., 1989). In many cases, the amount of food is low because children are not fed often enough. Given the small size of their stomachs, infants can hold only 200-300 ml, or 1 cup, of porridge at a time. To meet their needs, children of this age need to eat five times a day but often eat only two or three times.

In other cases, the amount is low because children fill up on low-quality food. Weaning foods in Africa are prepared from starchy flours, such as maize and sorghum, that are thick when boiled with water. The child fills up on a small amount, but the energy density of the food is less than a third of what is required. For example, the liquid pap eaten by Nigerian children is so low in energy density that children would have to eat approximately 3 liters of it to obtain their requirements. In most developing countries, children receive cereals and legumes but rarely wheat or rice, which would provide the most energy and enough protein. Although fat-free diets are currently popular in industrialized countries, the problem in developing countries is too little animal fat and oil. In many countries, such as Ethiopia and the Philippines, fruits, vegetables, and fish are available but are not often given to children (Bekele, Zewdi, & Kloos, 1993; Latham, 1983). Recall that foods rich in energy, protein, vitamins, and minerals are needed at this age of physical and mental growth.

The contamination of weaning foods is a major problem. In some places, 41% of the weaning food was found to have *E. coli* bacteria, especially food that was made in the morning and stored for use throughout the day. Without a refrigerator, mothers should make fresh porridge more often. In addition, many rural areas do not have protected water sources, so the child's drinking water is contaminated. It is not surprising that the age of weaning is also the age when diarrhea peaks. Contaminated food and water are only one source of bacteria and viruses. Children at this age also begin to move around on the ground and to suck fingers or utensils on which there is contaminated material.

There are many reasons that mothers do not feed enough nutritious solid foods to their children starting at 6 months. In some cases, it is because they barely have enough food to feed the older children and adults. In other cases, they do not know how to make available foods palatable and digestible for young children. Punjabi mothers, for example, were shown how to crumble chappatis made from wheat or maize into a little hot sweet tea to create a porridge, and how to mash potatoes and other vegetables. These foods were eaten daily by adults but rarely given to children under 18 months (Cowan & Dhanoa, 1983). Many cultures prohibit children from eating animal protein, fruit, and green vegetables because they are thought to cause illness (Lepowsky, 1987). To begin to understand why mothers feed children certain foods and avoid others, we are finding out from them what they mean by health and illness. Among the Yoruba people in Nigeria, for example, a healthy child is one who is light enough to carry to market, active, and not sick (Bentley et al., 1991). In other cultures, such as in East Java, foods are given to correct a "hot-cold" imbalance in the child (Launer & Habicht, 1989). To be effective in changing feeding habits, nutrition education must work within the cultural framework familiar to mothers.

How then do mothers know when their children become malnourished? The answer is that they usually don't. They are surprised when informed by health workers and may take it as a personal insult. Chronic mild to moderate malnutrition leads to stunting, and shortness is not an obvious cue for mothers or perhaps anyone without a Road to Health chart. Wasting is more salient (Roy et al., 1993). Even then, mothers may not identify the cause as lack of food. Mothers of children under 5 living in Karachi were shown a photograph of a marasmic child and asked about the problem, the cause, and the cure (Mull, 1991). The mothers called it the disease of dryness and thinness. Only three mothers said it was caused by lack of food, to be cured by feeding or medicine. Most said it was caused by a shadow cast by an unclean woman and was extremely contagious; it was to be cured by amulets and prayer.

Traditional beliefs about feeding and illness are held not only by mothers but also by the healers they turn to when their children become ill. Most healers believe in supernatural causes, and their cures attempt to appease the gods or to balance the cold-hot state of the person (e.g., Odebiyi, 1989). For dysentery, they suggest avoiding soups, which loosen the stools, and hot foods, which irritate the stomach. For worms, they suggest avoiding meats, fat, and sweet foods, which the worms like to eat. Traditional beliefs tend to focus on foods to be avoided by women, children, and sick people, often depriving them of the fats, proteins, and vitamins they need for growth and health.

The reasons for malnutrition may be somewhat different in different regions. But all these reasons are considered by Ramalingaswami, Jonsson, and Rohde (1996) as they try to understand why the rate of malnutrition is twice as high in South Asia as in sub-Saharan Africa. The regions do not differ much in poverty, agricultural production, inequality, diet, and safe water. The authors conclude that the important difference is in the inferior status and role of women in South Asia, who must please their husbands and their husbands' mothers rather than their husbands and their husband's children.

## HEALTH AND PSYCHOSOCIAL CONSEQUENCES OF MALNUTRITION

### Mortality and Morbidity

It is now generally accepted that malnutrition contributes to about half of the 12 million deaths per year of children under 5 years in developing countries. Malnutrition contributes directly, when children are severely malnourished, but more often indirectly, by making children susceptible to disease. In developing countries, 101 children out of 1,000 die before their fifth birthday (UNICEF, 1996). Death rates are particularly high in sub-Saharan Africa and South Asia, at 177 and 124, respectively. Half of these deaths are due to diarrhea and pneumonia, which are exacerbated by malnutrition, and 16% to vaccine-preventable diseases such as measles, whooping cough, neonatal tetanus, and tuberculosis. Mild and moderate forms of malnutrition are in this way indirectly implicated in childhood mortality and morbidity.

Specific nutrient deficiencies result in specific health problems (see Box 6.1). Vitamin A deficiency leads to xerophthalmia and perhaps blindness; it is also thought to have a general effect on decreasing resistance to infections such as diarrhea and respiratory infections. Iodine deficiency leads to mental retardation and lethargy; and iron deficiency leads to lowered work capacity and increases the chances that a pregnant woman will miscarry or deliver a low birth weight baby.

### Mental Development

It is now becoming clear that energy-protein malnutrition can also reduce the child's capacity to learn. Deficits in mental development are assessed by observing children from the first year through adolescence on tasks related to verbal, perceptual, memory, and school skills (literacy, numeracy). The age at which malnutrition began, its duration, and its severity are important factors to consider. If the fetus does not receive enough nutrition in the very early weeks, it will have severe problems. However, most instances of fetal malnutrition occur in the third trimester, and although the newborn will have a low birth weight, its long-term mental development need not be impaired. If children suffer a severe case of malnutrition as a result of illness and are treated in the hospital, they usually regain their weight and activity level but do not fully regain their mental skills (Galler & Ramsey, 1987; Grantham-McGregor, Schofield, & Powell, 1987). Remember that even though their severe condition may have been short term, if they returned to a poor family, they probably continued to live with mild or moderate malnutrition.

In fact, as I indicated previously, the most prevalent form of malnutrition is chronic mild to moderate malnutrition. It begins in the second half of the child's first year and becomes quite evident when children are 2, 3, and 4 years of age. Most of the evidence for adverse effects on mental development are concentrated in this group. Weight and height for age indicate the degree of chronic malnutrition, and the Bayley and Griffith scales evaluate mental development. Items tapping verbal skills might require the child to point to objects such as "a chicken" or "your nose" and to follow verbal commands such as "Clap your hands, then touch your nose." Items requiring eye-hand coordination include using a stick to get an out-of-reach object. Both the Bayley and the Griffith also have items assessing motor development, such as standing and climbing. There are a number of problems to consider before we use such tests in developing countries, such as translating them into the local language and training nonprofessional testers. Also, because the test has probably only been used with selected samples of children in the country, there are no median scores or standard deviations from a representative sample. Consequently, we use the number of items the child was able to accomplish without comparing it with a country norm or standard. More difficult is the requirement that we modify items and materials to reflect the child's home environment without altering the difficulty level of the skill. For example, instead of asking the child to name objects or pictures that include a watch, scissors, pencil, and purse, we included lamb, banana, pants, and sickle. Items that require timing the child's response are not even relevant in a village where watches are rare. Children approaching school age might be given tests that emphasize reading readiness, understanding of numbers, and cognitive skills such as categorizing.

Using these tests of mental development, researchers in Africa, Latin America, and the Caribbean have shown that preschool children with low weight and height do not perform as well as their well-fed counterparts. For example, we found that almost half of our sample of rural Ethiopian children were underweight, mostly in the mild to moderate range as a result of stunting but not wasting. Children with lower weights and heights for their age completed fewer Bayley items than did children with higher nutritional status (Aboud & Alemu, 1995). Similarly, children of 30 months living in rural Kenya performed less well on verbal comprehension and production items and on visual-motor coordination items if they were underweight for their age (Sigman, Neumann, Baksh, et al., 1989). In Kingston, Jamaica, stunted children between 9 and 24 months of age had lower scores on the Griffith scales than did nonstunted children before intervention started (Grantham-McGregor, Powell, Walker, & Himes, 1991). Even children in the early school years may be at a disadvantage in vocabulary and analytic skills as a result of malnutrition (Sigman, Neumann, Jansen, & Bwibo, 1989). Thus, although the first 2 years of life are considered critical for growth and development, nutrition throughout childhood is important for mental activity. In some cases, daily food intake is also related to mental development, but in regions where infection is high, not all food is used for growth. In these cases, height and weight are better predictors of mental development than food intake.

Correlational studies, like those just described, examine the relation between nutrition and mental development without disturbing the normal patterns of life in the community. Such studies can show how the effects of long-term malnutrition accumulate, and how the broader family and community context contributes to mental development. For example, we find that the mother's education level, even a mere 4 years, influences both her child's nutritional status and her child's Bayley score. We also find that there are other routes to healthy mental development, such as being raised by a mother who verbally responds to her child's overtures. This information is important for developing long-term strategies for child growth and development. But back to the question of how nutrition itself affects mental development. With correlational studies, it is possible to control the contribution of mother's education and socioeconomic differences with statistical procedures. When this is done, most studies continue to find smaller but significant contributions of nutrition to mental development (for reviews, see Gorman, 1995; Simeon & Grantham-McGregor, 1990; Wachs, 1995). The question of how family context contributes will be discussed shortly.

Another way to determine the effects of nutrition on mental development, while minimizing differences due to social and economic factors, is to give supplementary food to certain children or certain villages and compare their development with others (see Box 6.2). If children are randomly assigned to receive the nutritious or nonnutritious food or drink, then social and economic differences will, ideally, be matched in the two groups. In Guatemala, Colombia, and Jamaica, food supplements have enhanced stunted and underweight children's motor development in the first 2 years, verbal and eye-hand performance in preschool years, and school-related skills such as literacy and numeracy in adolescence (Grantham-McGregor et al., 1991; Pollitt, Gorman, Engle, Martorell, & Rivera, 1993; Super, Herrera, & Mora, 1990). Memory and reaction time tests are not improved with supplements. The supplementation studies have been summed up as follows by Simeon and Grantham-McGregor (1990): Supplements did not bring the children up to the anthropometric reference levels, "so that small improvements in [physical] growth were accompanied by small improvements in [mental] development" (p. 18).

Certain groups of children might benefit more than others from supplementation, especially if it lasts for many years. When extra calories and proteins are provided to the whole family, as they must be, children benefit not only from the supplement but also from a more lively, stimulating family. In addition, the supplement was used to greater effect by children with lower SES, perhaps because they were initially performing far below their potential and so had more gains to make (the catch-up effect). It was also used to greater effect by children who stayed in school longer, because formal schooling gave them the opportunity to use their mental resources (capitalizing on one's resources). It has greater effect when given early in the child's life but may lead to some gains on school attendance and performance when given in a school feeding program (Levinger, 1986, Case 7 in the chapter on health education and promotion).

Iron-deficiency anemia also results in poorer scores on the Bayley Mental Scales. Evidence from supplementation studies does not provide a clear answer on when treatment or preventive doses of iron should be given for maximum benefits. Only one study has found that a low daily treatment dose of iron, given at home for 4 months, brought up the Bayley Motor and Mental scores of children under 2 years (Idjradinata & Pollitt, 1993). Iron supplements are clearly beneficial for children over 2 years. Before concluding that this is a quick and easy remedy, remember that iron may place a person at greater risk for malaria and that high levels of iron are toxic.

Socioemotional Development

Another aspect of mental development is sometimes referred to as socioemotional development. The first, and perhaps most important, emotional relationship in our lives is the one we have with our mother. The quality of this child-mother bond, or attachment, varies on an important emotional dimension called security. Children who are securely attached to their mothers receive not only pleasure from her presence but also comfort when they are tired, sick, or afraid. More important, a secure attachment provides the child with a feeling of confidence or assurance especially during the second year when novel things are explored. Thus the benefits of attachment for young children can be seen in the comfort it gives them during times of stress as well as the confidence to explore novelty.

Without this conception of a secure attachment, we might have mistakenly inferred that malnourished children, because they spend so much time close to their mothers, have a strong attachment. A Chilean researcher, Marta Valenzuela (1990), used a procedure initially developed in Uganda to find out whether malnourished children were strongly attached. Called Ainsworth's Strange Situation, the procedure is generally used with children between 12 and 24 months who have already spent 1 year developing an attachment and, with that "under their belt," are beginning to explore. The Santiago children were between 17 and 21 months. Each child was brought by his or her mother into a room with some new toys, and then an unfamiliar woman entered. There are eight steps to the procedure, two of which are revealing. In the first,

> ## BOX 6.2.
> ## SUPPLEMENTS ARE NOT ENOUGH
>
> Giving extra food to young children has, in the past, been a strategy for improving nutritional status and testing its effects on health at the same time. In 1969, the Institute of Nutrition of Central America and Panama (INCAP) supported a major longitudinal study into the effects of food supplements on the physical, mental, and social development of children. Ernesto Pollitt and his colleagues (Pollitt et al., 1993) studied mental development. Four villages in Guatemala were selected based on the finding that 80% of the preschoolers were underweight. Children and pregnant mothers were eating less than the recommended diet of calories and protein. Two of the villages were given *Atole*, a milk-based drink with 11.5 g of protein and 163 kcal of energy. The other two villages were given *Fresco*, with only 59 kcal. The drinks were made available on a voluntary basis to whoever came to the feeding station twice a day for 7 years. They collected information on children whose mothers received the supplement while pregnant and who themselves received the drink. Workers recorded how often each child took the supplement, and those who took Atole grew more in height and weight than those who took Fresco. Some children received the supplement only after their second birthday, and although they benefited, they did not develop as well as those who had had the supplement early.
>
> Not every eligible person came regularly to get the twice-daily drink because it was voluntary. Even during the peak years, the average number of drinks per person was 200. Why did some come and others not? The mother's perception of the nutritious value of the drink may have affected her motivation to attend with her children. The only socioeconomic variable that predicted attendance was the mother's years of schooling; mothers with less schooling came more often with their children, perhaps to make up for less food at home.
>
> Infant motor and mental tests were given to children under 2 years of age. The supplement improved scores on the motor test but not on the mental test. Children reached the motor milestones of crawling, walking, and climbing earlier if they had Atole rather than Fresco. During the preschool years, from 3 to 6, children with the Atole supplement benefited in their verbal skills, arithmetic, and basic knowledge; they were on average 8 months ahead of

> the Fresco children in these cognitive skills. Ten years later, when the children were 13 to 19 years of age, the Atole children had better literacy, numeracy, reading, and knowledge scores than the Fresco children.
>
> Two context variables influenced how much the children benefited from the supplement. One was socioeconomic status. Children from lower socioeconomic status benefited more from Atole, and so socioeconomic status no longer influenced their performance on the tests. However, performance of the Fresco children was, as usual, affected by their parents' economic status. In other words, the food supplement compensated for constraints usually imposed by being raised in a low-socioeconomic-status family. The second context variable was schooling. Atole children who did not attend school showed little benefit from the supplement. However, Atole children who stayed in school benefited the most. Thus the food supplement had its greatest effect on mental development in conjunction with the stimulation and opportunities provided by formal education. The conclusion that supplements are not enough is supported by Grantham-McGregor and colleagues (1991) in Jamaica. Malnourished children who played and talked with a community health worker for an hour every week at home made better use of the food supplements than children who had food alone.

critical step, the child's exploration of the new toys is observed. Some children are wary of the strange situation and too distressed to explore the toys; others are wary at first but gain a feeling of security from their mothers' presence, enough to move away from her and explore the toys. In the second critical step, which comes later, the mother returns to the room, having left for several minutes. Most, but not all, children are upset by their mother's departure; some then show pleasure at her return but others are too distressed or angry to be soothed. Those who explore and show pleasure at their mothers' return are considered to be securely attached; those who are unable to explore or to be soothed by the mother's return are considered insecurely attached. Children who were mildly or moderately underweight were not securely attached to their mothers. Only 7% were securely attached compared with 50% of the nutritionally healthy children. Unable to regulate their own emotional distress or be soothed by their mother's comforting overtures, the malnourished children remained apart yet irritable.

The social and emotional problems of malnourished children appear to persist into the early school years when children are expected to interact with peers. However, there are too few studies at this point to draw any firm conclusions. After several years of *Atole* supplement, the Guatemalan children showed more social responsiveness to their peers, more group involvement, more happiness and anger, less anxiety, and better control over their own frustration and impulses (Barrett & Radke-Yarrow, 1985). Yet in a recent Kenyan study, only a few social skills such as leadership were related to current nutrition, but none to past nutrition (Espinosa, Sigman, Neumann, Bwibo, & McDonald, 1992). Although no conclusions can yet be made on the social development of malnourished or supplemented children, it is important to remember that social skills are as valuable as reading and arithmetic.

## Three Routes From Malnutrition to Development

Three hypotheses have been proposed to explain the poorer mental and social development of children with protein-energy malnutrition. Each emphasizes a specific process:

1. Biological
2. Exploration
3. Social stimulation

The biological route is implicated if malnutrition leads to biochemical and anatomical changes in the brain that affect its functioning. Studies with animals undernourished in their early years show a reduction in glial cells, which are responsible for myelinization of the axon, resulting in slower transmission of nerve impulses. They also show a reduction in synapses and in the biochemical substances needed to transmit impulses from one nerve to another (Bedi, 1987). Many aspects of brain development take place during the last months in utero and in infancy. Inadequate food intake at this age can have very detrimental effects. Other aspects of brain growth, such as the number of neurons and synapses, show improvement when more food is provided at a later age. If this were the only route by which nutrition affects mental development, then improvements in nutrition during the preschool and school years would be less effective, and we know this is not the case.

The exploration hypothesis is that malnourished children are lethargic and passive and so deprive themselves of the stimulation needed for mental and social development. Active, healthy children are curious; they watch novel displays more than familiar ones, they smile and wave at people to get a reaction, they manipulate objects, they ask questions, and they play games with friends. Exploration takes different forms at different ages and perhaps in different cultures, but the common feature is that the child's action brings new information. We have suggestive evidence that malnourished children explore less, but there is no clear confirmation that lowered exploration accounts for poorer mental development. Current food intake is a better predictor of exploration than is height. For example, undernourished preschoolers tend to talk and play less than well-fed ones; they are less engaged and active when playing with peers. They become more anxious in the presence of unfamiliar people and toys, and are unable to regulate their emotional distress enough to explore and learn from the novel stimulation (Barrett & Radke-Yarrow, 1985; Meeks Gardner, Grantham-McGregor, Chang, Himes, & Powell, 1995; Sigman, Neumann, Baksh, et al., 1989; Sigman, Neumann, Jansen, & Bwibo, 1989; Valenzuela, 1990). Thus the malnourished child deprives itself of important social and environmental stimulation. Furthermore, passive and isolating behaviors may become a habit even after food intake increases, and there may be long-term effects on the child's social and problem-solving capabilities.

The third route from malnutrition to development is through social stimulation from other people. One suggestion is that malnourished children are frequently irritable and unsoothable and so receive less attention from their mothers. The other, more promising, suggestion is that malnourished children evoke caring practices that are meant for less mature children. To illustrate, mothers more often pick up and carry young children, whereas they are more likely to converse with older children. We find that wasted, but not stunted, children, as well as those recovering from an illness, are more likely to be picked up and carried; Kenyan mothers similarly have more physical contact with underweight children. Picking up and holding a child, particularly when the child has not signaled the need for physical contact, appears to be detrimental to the development of eye-hand coordination, a component

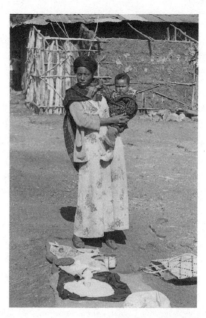

*In infancy, children need to be held and carried often, but by the second year, they need freedom to initiate their own motor and social explorations.*

of mental development (Aboud & Alemu, 1995; Sigman, Neumann, Baksh, et al., 1989). Perhaps this kind of infantile care prevents children from developing their own fine motor abilities.

Mothers provide more beneficial stimulation when they talk in response to their child's signals. There is little evidence that mothers respond less verbally to wasted or stunted children, although they do talk more to fussing, crying children ("the squeaky wheel gets the oil"). Other than reacting to fussiness in the child, the Ethiopian mothers we observed were more responsive as a function of their own beliefs about child development, such as recognizing that even infants can understand words and communicate needs. Furthermore, mothers' verbal responsiveness, although not related to their child's weight or height, does appear to influence mental development (Aboud & Alemu, 1995; Sigman et al., 1988; Super et al., 1981).

In conclusion, the three routes by which malnutrition may impede mental and social development have provoked a good deal of insightful research. The research shows that chronic malnutrition at even mild or moderate levels can reduce cognitive and social functioning. Malnutrition can affect brain development, but more research is needed to determine the reversibility of these effects in children. Current malnutrition appears to result in less active and less emotional involvement with the social and physical environment as well as in more anxiety. Socially and emotionally secure children may, in turn, learn more through confident exploration of their environment. Caretaker behavior does seem to affect mental development, but it is not clear what child cues are used by the mother and whether she withholds stimulation or provides more to compensate. With the little research available, it appears that social and physical aspects of the environment have an important but separate effect on mental development, adding on to the benefits of nutrition. Opportunities for exploration, conversation, and schooling can to a certain extent compensate for the early effects of malnutrition (Gorman & Pollitt, 1996; Werner, 1989).

You may wonder how it is possible to study child feeding and mother-child interaction without including the broader social and cultural context. The simple answer is that all research is limited to a few influential inputs. The studies previously discussed focus on the inputs of nutrition, family, and school by letting these vary among children who share a similar culture. This is not to say that culture has no bearing on growth and development, but one study cannot look at all the contributing factors. One can, however, compare the results of such studies from different cultures. For example, mothers in Kenya and Egypt seemed to have different ways of caring for their children; Kenyan mothers who fed their children well were less likely to be verbal in their responses, whereas Egyptian mothers were more likely to be verbal (Wachs et al., 1992). Cultural groups have different goals for their children and use different strategies to promote these (e.g., LeVine et al., 1994; Whiting & Edwards, 1988). However, the way a mother interacts with her child may also depend on her own beliefs about child development and her role as a mother.

Generally speaking, rural mothers in developing countries spend most of the day involved in household management and agricultural activities. Their role as a mother is to feed and clean their children and protect them from harm and illness. Their beliefs about child rearing and child development are, not surprisingly, derived from the culture in which they were raised. Because of the different cultures they came from, even second-generation mothers in Israel provided different kinds of care and stimulation to their children; Kurdish mothers emphasized motor development, whereas Yemeni mothers provided verbal and physical stimulation for intellectual growth (Frankel & Roer-Bornstein, 1982). On average, mothers in our Ethiopian sample expected late development of social and language skills in their children. They were asked at what age they expected a child to begin to communicate with sounds and gestures, and to understand words spoken to it. These and other communicative skills were not expected until the third year. However, there were differences among the mothers, even though they lived in the same small farming village. Some mothers recognized that children could communicate and understand at 6 months, and others pegged these abilities at 4 years. Those who expected late development were less verbally responsive to their child: What is the point in wasting words that won't be understood? The question as to where mothers get their child-rearing and child feeding practices is a valid and complex one.

## TREATMENT AND COMMUNITY PREVENTION PROGRAMS

Treatment for severe malnutrition is usually given at a clinic and involves not only supplementing the diet with 150 to 200 kcal per kg of body weight per day along with milk and vitamin A but also treating dehydration and infections. For a very young infant, the mother may be encouraged to relactate and breast-feed her child. The decline in breast-feeding has been observed most often in urban centers, where hospital staff and formula manufacturers explicitly encourage new mothers to use bottles. The baby-friendly hospital program begun in 1991 by UNICEF (1993) has been successful in banning the use of bottles and infant formula by hospital staff. The award was given to leading hospitals in 12 developing countries in the first year of the program and to many other hospitals in subsequent years.

Fortified Foods

Because deficiencies in vitamin A, iodine, and iron are so widespread, and only small amounts are needed, many countries have begun to fortify foods with these substances. Iodized salt is the most common way to provide iodine in regions where it is lacking. There is little controversy about this approach, which has been used for a long time in industrialized countries. Extending this solution to vitamin A and iron is now being considered in developing countries where deficiencies are widespread. The common approach is to put vitamin A in sugar and iron in wheat flour. Some countries are concentrating on foods for young children; Mexico is fortifying a chocolate drink mix with both vitamin A and iron. Others such as Venezuela are fortifying maize flour with both nutrients. The strategy is to find a common food, such as salt, sugar, or flour, that most people buy and use regularly. The cost of the added nutrient is minimal. Although many countries are now fortifying salt, sugar, and wheat flour, it has yet to be determined how much of this food is reaching the young children of subsistence farmers. Another strategy is to provide vitamin A capsules every 6 months to young children. A comparison of capsule distribution with vitamin A-fortified MSG (monosodium glutamate) showed that both were effective in reducing the clinical signs of xerophthalmia in the Philippines and Nepal, but that fortifying MSG was more acceptable to the community and less expensive (Latham, 1983; Pant et al., 1996). These projects also promoted home gardens for growing vegetables and fruits; the general nutrition of these children improved, but the disadvantages were cost, time, and effort.

Food Supplements

When the community as a whole lacks food, as happens in drought-prone areas of sub-Saharan Africa, food relief is provided in the form of grains and oil. An early warning system has been created in some regions to monitor the availability and price of food in local markets. This allows relief workers to identify and prepare for food shipments before the famine takes its toll. Some NGOs provide food for work in areas where there is a shortage. They might buy staples in one region of the country to support agricultural production while using it as payment in a drought area. Another type of food program provides meals at school. Once again, the goal is to provide food supplements for children while financially supporting local agriculture. NGOs often take on this kind of development work.

In comparison, the previous studies described in Latin America and the Caribbean were not aimed at promoting healthy eating practices. They were aimed at finding out if nutritional status and mental development would improve with extra intake of protein and energy, and if the effects of early malnutrition were reversible. They were targeted at mildly and moderately malnourished young children. In this sense, they were community prevention programs, preventing severe malnutrition and poor learning.

In Colombia, instruction was given along with the food. Families were provided weekly food supplements of bread, oil, and milk to bring them up to the recommended intake requirements. In addition, a nutritionist taught mothers how to prepare simple, nutritious foods for children. After 3 years, the children who received supplements since birth had better weight and height than children without supplements. They maintained their advantage for several years after the supplements stopped. But by this point, their diets were no different from the nonsupplemented children. They were eating the same amount of proteins and calories. Three years of intervention benefited the target children only but had no lasting effect on their diets or, by implication, that of their younger siblings (Super et al., 1990). Food supplements work in the short run, and we can now only guess at why they do not have more long lasting effects.

When food supplements are voluntary, it is interesting to examine why not all families avail themselves of the service. In Haiti, the directors of feeding centers reported that 30% of the needy families did not come because they failed to recognize malnutrition in their children or because of transportation problems (Coreil, 1987). The mothers who came were more interested in education, occupational training, medical services, and recreation than in nutrition. A Mexican program to supplement children's diet with alfalfa leaf nutrients failed within a few months. Although a majority of the children were malnourished and lacked iron and vitamins, the families were more eager to buy junk food than alfalfa, "the poor man's food." Additionally, the project never gained the support of the community or the church (Nelson, Jenkins, et al., 1989). There are lessons to be learned from failed projects—if only they were better publicized. Food in particular provokes strong attitudinal reactions from adults, who often assume that their children will react similarly. Advertisers know how to promote a product. Their

Instruction and Products for Weaning

Where malnutrition is endemic, communitywide programs are necessary to reverse mild and moderate levels of malnutrition. The best long-term strategy appears to be teaching mothers how to feed their children in the 6- to 24-month age period at little extra cost in money and time. As noted previously, there are several obstacles to be overcome: starting young enough, giving often enough, minimizing bulk, and maximizing calories and protein. Many manuals are available with recipes for infant foods (e.g., Cameron & Hofvander, 1983), but a great deal of manpower is needed to convince mothers of the need for weaning foods and to teach them how to prepare the foods within their means. Community health workers have been successfully engaged in this labor-intensive effort in India and Nigeria.

In the Punjab district of India, where grains are grown, 47% of the girls between 13 and 36 months were malnourished because they received no weaning food before 18 months. They were drinking only a little tea and breast milk. Mothers were shown how to use the chappatis, made from wheat or maize and eaten by the rest of the family, to make a weaning food. Crumbled and added to a little hot sweet tea, it made a nutritious porridge. Mothers were taught to use other vegetables and lentils that were part of the family diet to make a soup for the baby (Cowan & Dhanoa, 1983). A community health worker visited the children daily or every other day from birth to 15 months. Mothers were also taught about family planning, immunization, and diarrhea management with the salt-sugar solution. Among the children visited, food intake increased to 1,200-1,300 calories per day, and an adequate diet was attained by 82% of the boys and 70% of the girls.

In Nigeria, the problem was that children were given a bulky porridge that filled them up quickly but provided too few calories. *Eko mimu*, as it is known, is the traditional weaning food of this culture, and all children between 6 and 11 months were fed eko along with breast milk. Nutritionists and health workers wanted to provide an alternative to the low-energy eko, one that would have more nutrients per cup. With the help of mothers, the team of workers developed a new recipe.

They added toasted cowpeas, red palm oil, and sugar to *ogi* and malt flour to make a fortified eko that contains more than three times the amount of calories as the traditional one. However, the successful adoption of the new recipe required that mothers accept the use of a spoon to feed their child instead of forced hand feeding, and accept some increased time and cost in its preparation. They would also have to accept a heavier child to carry around. Social marketing was carried out in each village by 20 Teaching Moms, who are each responsible for teaching 10 village mothers (Bentley et al., 1991).

One of the side benefits of increased feeding is that it is usually accompanied by social stimulation. Only a few studies have used this opportunity to instruct mothers on the social and mental stimulation of their children. In Jamaica and Colombia, mothers were taught during weekly visits how to talk to their young children and encourage toy play. This training had longer term effects on the diet and nutritional status of the children than did supplementation alone. It also improved eye-hand coordination, verbal skills, and motor development when continued for 2 years. The effects of stimulation are greatest when combined with food supplements, but the effects are additive and do not depend on both being given (Grantham-McGregor et al., 1991; Super et al., 1990). Although more costly and time-consuming, nutrition education and home gardening are often more sustainable over the long term.

## STUDENT ACTIVITY

In 1974, delegates to the World Food Conference in Rome proclaimed the end of hunger within a decade. This obviously failed. Delegates to the 1996 conference called for cutting the numbers of chronically hungry people by half by 2015. Is this goal any more feasible? Set up a government committee or local NGO of students to devise an action plan to work toward this goal. Consider the chain of events from production to feeding practices. Are you going to bring in the tractors, chemical fertilizers, and irrigation wheels, or teach tool making and composting? (Remember that there is very little garbage, although "night soil" is a possibility.) Are you going to fortify and supplement or change eating habits?

# 7

## ALCOHOL USE AND ABUSE

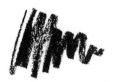

Alcohol is a legal drink in most places; it is sensibly and responsibly used and enjoyed by many adults. In most societies, drinking takes place in a social setting, where decisions are made, emotions are shared, and people relax with family and friends. The sensible drinker drinks moderately because there is either societal or personal control over the amount drunk. Moderate drinkers, for example, limit the number of occasions they drink and/or the quantity they drink to two or three drinks a day, or four drinks on a weekend. It is commonly accepted now that moderate drinking is actually beneficial to one's health; mortality rates are lowest for this group although the reasons are not clear. Because beer, wine, and distilled spirits vary considerably in pure alcohol (ethanol) content—from 3%-5% for beer, about 12% for wine, and more than double that for spirits or distilled liquor such as vodka and rum—one drink is somewhat equivalent to a mug of beer, a glass of wine, or a half jigger of rum (Miller, Heather, & Hall, 1991). This is essentially a North American and European perspective, the two regions where about 75% of alcohol is commercially produced and consumed (Walsh & Grant, 1985). Even in these regions there are national differences—with the wine-producing French and Italians consuming quantities daily with little public intoxication, and the Scandinavians drinking less frequently with more serious social problems.

There are at least two other perspectives on the proper use of alcohol. In some Moslem countries, drinking alcohol is forbidden, and devout Moslems throughout the world refrain from drinking alcohol. In developing countries, home-brewed beer is by far the most common beverage, accounting for 90% of all the alcohol available (Kortteinen, 1989). Home brew is produced from sorghum, maize, millet, or palm sap in Africa (Molamu, 1989; Peltzer, 1989) and from fruit, the aloe plant, and sugar cane in Latin America (Negrette, 1976). Its concentration is fairly low, around 3%-5% pure alcohol, and it is often sold by the women who make it. Furthermore, traditional drinking practices in rural areas often specify that only married men and elders of the community are allowed to drink. Thus alcohol previously was not usually a problem in developing countries; drinking was responsible and moderate.

Heavy alcohol drinking, however, is a major public health concern of most industrialized countries, including those in Europe and North America. Not only are there large numbers of alcoholics who drink excessively on a regular basis, but more women and adolescents have begun to drink since the 1970s. For example, between the ages of 18 and 20 years when male adolescents drink most in the United States, 51% drank at least four times per week and 50% drank on average five drinks per occasion (Kandel & Yamaguchi, 1985). The concern over adolescent drinking is not primarily a fear that the adolescent will become dependent on alcohol or even that he will move on to illicit drugs. Recent data show that sometime during the adolescent and young adult years, 35% of drinkers considerably reduce their intake; both the quantity and the frequency of drinking decline (Fillmore et al., 1991). The concern is over problems associated with heavy drinking, such as motor vehicle injuries, violence, delinquency, being expelled from school or fired from a job, and conflicts with parents.

Alcohol abuse is now spreading to countries where alcohol was previously not a problem because of its rare or controlled use. Japan, Mexico, South Korea, and now Kenya have been identified as countries with high alcohol consumption (Saunders, Aasland, Amundsen, & Grant, 1993; Walsh & Grant, 1985). This is often blamed on the international spread of modern culture, through industrialization and urbanization, which undercuts traditional norms for drinking. As young single people move into cities, away from their families, their lives becomes more stressful and peer oriented. Drinking practices change; with money, a job, and leisure time, young men and women can drink commercially made beer and spirits in bars with their friends. For example, between 30% and 40% of men who were "social" drinkers in Kenya averaged more than four drinks a day for a typical month (Saunders et al., 1993). Although men worldwide drink much more than women, 30% of Kenyan women also have four drinks a day. These people were not identified as alcoholics. Consequently, the treatments we have developed for alcoholics would not adequately tackle the problem. The host (drinker), the agent (alcohol), and the environment are all sources of the problem and will be considered in its solution.

## DEFINITIONS AND MEASURES OF PROBLEM DRINKING

International work on alcohol use and abuse reveals that extremely heavy drinkers around the world tend to have the same patterns of alcohol use and similar problems associated with overuse. However, there are cultural differences in the more moderate patterns of use. For example, in some countries such as Japan and Scotland, people drink smaller amounts daily and do not often experience problems as a consequence. On the other hand, in Mexico and Zambia, many abstain from drinking, and many drink large amounts on infrequent special occasions, with resulting domestic and other problems. In an attempt to focus on problem drinking, researchers and health workers tend to use two types of indicators:

- Heavy consumption (frequency × quantity)
- Alcohol-related problems, such as medical, social, personal problems

Although there may be a cutoff point to identify problem drinkers, it is important to remember that people fall on a continuum from no drinking to excessive drinking, with most of us in between the two extremes.

The extreme end of the continuum is alcoholism. Given that alcoholics consume more than half the alcohol available in a community, and that they are responsible for most of the social and economic problems, this index could be a valid indicator of the extent of the problem. However, another group of drinkers need serious attention before they become alcoholic. Thus the second set of measures attempts to identify hazardous drinkers, those who abuse alcohol but are not known alcoholics. A third set of indicators, for example, the annual per capita consumption of people 15 years and over, refers to the alcohol rather than the drinker. Public health measures aimed at limiting the availability of alcohol through price increases are based on this kind of indicator.

Alcoholism

The definition of an *alcoholic* initially used by the WHO (1952, reproduced in Vallance, 1965) was

> excessive drinkers whose dependence upon alcohol has attained such a degree that it shows a noticeable mental disturbance or an interference with their bodily and mental health, their interpersonal relations, and their smooth social and economic functioning, or who show the prodromal signs of such developments. (p. 348)

More recently, the criteria spelled out in the *International Classification of Diseases (ICD)* and the *Diagnostic and Statistical Manual (DSM)* include alcohol dependence as only one form of alcohol abuse. Other nonphysiological problems stemming from the excessive use of alcohol are more prominent. They include culture-specific social and psychological problems, such as problems in the job, school, family, and peer context. The current definition has therefore gone beyond the pharmacological definition of alcoholism in terms of an addiction to include behavioral patterns of drinking and its consequences for the drinker and others.

**Alcoholism** could be described as the excessive and regular use of alcohol leading to alcohol-related problems. **Alcohol abuse or harmful use**, the broader term, refers to the harmfully excessive and recurrent use of alcohol resulting in physical, personal, or social problems. One or more of the following alcohol-related problems are experienced within a 12-month period: (a) failure to fulfill major role obligations at work, school, or home, such as absenteeism from work due to hangovers, school suspensions, or marital problems; (b) recurrent use in physically hazardous situations such as when using industrial equipment or driving an automobile; (c) legal problems such as arrests; and (d) continued use despite persistent social or interpersonal problems exacerbated by the effects of alcohol, such as fights with spouse and friends. A common example is the heavy weekend "binge" drinking of young men, which leads to injury, family discord, or periodic absenteeism from work.

**Alcohol dependency** refers to more excessive and prolonged drinking, which affects the person at many levels and creates physiological dependency that manifests as withdrawal (symptoms of nonuse such as seizures and tremors) and tolerance (needing more alcohol to have an effect), craving alcohol, and curtailing normal activities to obtain alcohol. Three or more out of the seven criteria must be met for the term *dependency* to apply. When people refer to alcoholics, they generally mean those dependent on alcohol. Adolescents and young adults, although they may drink excessively, are not generally dependent on alcohol because they have not been drinking for a sufficiently long time to experience tolerance or withdrawal.

The term **alcohol intoxication** refers to a temporary state due to the recent consumption of alcohol that results in maladaptive behavioral or psychological changes such as aggressive or argumentative behavior, disinhibition, and impaired social or occupational functioning. Other signs such as slurred speech and uncoordinated movements are apparent. People differ in the amount of alcohol they need to drink before becoming intoxicated. For example, females develop higher concentrations of alcohol in their blood than males after drinking the same amount, because their body water-fat composition is different and they metabolize alcohol more slowly. One of the legal problems encountered by alcohol abusers is to have a record of intoxication, which therefore also has a legal definition, used to identify a person whose functioning is impaired by alcohol. Breath or blood analysis is often used to determine a person's blood alcohol concentration (BAC). The level at which a person is considered legally intoxicated in many places is 0.10% BAC—which means 100 parts of alcohol per 10,000 parts of blood, or 100 mg of alcohol per 100 ml of blood. At this level, a person's driving is usually affected and he or she has an unsteady gait. Even at lower levels such as 0.05 BAC, rational thought and muscular control are impaired (Davidson, 1985). Consequently, in some places, a BAC of 0.08% is the legal threshold for intoxication.

Usually, in a health care setting, the criteria described above would be considered during an interview with the patient. A diagnosis of alcohol abuse (harmful use if using the *ICD* classification) or dependency would be made if the patient expressed the listed problems. However, not all who abuse alcohol seek help for their problem. So it is important to find out how many people in the community have a serious alcohol problem. For this we need a survey questionnaire. Using the criteria specified by the *ICD* and the *DSM*, researchers have developed survey instruments with specific questions whose answers can be summed to obtain a total score for each respondent. The survey instruments include items that parallel the definitions. A score over the threshold indicates alcoholism.

The *Diagnostic Instrument Schedule (DIS)* is one such instrument, developed from the *DSM*, which identifies both alcohol abuse and alcohol dependence. It includes 21 items to be answered with a simple yes or no. The following are examples of items:

- Have you ever drunk as much as 20 drinks (the equivalent to 200 g of pure alcohol) or its equivalent in one day?
- Have you ever wanted to stop drinking but couldn't?
- Have you ever tried to control your drinking by making rules, like not drinking before sunset or never drinking alone?

As you can see, the items refer to "ever" having had the experience. Thus it measures what is called *lifetime alcoholism*, meaning whether one has at any time in one's life consumed the quantities and had the problems of alcoholism. The questions were recently answered by a sample of people, aged 18 to 65 years, who had gone to a large clinic in Kenya for problems other than drinking. Almost 40% met the criteria for lifetime abuse and/or dependence, which requires that two or more symptoms be experienced in one's lifetime (Nielsen, Resnick, & Acuda, 1989). Although rates differ across countries, the number and nature of symptoms appear to be very similar, indicating that the *DIS* may validly measure alcoholism across many cultures (Helzer et al., 1990).

To make the *DIS* more inclusive of international classifications and more cross-culturally relevant, a task force was set up by the WHO to develop a composite instrument. The *Composite International Diagnostic Interview* includes items from the *DIS* as well as the *ICD* and another international survey form, the *Present State Examination (PSE)*. A subset of these items comprise the *Substance Abuse Module (CIDI-SAM)* to identify cases of alcohol abuse and dependence. After inquiring about a particular symptom such as withdrawal, probes are used to determine the recency of the symptom (1 month indicates a positive symptom) and its severity. It identifies *current alcoholism,* meaning that the person is presently abusing alcohol, rather than lifetime alcoholism. Modifications for less industrialized countries include, for example, asking about failing to accomplish one's chores rather than absenteeism or loss of one's job. Field testing with nonclinician and clinician interviewers in 18 countries indicates good reliability (North America, Europe, Greece, China, India, Brazil) (Cottler et al., 1991). This instrument holds good promise for providing a standardized measure of alcoholism, thereby allowing for cross-cultural comparisons (Robins et al., 1988).

Hazardous Use of Alcohol

Those interested in the prevention of alcoholism have tried to define a level of drinking that is not considered alcoholism yet is not moderate and responsible. Saunders and colleagues (1993) refer to this as harmful or **hazardous consumption,** meaning that the person has an average daily consumption of, for men, six or more drinks in a typical month, or, for women, four or more drinks. Also, they defined **episodic heavy drinking** as having six or more drinks per occasion at least weekly, similar to alcohol abuse. Most of these people did not meet the criteria for alcohol dependence so they are not likely to have sought or received treatment. The value in identifying hazardous and episodic drinking is to provide brief, low-cost programs for people whose drinking creates problems on a much larger scale than that of alcoholics, simply because of their larger numbers. Such programs may prevent more severe alcoholism from developing.

Structured questionnaires were developed to assess hazardous drinking in a general population of clinic attenders (Saunders et al., 1993). Two of these questions are asked on most surveys of drinking: How often do you drink in a typical month? How many drinks do you have on a typical occasion? The first is the frequency question; the second is the quantity question. By combining frequency and quantity, one can calculate the level of alcohol consumption (Fillmore et al., 1991; Rootman

& Moser, 1984). To assess episodic heavy drinking, they also ask how often the person has six or more drinks on a single occasion. Finally, alcohol-related problems in health, domestic, legal, psychological, occupational, and social areas are assessed.

Survey questionnaires such as this have also been used extensively in industrialized countries to determine the use and abuse of alcohol by adolescents from 12 to 20 years as well as the problems they encounter from overuse. The questions may concern current frequency and quantity as well as lifetime use and discontinued use. Because use fluctuates considerably throughout one's lifetime, we want to find out whether early use leads to greater abuse in adulthood or to discontinued use when adult roles are adopted. In addition, some social scientists may conduct a more hands-on type of study, observing and recording activities in a drinking establishment. If drinking practices appear to be changing, these small-scale studies may help specify how social context effects changes.

After using these measures in six countries, the WHO team concluded that the frequency-quantity consumption indicators converge on a single cross-cultural concept of hazardous drinking, whereas the problems experienced as a result of drinking differ depending on the laws and norms of the culture (O'Nell & Mitchell, 1996; Saunders et al., 1993).

Country Levels of Consumption

Community levels of alcohol consumption present another picture of the level of problem and nonproblem drinking. When aggregated for a whole country, **per capita alcohol consumption** figures are usually based on what is commercially produced in the country plus whatever is imported minus whatever is exported during that year. The amounts are usually converted to quantities of 100% ethanol per capita population 15 years and over. Sometimes the figures are given for drinkers only, that is, excluding abstainers. Because this does not include quantities of home-brewed alcohol, which may be substantial in developing countries, the rates are not entirely accurate but are nonetheless considered to be a useful estimate of how much is consumed in a country. These figures can be calculated for the different beverages such as beer, wine, and distilled spirits (Walsh & Grant, 1985).

## INTERNATIONAL RATES OF ALCOHOL USE AND ABUSE

Few of the previously described indicators of alcohol use and abuse are available for more than a handful of countries. As a ballpark figure, we could take the findings from 18 sites around the world where the *CIDI-SAM* was used. Respondents were 590 adults from hospitals and outpatient clinics in North America, Europe, Brazil, Greece, India, and China. Overall, 25% of the adults had been heavy drinkers at some time in their lives. A "heavy drinker" was someone who ever drank the equivalent of 20 drinks of liquor in one day, daily drank at least 7 drinks for 2 weeks, or spent 2 months drinking at least 7 drinks a week (Cottler et al., 1991). Approximately 19% could be classified as dependent on alcohol and 6% as alcohol abusers. Of interest, 25% were abstainers, with the remaining 50% moderate drinkers. The current prevalence of alcohol problems in 15 health centers around the world is closer to 6%—the third highest of all mental health problems (Goldberg, 1995). The difference between lifetime prevalence and current (or period) prevalence is due to people who stop drinking heavily. In some studies, up to 40% of past drinkers have discontinued frequent use of alcohol (Fillmore et al., 1991; Giovino, Henningfield, Tomar, Escobedo, & Slade, 1995). We must remember that prevalence in the general population is bound to be lower than what is found at clinics; heavy drinkers often have health problems, so they might disproportionately fill the seats of a health clinic.

To identify countries where there might be an alcohol problem, investigators look at per capita consumption figures. Because beer is by far the most popular drink worldwide, statistics on its consumption are more available and allow for international comparisons. Amounts consumed in liters per person 15 years and over show that Australia, Germany, Czechoslovakia (combined), and Gabon consumed the most beer—180 liters and over in 1981 (Walsh & Grant, 1985). Other European and North American countries follow close behind in rank order. Latin American countries such as Venezuela, Colombia, Mexico, and Panama also have high rates of beer consumption. Among the East Asian countries, Japan and South Korea have lower, but rapidly rising, consumption rates. Three sub-Saharan African countries are lower still yet high among developing countries, namely, Kenya, Gambia, and Tanzania, whereas Sri Lanka, Egypt, and Morocco have low consumption (Kortteinen, 1989).

These statistics are supposed to include home-brewed alcohol in addition to what is produced industrially, although it is difficult to obtain accurate figures on the former. In some places, home brew is known to be produced and presumably consumed in large quantities. For example, up to 50% of self-employed persons in one Botswana district (Molamu, 1989) and 50% of the population of the Kombo peninsula in Gambia (Kortteinen, 1989) may be involved in producing and selling traditional beer or wine. It is often sold in an unlicensed bar run by the woman who makes the beer. Most of this beer would probably not make it into the per capita statistics.

Country differences can be compared using the *Diagnostic Instrument Schedule (DIS)*. This has been used in community surveys in the United States, where the lifetime prevalence of alcoholism was 13.4% in one sample and 17% in another (Compton et al., 1991; Helzer et al., 1990). The lifetime prevalence for men was 29% and for women, 4%. In Edmonton, Canada, the prevalence was 19%—31% for men and 7% for women. In contrast, the 6-month prevalence for the U.S. sites was only 9% for men, a quarter of the lifetime rate (see also Robins, Locke, & Regier, 1991). Rates are always higher for men than for women. Similarly high rates are found for other industrialized countries including Europe and Australia (Hauge & Irgens-Jensen, 1986; Moser, 1980).

Because alcohol use is high in industrialized countries, it often leads to problems associated with abuse and intoxication rather than solely dependency. The Household Survey in the United States and the Health Survey in Canada monitor drinking habits on a yearly basis. They find that by 18 years of age, almost 90% of males and 80% of females have consumed alcohol sometime in their lives. However, 50% of Americans and 55% of Canadians were current users, meaning they had consumed alcohol sometime in the past month (Giovino et al., 1995; Millar, 1991). As a result of widespread efforts to reduce alcohol consumption, the use of alcohol has been declining over the past 15 years. In Canada, 23% of male drinkers reported having two or more drinks per day, on average, in 1985, and this dropped to 16% in 1990. In the United States, the percentage of men drinking at this level dropped from 17% to 14%.

Developing countries show wide variations in their rates of alcoholism. India, China, and the North African countries are rarely mentioned in alcohol studies because drinking is not a problem. In Latin America, where per capita beer consumption appeared to be highest for Venezuela, Colombia, Mexico, and Panama, there are indications of alcohol abuse in those and other countries (e.g., Moser, 1980; Negrette, 1976; Pan-American Health Organization [PAHO], 1990). For example, in one Guatemalan study, 68% of the urban employed men drank frequently, and 30% drank more than six beers per occasion (Coombs & Lowe, 1987); 50% of traffic injuries involved alcohol. In Lima, Peru, a Spanish version of the *DIS* found that 35% of men and 2.5% of women had at one time been alcoholic (Yamamoto, Silva, Sasao, Wang, & Nguyen, 1993). Chile and Argentina report similar rates, although their preferred beverage is wine. Depending on the country and the urban-rural setting, rates are anywhere from 8% to 30%. Male abusers outnumber female abusers 10:1. Heavy drinking to intoxication is a socially approved way of celebrating a religious or civil festival among men. Low production and absenteeism are similarly tolerated postcelebration. The *DIS* was used in Puerto Rico, yielding a lifetime prevalence of 13%—25% for men and 2% for women (Helzer et al., 1990). Although part of the United States, the island shows the 10:1 sex ratio typical of Latin American countries.

In the region of East Asia, two countries—Japan and South Korea—were identified with rising per capita consumption. Lifetime prevalence rates using the *DIS* were 23% for South Korea, which is much higher than the 7% found in Taiwan (Helzer et al., 1990). In both countries, men alcoholics outnumber women alcoholics 14:1. Abuse is a greater problem than dependence. For example, in South Korea, 14% had sometime in their life abused alcohol but not been dependent on it, while 9% had alcohol dependence with or without abuse. This abuse is blamed on the popularity of social drinking parties after work, where coworkers challenge each other to consume large quantities. A similar phenomenon is found among Filipino men living in Los Angeles, of whom 30% were classed as heavy drinkers according to their frequency and quantity answers; most of them had drinking friends (Lubben, Chi, & Kitano, 1988). In contrast, 55% of the women abstained and a further 40% were infrequent or light drinkers. Thus, although rates in East Asia are generally low, men in some countries are beginning to follow the Latin American style of heavy drinking while women maintain the value of temperance.

In sub-Saharan Africa, Kenya, Gambia, and Tanzania showed rising levels of alcohol consumption. People in these countries also produce unknown quantities of home-brewed beer for use or sale. Small-scale surveys have been conducted in specific rural and urban settings in Kenya using a standardized measure such as the *DIS* (e.g., Acuda, 1985; Nielsen et al., 1989; Otieno, Owola, & Oduo, 1979). Some 40% appeared to be abstainers, and 30%-40% heavy drinkers. High prevalence is also reported in Zimbabwe (Moses, 1989) and Lesotho (Moremoholo, 1989), although standardized measures were not used. These studies may have been conducted in areas where alcoholism is a problem. A rate more representative of the general adult population could be as low as 3% (Moser, 1980), as in Nigeria, where it was 5.2% for men and 0% for women (Gureje, Obikoya, & Ikuesan, 1992).

Cross-country comparisons are provided by a study on hazardous levels of drinking among clinic attenders, using questions on frequency and quantity rather than a mental health instrument. Saunders and colleagues (1993) went to urban clinics in six countries with different cultures: Australia, Bulgaria, Kenya, Mexico, Norway, and the United States. They wanted to question only "social" drinkers, not abstainers or known alcoholics. However, the Kenyan clinic attracted some alcoholics, so I will try to adjust the figures to represent nonalcoholics. To identify binge drinkers, they asked how often one had six or more drinks per occasion at least weekly. Overall, 25% were binge drinkers; there were more in Kenya and Mexico, and fewer in Norway. To identify hazardous drinkers, they used an average daily intake of six drinks per day or more for men and four drinks per day for women. The following table shows the prevalence of hazardous drinking (see Table 7.1). For comparison, you can see how many of the same people fit the *DSM-ICD* criteria for alcohol dependence, which include withdrawal, tolerance, uncontrolled drinking, and major interference with roles.

These figures indicate that alcohol consumption is excessively high among some people even though they have not sought treatment for alcoholism. About 30% of the people in Kenya, the United States, Australia, and Mexico reported at least one major alcohol-related problem in the past year, such as domestic conflict, injury, arrest, or ill health. Many did not think they had an alcohol problem and had not sought treatment, although 22% thought they might in the future have a

*Alcohol Use and Abuse* 197

**TABLE 7.1** Percentage of Drinking Clinic Attenders Who Fit the Criteria of Hazardous and Dependent Drinkers

| Country | Hazardous Drinkers | | | Alcohol Dependence |
| | Men | Women | Total | Total |
|---|---|---|---|---|
| Kenya | 26 | 30 | 28 | 22 |
| United States | 17 | 10 | 14 | 11 |
| Australia | 18 | 7 | 14 | 10 |
| Bulgaria | 13 | 7 | 12 | 4 |
| Mexico | 16 | 3 | 10 | 18 |
| Norway | 6 | 1 | 3 | 5 |
| All Countries | 16 | 7 | 12 | 11 |

SOURCE: Adapted from Saunders et al. (1993).

problem if they kept drinking as they were. This 22% represents a group who would benefit from preventive programs.

Adolescent and Young Adult Drinking

The problem of adolescent drinking, already high in North America and Europe, is rising in many other parts of the world. The problem is that adolescents are starting to drink at a younger age, they binge drink in groups, and intoxication is associated with injury, aggression, and school or job failure. U.S. surveys indicate that by 15 years of age, more than half the students have tasted alcohol, and by 19 years, 90% have. This is not surprising given that beer and wine are legal and present in most homes. The problem occurs because, during this age span, the frequency and quantity increase dramatically from 3 to 9 times a month and from 1 to 4 drinks per occasion (e.g., Fillmore et al., 1991). Large-scale surveys of adolescents in North America show how the frequency of heavy drinking doubles in the last 2 years of high school. At 16 years of age, 25% of students said they consumed alcohol in the past month and 16% said they had had five or more drinks at a single sitting during the previous 2 weeks; by 18 years of age, 60% were current drinkers (in the past month) and 32% had at least one occasion of five or more drinks (Kandel & Logan, 1984; Oetting & Beauvais, 1990). The reasons usually given for heavy drinking are to have fun at a party and to experience the new and exciting sensations that come from alcohol (Binion, Miller, Beauvais, & Oetting, 1988).

Many people worry that these adolescent abusers will become alcoholics in the dependent sense, but most do not. Fillmore et al. (1991) found and analyzed a number of longitudinal studies in which the same adolescents were questioned over a period of time. Both frequency and quantity declined after 20 years of age, and one third of the sample had considerably reduced their intake. Adolescent drinking in these countries therefore is a form of experimentation and intended nonconformity rather than the beginning of a lifelong pattern of alcoholism. Once adult roles and responsibilities are adopted, such as having children and taking a job, young adults generally drink more moderate quantities and drink less frequently. If young adults do not restrict their drinking, then not only they, but also their families and communities, suffer (e.g., Brady, 1990; Brunswick, Messeri, & Aidala, 1990).

Even if drinking declines with age, the damage may have been done during adolescence, for example, if the adolescent sustains a motor vehicle injury, acquires a police record for assault, or fails high school. One out of every four current drinkers aged 15-24 experience an alcohol-related problem with their physical health, their friends and families, or their studies, and 26% of adolescent males said they combined drinking and driving (Eliany, 1992). Adolescent binge drinking can become a future liability.

In many developing countries, young people cross the threshold into adulthood at 15 years of age. They are considered ready to take on adult roles such as marriage and employment at this time. Furthermore, many traditional cultures limit drinking in young people. A number of modern, urban activities delay or alter these roles and responsibilities, creating more available money, alcohol, peers, and leisure time. Also, in certain countries, group intoxication seems to lead to more serious and destructive problems, such as violence, rape, and car accidents. So although the magnitude of the problem, relatively, is not large, the consequences for that context may be. In Nairobi, Kenya, 55% of those between 10 and 29 had tasted alcohol, yet only 11% of the males and 4% of the females were alcohol abusers or regular drinkers, drinking on 3 or more days a week (Acuda, 1985). Rates were higher in urban youth who had left school. A study in Zimbabwe found that although 43% of upper-level students abstained from drinking, 35% frequently drank to intoxication (Chambwe, Slade, & Dewey, 1983). Similarly high rates of binge drinking have been reported for Papua New Guinea (Marshall, 1988, 1991) and Lesotho (Meursing & Morojele, 1989) among youth who drink large quantities of beer at parties with friends and whose family drink. These young men stated that the fun of drinking is to get drunk. Anthropological studies in the Federated States of Micronesia show that 43% of men use alcohol regularly; drunken, violent behavior is expected between the ages of 15 and 35 years. Many boys under 15 start by sniffing gasoline and then progress to alcohol combined with other drugs. The problem, then, is not dependency on alcohol but the antisocial and destructive consequences of group intoxication that affect a whole community. Whether they lack a history of legal and moderate use of alcohol or are simply rebelling against the traditional dictates of who drinks and how much is drunk, these young men create a serious public health problem (see Box 7.1).

## PERSONAL AND SOCIAL CONSEQUENCES OF ALCOHOL ABUSE

Physical and mental health problems result from prolonged dependence on alcohol. These include cirrhosis, fatty liver, chronic obstructive lung disease, cardiomyopathy, alcohol gastritis, tuberculosis, cancers, and mental disorders (Hurley & Horowitz, 1990). Concerning admissions to mental hospitals, 8.4% of Ugandan admissions had alcohol psychosis (Acuda, 1985) and 20% to 30% of Swaziland admissions were for alcohol- or drug-related psychosis (Malepe, 1989).

Within the family, alcohol problems lead to poverty, marital discord, child and wife battering, rape, home injuries, and child neglect. Domestic problems of this sort were the ones most often mentioned by hazardous drinkers in Saunders et al.'s six-country study (1993). When cases of domestic violence lead to severe injuries, they show up on police records and emergency room statistics. In about one third of the cases, alcohol is implicated (e.g., Haworth, 1989; Medina-Mora & Gonzalez, 1989; Roizen, 1989). Officials suggest that the actual incidence is much higher because patients are unwilling to report the cause of their injuries.

## BOX 7.1.
## WHERE "GETTING SMASHED" HAS DOUBLE MEANING

Binge drinking to the point of intoxication is a common pastime among young males in a number of locations around the world. Not only do they "get smashed" in the slang sense of being drunk, but they also are likely to injure or be injured as a result of fights, property damage, and vehicle collision. Mac Marshall vividly describes the trauma and destruction left in the wake of intoxicated youth on two Pacific Islands: Papua New Guinea and Chuuk (1988, 1991). Drinking beer is viewed as a symbol of modern masculinity and drinking to intoxication is the activity of choice for many young men between 20 and 35 years. In Papua New Guinea, up to half of motor vehicle injuries and deaths are due to being "smashed"; wife battering, tribal fights, and bar brawls are also common. In some cases, people have poisoned themselves by trying to get intoxicated on methylated spirits. Often the reasons given for drinking are to be happy, to be with friends, and to get up one's courage to talk to girls and fight with boys. There appear to be similar motives behind drinking in many Latin American countries where men drink to intoxication during celebrations. The festivity itself no longer seems sufficient to raise levels of happiness and reduce inhibitions. Alcohol in low and moderate amounts is indeed stimulating and will reduce anxieties. Higher levels, however, have an opposite effect and often lead to day-after industrial accidents. Soccer rowdies in Britain get drunk on beer before and during competitive soccer matches and then smash up the stands and fans of the opposing team. A similar incident occurred in my city when the favorite hockey team lost in a close match; led by a number of drunken youth, loyal fans went on a rampage down the main street, smashing the storefronts of other loyal fans. In the United States, 42% of all vehicular deaths involving drivers, passengers, and pedestrians in 1984 were related to alcohol; 42% of dead drivers were intoxicated (Hurley & Horowitz, 1990). A successful backlash against such unnecessary death and injury has come in the form of groups who advertise against drinking and driving. MADD, or Mothers Against Drinking and Driving, and SADD, or Students Against Drinking and Driving, have sprung up around North America to change drinking practices and laws. Their motto is "Don't drink and drive," not "Don't drink."

Yet it is within the community that problems due to alcohol become most visible. These include underproductivity at work, absenteeism, work-related injuries, crime, violence, death and injury due to motor vehicle accidents, and the cost of services to treat alcoholics. For example, in the United States, blood alcohol counts revealed that 43% of dead drivers during 1984 were intoxicated at a level equal to or greater than 0.10%, and 42% of all motor vehicle deaths to drivers, passengers, and pedestrians were related to alcohol use where the BAC was greater than or equal to 0.05% (Hurley & Horowitz, 1990). Records from Papua New Guinea between 1976 and 1980 showed that 85% of dead drivers showed signs of recent alcohol consumption, and 53% were legally intoxicated (Marshall, 1988). In Botswana, Kenya, and Mexico, 10% to 20% of all motor vehicle accidents involved alcohol, and the rates are rising (Haworth, 1989; Medina-Mora & Gonzalez, 1989; Molamu, 1989). The risk of injury is usually greater for pedestrians than for drivers in developing countries. The WHO (1980) reported that problems of health and social disruption are consistently rising in many countries due to increased drinking. The cost of dealing with these disruptions is particularly high for developing countries, where personnel is scarce and resources are being diverted from other needs.

Homicides and injuries resulting from aggression are commonly associated with drinking in the United States and Latin America. In fact, of all the traumas seen in emergency rooms, injuries from assaults and fights are the ones most likely to be preceded by heavy drinking (Medina-Mora & Gonzalez, 1989; Roizen, 1989). For example, in Venezuela, 56% of homicides were associated with drinking.

Controlled studies show that the effects of alcohol on aggression depend on the dose (quantity and strength of the alcohol) and on psychological aspects of the drinker. Small doses tend to lead to less aggression than usual, whereas large doses lead to significantly more aggression (Geen, 1990). The dose-response relationship has been outlined by Davidson (1985) as follows: With a dose of 1 oz (or 30 ml) in a person weighing 150 lb, the blood alcohol count would be 0.03 or 30 mg of alcohol per 100 ml of blood. Such a level of intoxication leads to feelings of stimulation and disinhibition. With a dose of 2 oz and 0.05 BAC, the drinker would experience impaired rational thought. A dose of 4 oz with a BAC of 0.10 is the legal definition of intoxication in many countries. When intoxicated, rational thought and the ability to inhibit aggression are minimized. Intoxicated people tend to misinterpret others' facial cues, perceiving them as angry and threatening when in fact they are not; they also respond more aggressively to these misinterpreted cues. Peer pressure can easily encourage aggression in an intoxicated person but cannot easily restrain it. This is illustrated by the violent weekend behavior of gangs of young intoxicated men in Papua New Guinea (Marshall, 1991) and the barroom brawls common in other places. Strong social norms against aggression, however, are effective in inhibiting aggression, even in drinking situations.

Characteristics of the drinker also contribute to aggression. Regular heavy drinkers are not more aggressive after having a strong drink, but moderate drinkers are. So moderate drinkers and binge drinkers are more prone to violence when intoxicated. The drinker's expectancy that alcohol and aggression go together is also pertinent. If the culture does not promote this expectancy, then alcohol and aggression will not occur together. Neither the pharmacological aspects of alcohol nor the psychological aspects of the drinker by themselves can explain why drinking and violence co-occur; both must be present (Bushman & Cooper, 1990; Murdoch, Pihl, & Ross, 1990).

A study on the effects of rational thought was carried out by Peterson, Rothfleisch, Zelazo, and Pihl (1990) to determine which aspects of thought are impaired at different levels of intoxication. The researchers were able to rule out the effects of expectancies about intoxication by misleading people about the amounts of alcohol they had consumed. Some were given a high dose of 1.32 ml of 95% alcohol per kg of body weight; 15 minutes after drinking, these people had a BAC of 0.093, close to the 0.10 legal threshold. Others were given a moderate dose of .66 ml; their BAC was 0.044. Others were given a low dose of .132 ml, and their BAC was 0.003. Tests of cognitive functioning were administered at this time, and the scores indicated that those with the high dose performed significantly worse than the others on measures of planning, perceptual organization, verbal and visual memory, and word fluency. However, the dose had no effect on measures of general IQ. These results point out that although general knowledge and thought were not impaired, rational thought, which requires planning, organization, and memory, was affected.

## RISK FACTORS FOR ALCOHOL ABUSE

Research comparing drinkers with nondrinkers aims to discover why the former are more vulnerable to alcohol abuse. Prospective designs compare people at risk for alcohol abuse (e.g., sons of alcoholics) with people at low risk. Identifying the characteristics of those with drinking problems helps to tailor prevention programs for those who are likely to develop problems and focuses attention on possible causes of alcoholism. Characteristics that increase the likelihood of alcohol abuse fit into two groups: exposure and vulnerability. *Exposure* refers to variables such as the availability of alcohol, an individual's intake, its use by friends and family, and attitudes toward drinking. *Vulnerability* refers to characteristics of the person that make them at greater risk for problems, such as age, gender, antisocial personality, and family history.

Research has shown that exposure is an important risk factor for developing alcohol problems. To a certain extent, the number of drinking outlets, the price of alcohol, and the drinking pattern of friends and family affect the likelihood that a person will drink (Kortteinen, 1989; Meursing & Morojele, 1989; Moser, 1980). Consequently, prevention programs are sometimes directed at reducing the number of outlets and the times at which people can buy alcohol, and increasing the price of alcohol and the age at which it can legally be bought. When alcohol becomes less available, everyone drinks less.

The two most common risk factors that make a person more vulnerable to drinking problems are gender and age. Universally, men drink more than women and have more problems with drinking (WHO, 1980). In general, men are five times more likely to be alcoholic than women (Pihl & Peterson, 1992), although in some countries, such as the United States, Scotland, and Australia, the ratio is 2:1, and in developing countries, the ratio is likely to be 10:1 or higher (Helzer et al., 1990; Moser, 1980).

Age is another risk factor in that alcohol problems are most likely to surface in the 25 to 45 age group. Because alcohol dependence requires prolonged use, most institutionalized alcoholics are in their forties (Davidson, 1985). However, there is growing concern about the high rates of drinking in young males in their late teens and twenties, for whom alcohol abuse and binge drinking is becoming more common. Because many people move in and out of problem drinking and because dependence and abuse commonly occur in different age groups, prevention programs must be directed at young people to encourage abstinence or sensible drinking.

Family variables are consistently found to be risk factors for alcohol problems. Heavy drinkers, for example, are more likely to have a family history of alcoholism and marital discord (Davidson, 1985). The family connection may operate through several mechanisms. Children may learn by watching parents that drinking is a way of solving problems; children may inherit a predisposition for uncontrolled alcohol abuse from parents; or family problems may create anxiety, depression, and hostility that are relieved with alcohol (Walker, Lambert, Walker, & Kivlahan, 1993). More precisely, there appear to be two types of alcoholics (see reviews by Pihl & Peterson, 1992; Wallace, 1989). Type I alcoholics are either male or female. They are able to abstain from alcohol on a day-to-day basis, but they lose control over their drinking and their actions when they do drink. Type II alcoholics are exclusively male, their alcohol problems begin in the early teens, they are involved in violence and criminality, and they are very likely to have a father and grandfather with Type II alcoholism. This constellation of characteristics along with the results of adoption studies has led many researchers to conclude that Type I alcoholism is caused by a combination of genetic and family environment factors, while Type II alcoholism or its personality predisposition is almost entirely genetic.

Behavioral models of alcoholism have stressed the reinforcing properties of alcohol, which may affect Type I and II alcoholics differently (Pihl & Peterson, 1992). Type I alcoholics may be motivated by the stimulating properties of alcohol, in that it arouses the pleasurable activity systems of the brain, leaving the person with subjective feelings of euphoria, energy, and power. This was supported by a study of risk factors for drinking in Californian adolescents, in which those who were unhappy and blamed themselves for failures were likely to drink more (Scheier & Newcomb, 1991). Alcohol may reduce their anxiety and depression.

Type II alcoholics appear to be motivated to consume alcohol because it reduces their overreaction to stress and allows them to feel less inhibited about expressing their aggression. As children, they have personality and social problems such as conflicts with parents and peers, aggression, impulsiveness, and hyperactivity (Pihl & Peterson, 1992; Pihl, Peterson, & Finn, 1990). These children are unable to control or regulate their heightened reaction to stressful situations; they become anxious and respond with impulsive actions. In a series of studies with sons of male alcoholics, who at the time of study were not themselves alcoholic, Pihl et al. (1990) consistently show that these sons are overly reactive, physiologically and motorically, to novel and threatening situations, and that alcohol reduces their hyperreactivity and anxiety. Thus, for the nonalcoholic sons, as for alcoholics themselves, alcohol consumption was a way of reducing the unpleasant hyperreactivity and anxiety. This research confirms beliefs that people who abuse alcohol also have other emotional and social problems, such as depression, anxiety, conduct disorders, failure at school, and conflict with parents and other authority figures (Donovan & Jessor, 1985). They seek friends with similar problems, and thereby set the stage for their introduction to alcohol and other antisocial means of resolving their problems.

## ALCOHOL PREVENTION PROGRAMS

Long-term treatment of alcoholics takes place in addiction or psychiatric centers as well as in self-help groups such as Alcoholics Anonymous (e.g., Guatemala; see Coombs & Lowe, 1987). The treatment programs are considered somewhat costly relative to their effectiveness. They are often successful in reducing alcohol intake and alcohol-related problems (e.g., with family and job) but less successful in promoting abstinence. In fact, brief interventions in primary health care settings are often just as effective. Giving a self-help manual to hazardous drinkers along with a mere 15 minutes of counseling can reduce alcohol consumption by one third (Bien, Miller, & Tonigan, 1993). Alcoholics Anonymous (AA) is a self-help group that provides social support for alcoholics who want to stop drinking; membership is often required as part of treatment at a health service. The group is run entirely by former and current alcoholics who want to stop drinking. The two preconditions for joining are that the alcoholic admit to his or her problem and promise to abstain from drinking as the only way to break the addiction. At local meetings, members publicly admit to their problem and describe how it has affected their lives. Each member pledges to go at any time of the day to the aid of any other member who is tempted to drink. Studies of alcoholics who have not attended any treatment program show that over time 43% reduce their drinking and 13% become abstinent (Davidson, 1985). To be considered effective, a treatment program must exceed these figures.

The preferred approach, however, is prevention. This typically takes one of two forms: either control or education. *Control* refers to limiting the availability of alcohol through government controls. *Education* refers to reducing the demand for alcohol through education. Control manipulates the interaction between agent and environment; education attempts to influence the host. Few countries have taken the path of India, where a clear policy of control is or was part of the constitution.

Controlling the Availability of Alcohol

Control over the availability of alcohol has been tried with success in many developed countries. Because the state is the only authority able to enact and enforce laws restricting the sale and distribution of alcohol, partial or full state monopolies are common. Government controls sometimes take the form of controlling production, but more often only the distribution. Alcohol pricing and advertising can thereby be tailored for public heath benefits rather than for profit. Distribution outlets may be located so that no neighborhood has an excess of outlets and so that schools and hospitals are not adjacent to outlets. Times of purchase may be restricted so that alcohol cannot be bought late at night or on certain holidays. The size of bottles may be controlled because people tend to finish the bottle, whatever its quantity. Increasing the price of alcohol is a very effective means of controlling its use, in that consumption even among heavy drinkers will decline with increases in the cost. This extra revenue can be put back into the health care system. Another common restriction is the age at which one can legally buy alcohol. These controls are reasonable ways of reducing consumption. At the same time, control bodies must take into account the demands of moderate drinkers as well as the need to increase state revenues and provide employment through the sale of alcohol (Bucholz & Robins, 1989; Moser, 1980).

In developed countries such as Canada, Finland, Germany, Norway, Poland, Sweden, and the United States, state control over some aspect of the availability of alcohol has been an effective way of reducing consumption and alcohol abuse. The major problem in developing countries is the control over traditional, noncommercial production and consumption of alcohol. First, governments do not always have the economic or political will to control this aspect of the economy because of the employment it provides. Second, controls may not be feasible given the widespread production of alcohol in rural areas; imposing unenforceable state control simply invites illegal distribution. Third, it is highly popular among the local population who use it for social functions and do not therefore view it as an intoxicant. Each country must therefore determine how controls will be accepted by the population before implementing government controls. A more favorable climate for both popular support and for state controls can be created by a government if it first gets involved in the production of traditional brews. This increases the demand for locally produced grains and leads to other economic spinoffs such as secure employment, exports, and state revenues (Kortteinen, 1989). State control over advertising may be the only acceptable avenue in Latin America (Negrette, 1985); in some countries, it has been entirely banned. Advertising alcohol on billboards and magazines repeatedly exposes children and adolescents to the products. The use of image-oriented advertising, in particular, appeals to adolescents and young adults who identify themselves in terms of the fun-loving, good-looking young people portrayed in the ads (Covell, Dion, & Dion, 1994). But attempts to impose too much control over production, distribution, and advertising can be undercut by domestic networks, as they have in Costa Rica (Negrette, 1985).

Work- and Family-Based
Education Programs

The second thrust of prevention programs is aimed at educating people in the responsible use of alcohol. Mass media campaigns are regarded as ineffective if they emphasize the negative consequences and affect only one's knowledge of alcohol use rather than personal attitudes (Moser, 1980). Campaigns directed toward specific targets such as drivers, youth, abusers, and employees have been more effective. For these programs, specific personnel need to be trained. For example, an employee assistance pilot project was begun with nine Guatemalan companies (Coombs & Lowe, 1987) and gave intensive training to managers and health personnel who assessed and discussed drinking practices with workers. The result was a reduction in on-the-job drinking and absenteeism as well as improved treatment of abusers.

Another strategy has been to work with families of problem drinkers. Al-Anon and Alateen are two community groups in which spouses and children of alcoholics meet to discuss their problems and learn new ways of coping with the economic and social disruptions. Because alcoholism often runs in families, these groups may also help prevent children from turning to alcohol to solve their problems, only one of which is an alcoholic parent. Also, because alcoholism presents a severe burden that most families cannot cope with on their own, the responsibility of the whole community should be addressed and strengthened to deal with these cases.

Finally, youth education programs have been tried with some success in schools in four countries: Swaziland, Chile, Australia, and Norway (Perry & Grant, 1988). The five 1-hour education sessions dealt with the social and physical consequences of alcohol use, positive attitudes toward abstaining, and practice in refusing alcohol under peer pressure. In comparison with the pretest, those who took part in the sessions subsequently showed less use of alcohol, better knowledge of its consequences, and more positive attitudes toward abstention. The most successful groups were those led by peers who had been previously trained rather than those led by teachers. They showed significantly more change than control groups who had no education program, and in many cases showed more change than groups led by teachers. Because drinking is a peer-oriented behavior, peers may have more influence than adults in reinforcing and modeling the behaviors associated with responsible drinking. In the United States, Girl Clubs have been training young adolescent girls to be more assertive with their persuasive boyfriends. The girls are trained to be trainers of other girls, thereby giving them status as responsible "teachers" of younger girls. Through discussion and practice, they role-play situations where boys try to persuade them to drink—and their replies are not always a polite "no, thank you" (Chaiken, 1990). This is an example of the Life Skills Training program that teaches behavioral skills to increase personal control over one's life. Other successful school programs try to improve self-discipline and school performance, thus minimizing the chances a student will become alienated from school values, school authority, and achievement-oriented peers. When parents were involved in the school programs, their effectiveness improved further (Bry & Greene, 1990).

Sensible and responsible drinking is the goal of most prevention programs. Although many risk factors, such as being male, rapid urbanization and other life stresses, family predispositions, and cheap alcohol set the stage for heavy drinking, they do not constrain one to drink. Even the so-called gene for alcoholism does not force one to drink any more than hanging out with a drinking crowd forces one to conform. Families, communities, and health services have a role to play in providing constructive means for solving personal and social frustrations as an alternative to drinking.

## STUDENT ACTIVITY

Collect evidence on prevention programs from a specific region of the world or country. Using this evidence, have a debate with three students on each team: Resolve that government control is more effective than education programs in reducing the negative problems associated with alcohol abuse.

# 8

# HEALTH EDUCATION AND PROMOTION

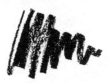

The attempt to introduce new ideas and health behaviors to a community is a difficult process, now recognized by most as the key to sustained improvements in health. Without intending to lay blame, it is fair to say that everyone has room for improvement in their health behaviors. Thinking of a few that we should have adopted, but did not, is a humbling experience. Our only satisfaction is that we are in the company of multitudes. We still have no simple recipe for changing health behaviors, even when we know the benefits. Health professionals have attempted to change behaviors; in developing countries, we try to encourage adults to immunize children, use family planning, drink clean water, use latrines, start infants on weaning foods at 6 months, and avoid risky sex. In industrialized countries, concerted efforts abound to change eating, drinking, smoking, and exercise behaviors (e.g., Young, Haskell, Taylor, & Fortmann, 1996). Our strategy will be to analyze some of these interventions to find out which procedures work and which do not.

Many different routes are available to promote health and prevent illness in a community, and the terms used by professionals reflect these different routes: *education, information, communication, promotion,* and *empowerment.* The popular phrase today is **health promotion,** which refers to political, social, and educational action that enhances public awareness of health, fosters healthy lifestyles and community action in support of health, and empowers people to exercise their rights and responsibilities in shaping environments, systems, and policies that are conducive to health and well-being (Dhillon & Philip, 1994). Thus health promotion experts recognize the need for strategies on three fronts:

political, which means advocating resources and accessibility;
social, which means developing community systems that support health behaviors as a norm and mobilize for action; and
educational, which means equipping people with knowledge, attitudes, and skills to make decisions and act.

Of the three strategies, this chapter will focus on the educational strategy. It generally entails activities aimed at building people's capacities to improve their own and others' health within a social framework such as the family or community. Because of the nature of health problems and social life in developing countries, most education interventions are family- or communitywide attempts to prevent health problems in areas where they are endemic (Winett, 1995).

## CONCEPTS AND COMPONENTS OF HEALTH EDUCATION

Hubley (1993) defines **health education** as

a process with intellectual, psychological and social dimensions relating to activities that increase the abilities of people to make informed decisions affecting their personal, family and community well-being. This process, based on scientific principles, facilitates learning and behavioral change in both health personnel and consumers, including children and youth. (p. 17)

Regardless of whether we take Hubley's definition or someone else's, three ideas capture the essence:

- People perform activities that are intellectually, psychologically, and socially engaging.
- People acquire abilities to make informed, healthful decisions.
- People work toward the goal of acting on their decisions.

The objective of this chapter is to learn how to analyze specific projects that were designed to change people's abilities to make informed decisions and act on them. We will take an inductive approach—analyzing specific cases of health education and extracting the elements of a successful project—before looking at the theories. The case studies will first be described with information about the health problem in its context, the intervention, and an evaluation of how much actually changed. Our analysis of each case will then focus on four key questions that highlight criteria relevant to the success of an intervention. Through this analysis, we can perhaps identify strong and weak points that contributed to successes and failures. The four key questions are as follows:

*(1) Who, what,* and *how much change* is targeted? People whose decisions and actions make a difference to a family's and community's health are usually the targets of the intervention. Perhaps other participants will be included if they provide social support. The abilities to make and act on informed, healthful decisions involve a range of personal and social resources. Educators will identify one lacking resource that is the major block for that target group in their ability to make healthful decisions. If people are well informed, then the block may be lack of skill, lack of confidence, lack of interest, fear of being different, and social isolation. Theories provide some other suggestions. These are usually found in the boxes that are connected with arrows in various models. They include the perceptions of personal risk, expectations about the consequences of the action, knowledge about causes and prevention, attitudes toward the action, economic and social barriers to performing the action, and social norms (e.g., Ajzen, 1988; L. Green, Kreuter, Deeds, & Partridge, 1980; Janz & Becker, 1984; Rosenstock, 1990). Barriers, or problems that

arise and prevent people from making and acting on decisions, are the most important among these factors. Consequently, an important ability to develop is problem solving at the family and community levels. Some health educators emphasize two areas: the skill to perform the action and the willingness to perform the action (Graeff et al., 1993). We must remember that before the intervention, people have made sense of their world; they have a full day of activities and a coherent lifestyle. Change means adding new actions and investing extra mental energy, and perhaps modifying or eliminating old ones. Change is stressful.

*(2) What activity* is carried out as part of the intervention? Not everyone agrees that the health promotion activity must engage people intellectually, psychologically, and socially. There is mounting evidence that an intervention addressed to one's intellect alone will fail. The cases will be examined to see if and how the activity accomplishes three key objectives: fostering ability, motivating willingness, and tackling barriers. Communication is one common activity (Hubley, 1993; WHO, 1988).

*(3)* What procedure is used to help *translate abilities into action?* This component concerns motivation and willingness. People may have the capabilities to act differently but an explicit mechanism is often necessary to move them from ideas to action (Graeff et al., 1993).

*(4)* What procedure is used to help *sustain* these changes? One possibility is to involve the beneficiaries in the project design, implementation, and evaluation. Another is to transfer leadership skills to a local institution and to change government policy.

It will be important to link these procedures to the outcome of the intervention. We want to know if the procedure worked—if it led to improvements in ability and behavior. If at least some people changed, then there is reason to believe it might effect change in other people. There are no guarantees, though, that a program successful in one place will be successful everywhere because people's capabilities, willingness, and life contexts vary considerably. If a program works in several places, however, it is worth extracting its general principle and applying it flexibly in other contexts. Eventually, we may be able to integrate the best strategies of different programs.

## CASE 1: FAMILY PLANNING IN ETHIOPIA

Almaz Terefe and Charles Larson (1993) tried to increase the use of modern contraceptives through home visits that included the husband. At the time, only 2% of childbearing women in Ethiopia used modern contraceptives, and no family planning outreach program was operating in the targeted district. A trained traditional birth attendant made initial visits to every second house and enrolled married women between 15 and 49 years who were not currently using contraceptives. Then a health assistant known to the community made the educational visit, accompanied by the birth attendant. In half the cases, both the husband and the wife were requested to be present; in the other half, only the wife's presence was requested. The purpose was to see if the husband's presence facilitated the decision to use modern contraception.

The session started with a discussion of the family's health and the wife's reproductive history. The health attendant used this as an entry point to present the advantages of family planning as a means of preventing unwanted pregnancy and birth, of spacing births, and of controlling family size. This was followed by an explanation of alternative contraceptive methods and a discussion of the relative efficacy of modern contraception versus traditional methods. The health assistant made a second visit if requested. Couples intending to start contraception were given their choice of methods at the end of the session along with information about follow-up. Two months and twelve months later, the assistant returned to determine if the couple was using contraception.

The education was quite successful, given that it included only one or two sessions and one type of communication. Of those women who received the education by themselves, 33% expressed an interest in starting contraception: At 2 months, 16.8% had started; and at 12 months, 17.2% were using one of the recommended methods (two thirds of these began after the 2-month check). This represents an improvement over the 0% using contraception the year before. Of those women who received the education with their husbands, 47% expressed an interest in starting: At 2 months, 25.8% had started; and at 12 months, 32.8% were using contraception (half of these began after the 2-month check). Thus when husband and wife heard the message together, they were more likely to start contraception.

*Who, what, and how much change was required?* Married couples were targeted, and the area addressed was knowledge about modern contraception. A baseline survey indicated that women knew about some forms of contraception but more about the barriers than the benefits; none actually used modern contraception. The knowledge change would not be stressful, but the behavior change would be. Adopting contraception would require visits to the clinic, taking a pill daily, and substantially altering the expected size of their family. All of these were personal changes, but as well it meant breaking with the family and community tradition to have as many children as one was fortunate to have.

*What was the educational activity?* The intervention consisted of a single face-to-face communication with a couple or the wife alone at home. Because it was a private session, the health workers could address not only intellectual questions but also psychological fears about side effects and sterility. In addition to overcoming psychological barriers, the intervention overcame an accessibility problem by making contraceptives available on the spot through two familiar health workers. The communication was intended to be "soft sell" persuasion; incentives such as the No-Birth Bonuses used in India (see Elder & Estey, 1992) were not offered. The strongest point of the intervention was its inclusion of both husband and wife, thus engaging the decision makers in a dialogue that could be continued after the session. Many couples probably had never actually made a joint decision to avoid contraception, so the session provided them with an opportunity to arrive at an informed decision together and act on it. The presence of two partners makes it more likely that they will recall the information, that they will address the uncertainties, and that they will overcome any reluctance to make a decision and act. In cases where the husband was not present, the wife must decide on her own whether to present the issue to her husband and must give him the information. Clearly some did, but they were at a disadvantage compared with wives whose husbands attended the session.

*How did education prepare the couple to make a decision and act on it?* Given that people in this district had little information about contraception and less access, the session appears to have provided favorable conditions for opening a couple's dialogue about benefits, barriers, and options within a private and supportive context. In addition, the intervention made contraceptives available through the birth attendant as soon as couples made a decision. Most of those who expressed an interest in starting contraception did begin in the year following the session. So these couples appeared not to have a problem translating intentions into action. Without an explicit mechanism to sustain contraceptive use, the change was maintained and even increased as more couples adopted contraception. The problem, if any, was in the motivational component—the willingness of couples to space and/or limit births. In countries such as India, Taiwan, and Thailand, incentives such as livestock, loans, and education have been successful in increasing the number of family planning acceptors (Elder & Estey, 1992).

## CASE 2: COMMUNITY NORMS FOR FACE WASHING IN TANZANIA

Trachoma is an eye infection spread by flies and by hand contact. It is common in children and over time can lead to blindness. Trachoma can be treated with an antibiotic ointment applied to the eye, but this is expensive and requires daily visits to the clinic. Moreover, the child is likely to get reinfected after treatment. The best solution is a regular face wash; the water does not even have to be clean because it will not be ingested. The organizers of this intervention gave an antibiotic treatment for trachoma to all the citizens of six rural villages in Tanzania; in addition, to three of the villages they gave community- and family-

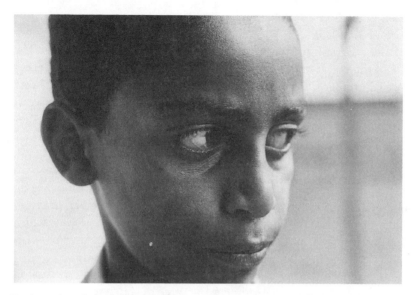

*Trachoma is a chronic disease of the eye, which may lead to blindness if not treated.*

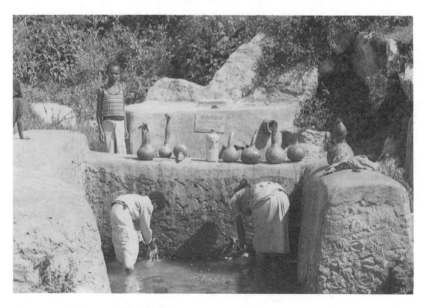

*Women and children often travel long distances to fetch uncontaminated water in containers of any shape and size.*

based education on preventing trachoma by washing children's faces (West et al., 1995).

Extensive preliminary research in this Tanzanian district showed that 60% of the children from 1 to 7 years of age had trachoma (McCauley, Lynch, Pounds, & West, 1990). Mothers said it took them at least 2 hours each day to fetch water, and they had higher priority uses for the scarce water, such as drinking, food preparation, washing dishes and clothes, and washing hands before meals. The social norm implicitly understood by everyone was that precious water and time would be wasted on a child's face. No woman wanted to be criticized for being wasteful. Furthermore, her action might be interpreted as vanity, provoking the "evil eye" from an envious neighbor. The decision was taken to implement education at the community level, where norms for face washing could be changed, and at the family level, where the problem of scarce water and time for chores could be addressed.

For 1 month during and after the antibiotic treatment, facilitators convened neighborhood groups in the three designated villages. Men and women discussed eye infection and made plans to implement face washing on a regular basis. To tackle the problem of scarce water, the organizers demonstrated how 30 people could wash their faces with the water from a small gourd. At a subsequent meeting, mothers helped each other solve problems that had arisen in their own attempts to wash their children's faces in the morning. The organizers tried to sustain the community organization by helping the village work on other needs, for example, stocking a drug store. Field-workers visited individual families to help identify reusable water and time for face washing and to reward improvements (Lynch et al., 1994).

The intervention succeeded in two of the three villages. One, five, and eleven months after the intervention, children from 1 to 7 years were examined for trachoma and clean faces. In the treatment-only villages, trachoma dropped by 20%—from 64% to 44%—1 month after treatment, but by the end of the year was up again close to 60%. Only 26% of the children had clean faces, compared with 19% before treatment. Thus treatment alone did not eliminate the problem for long. In two of the consensus-building villages, trachoma dropped by 30%—from 60% to 30%—1 month later, and rose to 48% by the end of the year. Children were also more likely to have clean faces (up from 20% to 40%), and those with clean faces had uninfected eyes. One education village looked exactly like a treatment-only village in that trachoma rose after treatment and at no time was there improvement in face washing. This village had a very strong norm against trying to be better than others or different. The intervention did not succeed in creating a norm in favor of face washing.

*Who, what, and how much change was targeted?* Even though the major beneficiaries were young children, the whole community was the focus of this intervention. Three areas were identified: knowledge about the benefits of face washing in preventing trachoma, a norm (social consensus) in favor of washing children's faces regularly, and solving the family's problem of how to allocate scarce water for washing faces. The intervention called for a number of changes in the mother's daily routine and the value she placed on water, eyes, and child hygiene. Imagine being asked to do something foolish and wasteful with your money on a daily basis, like throwing it into the river, and you might come close to the feelings experienced by these mothers. Perhaps finding water was not as big a problem as the mothers initially thought, because they could use recycled water. The major change was therefore to reverse the social norm concerning washing a child's face. Norms are powerful determinants of behavior whenever the behavior is performed in public view and people are dependent on the approval and goodwill of their neighbors. How many people must change to reverse a norm?

The education activities engaged people at intellectual, psychological, and social levels. At the intellectual level, mothers learned about the relation between eye infection, blindness, and an unclean face; they also applied their problem-solving skills to solve their own and their neighbors' difficulties in allocating water and time for household chores. They were engaged emotionally through discussions of eye and other problems they felt strongly about. They were engaged at the social level by interacting with neighbors and family to discuss the new behavior, eliminate criticism from neighbors and husbands for face washing, and build a new norm. This was seen as necessary to overcome the major social barrier to face washing; it was essential to motivating a mother to be willing to regularly wash her child's face.

*How were the knowledge and the norm translated into regular face washing?* Field-workers visited mothers at home to praise them for improved face washing. To work, washing a child's face had to become a habit that the mother would perform as part of another daily chore, such as washing her hands before a meal. That would minimize the mother's use of precious resources, including mental energy and water. Even in the two amenable towns, at most 52% of the families translated talk into action, as evidenced by clean faces 1 month later. Maintenance was less of a problem; those who had the habit at 6 months seem to have kept it for the year.

Thus, using community- and family-based education to build a social norm and to solve water allocation problems, Sheila West and her colleagues in Tanzania increased face washing and reduced trachoma in children. The problem lay less with acquiring a new skill and more with willingness. Initially it seemed to mothers and observers that water scarcity was the major barrier, but this was solved with new knowledge and family problem solving. The major gap was in translating knowledge and norms into action, and sustaining the action.

## CASE 3: INTERACTIVE RADIO FOR CHILDREN IN BOLIVIA

Diarrhea and other child illnesses are common in Bolivia and other developing countries. Children living in urban, suburban, and rural areas of Bolivia were the target of a school radio program to promote good hygiene, sanitation, and water practices (Fryer, 1991). As part of the international Child-to-Child program, its focus was on primary school children (Bonati & Hawes, 1992; Patil et al., 1996) because children are often caretakers of younger siblings; they are involved in household management and so can pass on relevant health messages to other family members; they influence their peers; and they are the parents of the future. A book titled *Children for Health* (Hawes & Scotchmer, 1993) provides health facts and activities for children that encourage learning through action. For example, children treat cuts and burns, make simple picture-word books and puzzles for younger children, and measure the arm circumference of their younger siblings.

Radio instruction followed by small group discussion has been used for a long time in India to bring about changes in agricultural and other practices. Michelle Fryer's school radio programs add a new feature—they are interactive and participatory, requiring children constantly to respond to questions, write concepts in their notebooks, sing songs, and role-play while the program is on the air. The radio teacher communicates information via stories and by giving the correct response to questions after children have had the opportunity to answer. Children take some action (verbal or written) on average every 25 seconds. For example, the radio teacher asks, "Children, how much liquid should you give a young child with diarrhea?" There is a 4-second pause for students response. Then the radio teacher says, "One liter each day." Then, "If you believe that you should continue feeding a child with diarrhea, raise your hand." Children should raise their hands. Then, "Lower your hands, and let us ask grandmother how she cares for young children with diarrhea," followed by an interview with grandma.

The Bolivian Child-to-Child project developed audiocassettes on good sanitation and water practices that combined a 25-minute interactive radio program with a 20-minute teacher-led discussion. The project prepared cassettes and teacher material for 10 sessions offered once a week to fourth- and fifth-grade students. Preliminary research identified common health beliefs and practices of children and adults in the communities. The content of the radio instruction therefore included concepts and actions that addressed local problems, although they appear to be the ones commonly experienced in most developing countries (see *Children for Health*, Hawes & Scotchmer, 1993; and *Facts for Life*, Adamson, 1993). For example, one learning objective was that children be able to know, explain, and demonstrate ORS preparation. Teachers were given a 1-day orientation along with materials for hands-on activities and homework exercises to be carried out with one's family. In 1990, approximately 10,000 fourth- and fifth-grade students in 250 schools participated in the radio lessons.

The program was evaluated with a 47-question test of students' knowledge given before and after the program. Posttest scores on a sample of 913 students showed a definite improvement, particularly in home management of diarrhea, where often 80% of the children gave correct answers. Parents and teachers commented on the improved attitudes and health behaviors of the children, but these were not assessed in any formal way.

*Who, what, and how much change was targeted by the radio program?* Children from 8 to 13 years of age in grades 4 and 5 were targeted because of their value as sibling caretakers, communicators, and future parents. The abilities included 10 or so health behaviors, along with related knowledge and attitudes. These behaviors were chosen because they commonly were not performed. Consequently, new behaviors had to be adopted and sometimes old habits had to be broken. Children who squatted anywhere would have to remind themselves to go the extra distance to a latrine or bury their waste. However, program planners followed HealthCom's criteria for behavior change by choosing ones that minimized negative readjustment, namely, that were compatible with existing practices, easy to do, and had observable and immediate benefits (Graeff et al., 1993).

*What activities were performed to foster these abilities?* The main activity was mass media communication geared to children's capacities with the high level of interaction usually found in face-to-face communication. For example, children were asked questions; they gave their answer as a group and then heard the correct answer from the broadcaster. The activity primarily engaged their intellectual and psychological processes, including thinking, problem solving, sensory stimulation, memory recall, motor activity, and emotions. The social dimension was confined to interactions with the radio teacher and peers in the classroom. There was a mechanism to translate knowledge and attitudes into action, but this did not often occur. Homeroom teachers were given instructions and materials for student activities after the broadcast, such as cleaning up the school grounds and measuring salt-sugar teas. But teachers, we are told, did not use the guide or understand how to reinforce the message after the broadcast. They were not used to the learner-centered style of teaching, and the material was new to the curriculum. Some teachers were more active, helping children construct a water purification system for their school as described in the lessons. Maintenance of the new knowledge and practices would depend on whether children continued to hear the radio programs. Ten sessions by themselves are not likely to result in sustained change.

The interactive radio program developed and tried in Bolivia seems to have produced changes in children's knowledge and perhaps attitudes. The weak point was in translating this into action within the family context. Teachers in developing countries often have low confidence in their ability to teach a new subject, particularly when it requires a new learner-centered style. How could they organize a class of 60 children to practice making salt-sugar teas? Homework exercises were developed, but teachers did not follow through on these either. These problems are not unsurmountable, but they were not sufficiently addressed in this project. Children are generally willing and able to change quickly, and if they attend school, they are a captive audience for such programs.

## CASE 4: DYADIC PROBLEM SOLVING ON CHILD FEEDING IN THE PHILIPPINES

Cynthia Ticao (Ticao & Aboud, in press) developed and evaluated a nutrition education program that focused on problem-solving skills. Pairs of mothers living in the Philippines were given a trial session in which they discussed solutions to child feeding problems with a friend, after which they met their partner for four more weekly sessions. The mothers had a fairly high literacy level (grade 9 average) and lived in a rural coastal village, but more than two thirds of their children were underweight. Focus group discussions with mothers in an adjacent village indicated that they often knew how and what to feed their children but did not feed them properly because problems stood in their way. They identified 10 common problems; for example, the child does not like vegetables, the child cries or fusses at mealtime, the child asks for seconds but no more food is available, and the child wants to buy junk food that is not nutritious. Feeding an underweight child is not always as straightforward as it may seem; they are not necessarily compliant eaters with good appetites. The intervention therefore focused on problem-solving skills within a supportive social relationship to deal with family and environmental barriers.

Mothers of children under 6 years were individually interviewed about their solutions to the 10 problems. During the trial session, mothers worked in pairs with another mother friend from the community, discussing their solutions to two problems. When the discussions were over, each mother privately gave what she thought were the best solutions. The discussions were tape-recorded to find out how the problem-solving process unfolded and whether the mother's final best solutions came from her own ideas or were borrowed from her friend. Because mothers solved these problems with a friend rather than a health professional, it was important to find out if they were working out solutions that were feasible and effective.

Ticao evaluated the trial session by examining the quantity and quality of solutions mothers proposed during the discussion and judged to be best afterward. The mothers came up with more solutions after the discussion than they had before, and the solutions were of better quality using the criteria of efficacy and feasibility. Furthermore, the source of a mother's final best solutions came from her own problem-solving efforts during the discussion and not from her friend. Mothers whose friends had similar initial solutions produced more and better solutions after the discussion than mothers whose partners had different initial solutions. When the trial session was over, mothers met their friends at a convenient time and location to discuss problems related to meals and snacks, self-feeding, and fussy eaters. The mothers showed improvements in their problem-solving skills and knowledge, and their children improved in nutritional status; but so did a group of mothers who did the problem-solving exercises alone. That is, the problem solving was beneficial whether it was done alone or in a dyad. The mothers kept records of their own behavior by tallying the frequency with which they gave a nutritious snack or asked about the child's hunger. Dyadic and solitary mothers showed similar levels of good child feeding practices.

*Who, what, and how much change was targeted?* Mothers of underweight preschool children were the focus of the intervention. Improving on the number and quality of mothers' child feeding solutions was the objective. The women voiced common problems, but children and families are different, so the solutions might be expected to take different forms. The change required was not great, as mothers created solutions at their own pace. Generally, the mothers had all the required problem-solving skills, although they had not been using them explicitly to solve feeding problems.

*What activities were conducted to foster this ability and to motivate willingness?* The only activity was to delineate problems and discuss solutions with a friend. The final step was to reconsider these solutions and identify one or more of the best. The social benefits of talking with a friend were counted on to motivate willingness. However, by the third or fourth session, not all were so willing to meet. Perhaps that is why their final knowledge and solutions were no different from the solitary mothers', which were fairly good. The activities engaged mothers psychologically and socially.

To translate the solutions into action, mothers kept daily records of their feeding practices relevant to the topic of the week (e.g., snacks). They could see how well they were using their own solutions. There was no explicit attempt to maintain the problem-solving strategy longer than the 6-week intervention.

Unlike other interventions, this one gave mothers the opportunity to tackle their own social and environmental barriers with a friend rather than a professional. The process of arriving at a good solution may have been more circuitous but perhaps also more effective in the long term, because people tend to prefer and recall their own solutions rather than someone else's. Better solutions were produced in the dyads, but there was no assessment of whether mothers continued to use the problem-solving process or try these solutions in their daily lives.

## CASE 5: MOBILIZING STUDENTS
## FOR SANITATION IN BANGLADESH

Although 80% of Bangladesh's population had access to safe water by 1990, only 26% had a sanitary latrine. UNICEF and government health officials initiated the promotion of two types of latrines: the cement ring-slab and the hand-dug hole with wooden foot rests. They sent field-workers to meet with groups of 20-25 families to discuss sanitation, immunization, and family planning. Several months later, workers met with leaders from the villages to discuss the benefits of sanitation, ways of promoting it in the community, and construction of the two types of latrines. This campaign, using large group instruction, led to no noticeable increase in the construction of latrines. At this point, high school students were mobilized to help the community build latrines and persuade people to use them (Bilqis, Zeitlyn, Ali, Yahya, & Shaheed, 1994).

The turning point arrived several months later, when the district commissioner announced an incentive: The school that achieved the highest sanitation coverage in its catchment area would be rewarded with a contribution toward its development fund. Teachers then organized groups of students to communicate the message to their villages, to build latrines for their families, and to help others to build latrines. The administrative head of the district issued an open letter to the people and to institutions asking them to help each other build latrines and warning that fines would be imposed if they did not. Thirteen months later, one boys' high school, one girls' high school, and one religious school won awards for the most latrines in their area. A small survey conducted at this time indicated that 73% of the households now had a sanitary latrine. When asked about the benefits of latrines, all respondents in a household survey gave appropriate responses, but the most common were that latrines prevent animals from spreading human feces around and prevent diarrhea and other diseases. Most people said they had heard the message from students, not from local leaders, and the majority said that these views were now their own.

*Who, what, and how much change was targeted in this campaign?* The objective was to reach all families in the district, with high school students as the vehicles for communication and action. The change was to build a sanitary latrine and use it. Building a homemade latrine does not require many new skills for an adult; it may take an hour of work, a shovel, and a wooden platform. To use it entails other problems, especially for children who are understandably fearful of the unstable homemade ones.

*What activities were planned to foster the ability and motivate willingness?* Students were taught how to construct latrines and why latrines were beneficial. They passed this skill and information on to the people they visited. Many people did not know how to build a latrine, so the skill was an important component. However, these two abilities had been promoted earlier in meetings with families and institution representatives, to no avail. The motivation was lacking. People generally feel secure in doing what is familiar and doing what everyone else is doing.

The real impetus came in the form of the district commissioner's offer of a reward to the school and community with the most latrines. He also reminded people of a law legitimizing fines for households without latrines. Using the language of behavior analysis, the commissioner created two powerful consequences for building latrines; both positive and negative consequences motivated willingness on the part of principals, teachers, students, and families. The commissioner's offer of a reward gave principals a reason for wanting to act, and they, in turn, through their position of influence, propelled others into action. Schools already have a structure of leadership, and students are used to taking instructions and acting on them. This, then, was the mechanism for translating abilities into action. The major worry of the population now is whether they can construct a second latrine when it is needed. Although people resent the threat of fines (the negative consequence used), laws often change behavior enough so that the law need never be enforced.

The strength of this intervention, created by the commissioner of the district, is in motivating a willingness to build and use latrines—the ingredient needed to translate ideas into action. He set up a competition among schools; three received the prize but everyone received the health benefits. A combination of incentives and fines has been used in many places—to promote family planning, use of seat belts, and safe driving, to name a few.

## CASE 6: HOME MANAGEMENT OF DIARRHEA IN GAMBIA

The Health Communication for Child Survival group and the Gambian Ministry of Health started a project to educate rural mothers in the proper treatment of infant dehydration due to diarrhea (Rasmuson et al., 1988). As in many countries, Gambian mothers often withhold food and fluid from children with diarrhea in a mistaken attempt to stop the diarrhea. This leads to dehydration and death in up to 20% of the sick children. UNICEF estimates that 8,000 children around the world die from diarrheal dehydration every day. The campaign therefore had to be powerful enough to overcome this common practice and the beliefs accompanying it. It also had to teach a new skill—that of mixing a water-sugar-salt solution and feeding it to the child. The combination of water with salt and sugar in precise proportions was first discovered by researchers in Bangladesh and India as a way to get the sick child's digestive system to absorb water. Homemade versions and sachets of dry ingredients to which one adds water are being promoted worldwide. The sachets cost U.S.10¢ to produce and are generally obtained free of cost from a clinic or bought from a drug store. At the time this project began in 1981, mothers were giving the solution in only 4% of the cases; none actually made a correct mixture.

The first part of the project was to train mothers, village volunteers, and health center professionals in the correct mixing and administration of the homemade water-sugar-salt solution. Quantities for the three substances were given in terms of a commonly available soda bottle and its top. Mixing pictures were sent to professionals and volunteers who, in turn, were to distribute handbills to mothers. Preliminary testing ensured that the pictorial instructions were understood on their own. In addition, the volunteer workers taught mothers the skills of mixing the ingredients and then watched them practice. Volunteers received a social form of reward; from their houses, they flew Happy Baby flags indicating their expertise in mixing the solution and their willingness to teach others. Because radios were available in 60% of the households, the national radio station also broadcast information on how to interpret the mixing pictures.

To encourage mothers to learn the material and to motivate health workers to teach them, mothers in 18 villages could enter a mixing contest. Mothers who correctly prepared the solution and answered questions about administering it won prizes (a one-liter plastic cup and soap). Fifteen grand-prize winners were announced on the radio and they received a radio-cassette player. Five villages with the most mothers entering the contest received community prizes of food.

The results of the program indicated that within 9 months, more than 70% of mothers knew the correct mixing procedure compared with 0% at the start of the program. Of 800 rural mothers followed up for 2 years, 74% of the diarrhea cases were treated with the solution and 43% of the mothers continued to mix the solution correctly. Thus the program was very successful.

*Who, what, and how much change was targeted in the Gambia project?* Three groups of people were targeted: mothers, volunteer workers living in villages, and professional health workers. They were taught how to make a homemade solution to prevent dehydration: 3 soda pop bottles of water, 8 capfuls of sugar, and 1 capful of salt. Thus a new skill had to be learned. In addition, the mothers had to understand when and how much mixture should be given and why it should replace their old habit of withholding fluid and food.

*What activity was undertaken to teach the mixing skill and motivate a willingness to learn and use it?* Copies of pictorial instructions were distributed to all three target groups. Health workers at the clinic and the community levels were trained to be trainers of others, and radio broadcasts also gave instruction. That part of the intervention focused on teaching the skill of mixing water, sugar, and salt. It was important because few mothers initially had the skill. Initially there was no motivation for the mothers to learn the skill or for health workers to teach them. To encourage their willingness, a contest was announced with prizes for each mother who correctly prepared the solution. In addition, 15 winners would receive grand prizes, and five villages with the most entries would win food prizes. The village prize made it more likely that everyone, not only mothers and volunteers, would get excited about learning the mixing skill. This brought in a social component.

The strength of this project lies in how it helped to translate the skill into action. The mechanisms were observational learning and reward. Local mothers showed other mothers, who then practiced making the mixture. The contest and rewards motivated mothers, families, and community leaders to learn and practice the mixing skill. This is one of the few programs to evaluate maintenance. When the project team returned 3 years later, they found that only 11% of diarrhea cases were being given the solution and only 21% of mothers knew how to mix it correctly. Thus even mothers who remembered were not giving the solution to their children. The team began another campaign designed to reinforce the skills that some mothers had learned and to teach new mothers about the ORS sachets (Graeff & Waters, 1994). The project raises disturbing questions about the sustainability of new health behaviors as well as what kinds of reminders and motivators are needed. The planners assumed that mothers would need rewards temporarily to learn the skill but that the benefits of recovering from diarrhea would foster willingness to use the solution in the long term. This was clearly not the case.

## CASE 7: SCHOOL FEEDING PROGRAMS

A *Guardian Weekly* article titled "Population Control That Really Works" (Mathews, 1994) stated,

> In the 1970s, the chief executive of this state in south India [Tamil Nadu] launched a free midday meal program for children in primary schools. The purpose was political populism—the result entirely unexpected. The number of schools and teachers had to grow—as vehicles for delivering the meals. A little girl became more valuable to the family by going to school and getting a nutritious meal (especially if she brought some home to share) than staying home taking care of younger siblings. The number of girls in school went way up . . . The midday-meal girls began to marry in 1985. In the next six years, the birthrate—which had declined slightly in the previous decade—dropped by more than 25 percent. (p. 15)

I was impressed by this. A nutritious meal plus a good education is bound to yield huge health dividends.

Researchers linking a mother's education with the health of her family find that as her years of schooling increase, so does

> her planning for a smaller family,
> the survival of her infants,
> the nutritional status of her children,
> the education level of her children,
> her future earnings.

Despite the obvious economic, psychological, and health benefits, many boys and girls still do not attend school and many do not achieve critical levels of basic literacy and numeracy, namely, completing fourth grade. Although school is compulsory, many governments do not have the means to enforce the law. Consequently, it is parents who decide. What influences if and at what age a child attends school? Do parents engage in a systematic cost-benefit analysis? Some of these influences appear in an analysis of seven African countries (Lloyd & Blanc, 1996) where enrollment rates are around 50%. Malnourished (stunted) children are often enrolled several years late, perhaps because they appear or act "young." Girls may be kept home to help with chores if there are younger siblings. When a mother is the head of the household, she is more likely to send her children, both boys and girls, to school. But the two major determinants are whether the household head, usually male, went to school, and the extended family's resources. To attract families in which neither parent went to school and in which resources are low, school feeding programs were tried.

Levinger (1986) describes a number of school feeding programs in Haiti, the Dominican Republic, Colombia, Sri Lanka, India, Kenya, and the Philippines. Generally these programs are very popular among both donors and recipient communities. Their goal is to improve the nutritional status of children while encouraging them to attend school, both of which will foster physical, mental, and social well-being. The provision of meals is not only an incentive for parents to send children to school but a source of energy for the mental and social activity required. Malnourished children often do poorly at school, both socially and academically, because they have problems with concentration, energy, coping with stress, and anxiety. Communities as a whole benefit because the program buys at least some of the food from local farmers and hires others to prepare and distribute it.

The programs vary greatly: They provide snacks such as a biscuit along with milk, breakfast, or lunch to children in primary school using donor-supplied food or local food. A great deal of community organization is required to consistently provide meals and sustain the service over a long time. Food must be bought from local farmers, stored in the community, prepared near the school, and distributed to children during school hours. In countries where fast foods are not an option and refrigeration is uncommon, the process of providing daily meals involves multiple steps and is labor intensive. A typical school might have 1,500 students in one half-day session.

The success of these programs has been evaluated in terms of school attendance, nutritional status, and cognitive development. Schools with food are compared with schools that do not provide food, or a longitudinal comparison is made from before to after the food program. The success of these programs varies widely; some show positive outcomes, and some show no change. Programs in countries where school attendance is already high, as in the Philippines and Colombia, are less likely to have an effect compared with programs in countries where attendance is low. It is not surprising that programs raise school attendance quickly, but nutritional status and cognitive development rise more slowly. Given the benefits of school attendance, this outcome alone justifies the intervention. The most successful programs are those that provide breakfast or lunch containing 30% of the minimum daily nutritional requirement and that target rural communities where many children are undernourished and would not normally attend school. Teachers generally report that children perform better after the meal, and some schools report higher grades among children who take the meals. But teacher reports on performance are not consistently related to participating in the feeding program.

The community benefits indirectly in that coordinated action is initiated and can be extended to other programs, and the feeding program is a stimulus to agricultural and economic activity. The family is affected by having children attend school; the children receive their main meal at school, but they are now unavailable for family work. However, in the long run, the benefit to children, particularly girls, is immense in that, as educated mothers, their children will be healthier.

Try to analyze this case. Who, what, and how much change is targeted by these feeding programs? Remember, it is not only the schoolchild who must change but also the family roles and relationships. What activities are undertaken to foster abilities, motivate willingness, and tackle barriers? Do school abilities transfer to health behaviors, and are these sustainable? The school feeding programs do not explicitly address the transfer and sustainability questions.

## LEARNING FROM SUCCESSES AND MISTAKES

The previously described case studies demonstrated some degree of success:

1. Spouses and friends acquired the information and social support they needed to make decisions about contraception (case 1), face washing (case 2), and child feeding (case 4), and many acted on their decision.
2. Children learned what they should do to maintain personal hygiene, environmental sanitation, water use, and how to prevent and manage diarrhea (case 3).
3. High school students dug latrines for their families and neighbors and taught people why latrines were beneficial (case 5).
4. Mothers learned how to mix an ORS solution and how to administer it, and began using it when their children had diarrhea (case 6).
5. Children were sent to school and ate well when breakfast or lunch was offered at the school (case 7).

In most cases, people acquired the personal resources—the knowledge, skills, and confidence—to make an informed decision about a health behavior. In some cases, they acquired social resources, such as family and community support. Often lacking in the potential beneficiaries was a willingness to make the change. Programs developed personal and social resources but did not transfer these to action. Perhaps the stress of change was a barrier in itself.

The most effective programs were those that explicitly motivated action, usually with incentives and rewards. According to applied behavior analysis (Graeff et al., 1993), there are a number of ways to help translate skill into action. The main one is by providing positive consequences. **Positive consequences** refer to the social, emotional, or material benefits that follow from the action: Receiving approval and recognition, feeling proud of oneself, receiving funds for the school or community, and noticeable improvements in a child's health are examples of things that people hope to obtain through their actions.

An important question is whether successes can be exported to a different place. Do we learn anything general from these cases, or are the solutions unique to their settings? For me, the real question is this: Under what conditions do these successes occur, and are the important conditions to be found in other places?

## TAKING THEORIES INTO THE FIELD

Would an analysis of health education theories provide a more general set of principles for guiding health education than this analysis of cases? Can they tell us what should be changed and how to bring about changes? There are at least three orientations to be found in current theories, as represented by a motto I have created for each:

> *Communication:* We tailor our message to you.
> *Health beliefs:* You are what you think.
> *Applied behavior analysis:* ABC is the recipe for action.

The health education cases we previously analyzed tend to lean toward one or two orientations. Most used a form of persuasive communication in which the style of presentation was as important as the health content. The health belief orientation tends to emphasize reasoning without suggesting how to engage action. The behavioral analysis alone targets action.

Persuasive Communication

Basically, **communication** involves the transmission of a message from one person to another. It can be face to face or mass media, auditory and visual; it can be informative, emotional, and persuasive; it can be positive (what to do and the benefits) and negative (what not to do and the disadvantages) (see Hubley, 1993). The innovative ideas presented in the message may persuade a few who then pass on the message to others (Rogers, 1983).

The content of a communication message usually engages the intellectual and/or emotional processes of a person. The intellect becomes engaged if the message informs about a health problem, a health behavior, or an available health service. However, another function of information is to trigger action at the appropriate time, such as a timely message to mothers that their babies are due for their third immunization or that the outreach team is in town. Messages appealing to emotions, such as pride, include social recognition and praise for people who have completed their child's immunizations, learned to used oral rehydration therapy, or built a latrine for their family. Persuasive messages consist of communications aimed at changing people's attitudes and actions. The intention to change those who receive the message becomes apparent in the use of information and emotion. Information is provided in the form of arguments as to why one should perform the proposed action and why one should not perform the alternative action. The action or attitude is described repeatedly. The emotions of the receivers are often aroused so that they will have more positive feelings about the proposed action and more negative feelings about the alternative, and so they will be energized into action. Because attitudes and actions are so difficult to change, information and emotion need to be combined in a special way to persuade the receivers to change.

A great deal of effort goes into preparing messages that are understood and accepted by the audience. For example, familiar analogies and concrete pictures are better than health jargon and symbols (Nichter, 1989). Of the seven cases just presented, the Gambian promotion of ORS and the Bolivian radio broadcasts made special efforts to tailor the style and content of their message to their audience. The discussions of Filipino mothers were by nature tailored to their friends, not because they intended to persuade but because the solutions they gave were relevant to both family contexts. The problem-solving discussions were emotional because mothers tend to talk passionately to friends about their children and because friends tend to boost each other's self-confidence.

A recent theory about persuasive communication proposes that a communicator first find out how "able and willing" listeners are to receive the message. If they do not have a lot of knowledge about the topic and are not particularly eager to find out, then the communication must have attention-getting qualities, such as being colorful, surprising, humorous, concrete, visual, and presented by a celebrity (Eagly & Chaiken, 1993).

Health Beliefs

The Health Belief Model of Rosenstock (1990) and Becker (Janz & Becker, 1984) emphasizes the intellectual dimension of health behavior. Recently it has added self-efficacy from social learning theory (Perry, Baranowski, & Parcel, 1990), and we might also add subjective norms from the theory of reasoned action (Ajzen, 1988). This theoretical orientation identifies the following beliefs as relevant:

1. *Perceived threat* includes two judgments: that one is susceptible to the illness (i.e., at personal risk) and that the illness is serious. If both are

judged to be high, then perceived threat is high, and one will be driven to act to avoid the threat.

2. *Outcome expectations* concern benefits of the specified action (e.g., effective, inexpensive) minus barriers to the action (e.g., costly, time consuming). If the outcome expectations of an action are high, one will take that action.

3. *Self-efficacy* is confidence that one has the skill and resources to perform the specified action. If one has self-efficacy, one can perform the action with confidence and pride, although not necessarily with skill or expertise. Practice enhances self-efficacy.

4. *Subjective norm* refers to one's perception that significant other people will approve of the action. If important people are expected to approve of the action, one will take that action.

Rosenstock (1990) recognizes that the theory has many shortcomings when it comes to planning how to change these beliefs in a particular context. The major limitations include the following:

- No mechanism is proposed to connect beliefs with action.
- No mechanism is proposed to change beliefs.
- The focus is narrowly on the individual; often the social environment also must change.
- Components could be additive or multiplicative; the distinction is important if one component is zero.
- Change is narrowly based on avoidance of threat, with no mention of desire to approach a rewarding healthy state.

The health education project for face washing in Tanzania focused largely on the health beliefs specified by this model—namely, the threat of trachoma, the expectation that face washing would prevent trachoma, and confidence that one could find the necessary water and time to wash every child's face. However, the organizers went one step further with respect to subjective norms; they tried to change the actual community norm, not simply the mothers' belief that others would approve.

### Applied Behavior Analysis

Applied behavior analysis as outlined by the HealthCom group (Graeff et al., 1993) targets specific behavior to be changed using principles of learning and performance. There are several steps. First, a behavior analysis is conducted to identify what health behavior should be changed. Criteria for choosing the target behavior include that it not be too complex or costly or lengthy, that it be compatible with existing practices, have high impact on health, and produce observable consequences. Second, the ideal behavior must then be broken down into its separate components to be learned step by step. Most health behaviors are not entirely new; people usually know some of the correct actions but need to learn more or to learn the correct timing or quantity. We have seen how important timing and quantity are when giving a child weaning foods or ORS. If the behavior is entirely new, then the person can learn through observing another before practicing. Third, once the person is able to perform some or all of the actions, rewarding consequences will serve to encourage further learning and performance of the new behavior. For this reason, the consequences of an action determine whether it will be performed or not. Positive consequences such as food and approval most effectively strengthen action when they immediately follow it, are salient, and are relevant to the person. They need to be concrete but not necessarily material. Praise and social recognition from one's family, the school, health workers, and community leaders were very effective in mobilizing Bangladeshi students to dig latrines. The promise of a monetary contribution to the best school's development fund was an incentive to school administrators. Gambian mothers were motivated with symbolic and practical rewards, such as a certificate of merit, a house flag, a personal mention on the radio, a bar of soap, and a liter cup.

The major problem to solve when applying behavior analysis concerns the lack of natural rewards for preventive health behaviors. The absence of disease is the big benefit, but it is unobservable. For example, child immunization leads to the absence of six deadly diseases for the following 5 or 10 years. This is not observable. Without sophisticated knowledge of the cause-effect relation between immunization and disease prevention, a mother would be unaware of the important consequences of immunizing her child. For this reason, planned artificial consequences must be provided during the health education project and then gradually other positive consequences will replace it to help maintain the behavior (Elder, Geller, Hovell, & Mayer, 1994; Graeff et al., 1993).

Although the theory deals mostly with behavior and its consequences, the antecedents of behavior must also be examined. Antecedents are things that trigger action; they do not force the action to happen but they inform the person that an action is now required. Examples are seeing a health worker demonstrate making ORS, seeing a handbill that pictures the substances and quantities for making ORS, seeing the ARI or diarrhea symptoms of a child, talking about child spacing with one's spouse, seeing a pictorial reminder on one's wall of the next immunization session, recalling what one learned about weaning foods for one's infant, and deciding to dig a latrine. According to this theory, health education activities must encourage learning and performance of health behaviors by arranging antecedents and consequences of the behaviors. It is called the A-B-C chain: antecedents → behavior → consequences. Antecedents stimulate action; behavior includes skill and performance; consequences strengthen behavior.

I have described the ABC theory last because its simple structure incorporates and goes beyond the previous two. Antecedents are part of the context in which the health behavior occurs—the resources that enable one to carry out the necessary actions. The Health Belief Model addresses the question of effective antecedents—threats, self-confidence, expected outcomes, and social norms. But it does not go far enough in specifying action triggers in the environment—reminders, media messages, illness symptoms. The theory of persuasive communication addresses how one can change health beliefs, namely, by pictures or words that arouse ideas and emotions. But communication may be more persuasive if it conveys positive rewards and arouses feelings of pride after building on skills, rather than being directed at knowledge. Mothers in the Philippines who solved their child feeding problems together were not receiving expert communications on the proper foods to feed a child; what a mother heard from her friend gave both of them the confidence to come up with their own solutions. The mental life of an innovative idea is short when the idea comes from someone else (6 months for ORS instruction) but is longer when it comes from oneself. Applied behavior analysis connects the ABC components while placing emphasis on health behavior. The proof of the project is in the behavior.

## THE CASE FOR EDUCATION

Universal primary schooling is a goal that most governments and international organizations place at the top of their priorities. Promoting general education must also be part of a national health promotion strategy. Not only is a person's education related to his or her general development and health but an educated mother raises healthier children with greater chances of survival. What are the "pathways of influence" between a mother's education and her healthier child? A number of interesting papers have been written on this question (e.g., N. Adler, Boyce, & Chesney, 1994; Caldwell, 1980; Cleland & van Ginneken, 1988; Link & Phelan, 1996; Lloyd & Blanc, 1996). One pathway is that an educated mother is more receptive to health education. She has a reservoir of skills, knowledge, and values that make her more able and willing to change and maintain the change. In general, primary schooling provides a person with personal and social resources on a grand scale.

A girl who attends school and finishes grade 4 is likely to be somewhere between 10 and 14 years of age. Education might delay the age at which she marries and has her first child, but this does not explain her children's improved health status as much as we might expect. The social and economic resources she accesses are more important. As an educated girl, she is more likely to attract and be compatible with an educated boy, and more likely to have educated girlfriends. These are just two examples of her wider social network and the new models she identifies with, such as teachers. Primary schooling also enhances her own economic productivity and earning power. In addition, she is more likely to demand and maintain water and latrine facilities, a clean home, and clean children. Thus the social and economic resources available to an educated woman are substantial and she is more likely to use them effectively. For example, she will have access to peers who perhaps have different solutions to health problems and different norms for child rearing. She will have some options to choose from if she has been exposed to teacher mentors in addition to parents. The better educated in each society often have access to social connections, money, power, and knowledge that bring them into contact with health innovations.

The personal resources one acquires from primary schooling are also immense. In particular, one acquires literacy and numeracy skills, a background of knowledge, and a set of values. Functional literacy and numeracy require at least the completion of the fourth grade. A mother with literacy and numeracy skills is more likely to understand and recall instructions on a sachet of oral rehydration salts; she is more likely to understand that causes of events such as illness are not necessarily proximal or observable (e.g., Eisemon, Patel, & Ole Sena, 1987; Patel, Eisemon, & Arocha, 1988). Literacy and numeracy are more than just the skills to read and combine numbers; they create an awareness of symbols, that is, of things that represent abstract entities. I once witnessed a surprising demonstration of just how different the perspective of a literate person is from that of an illiterate person. The words *three little piggies* were read to an illiterate person, then the last word was covered. When asked what it now said, the reader answered, "Two little piggies." Each word was treated as a tally of pigs rather than a symbol. Similarly, the causal impact of germs is both abstract and delayed. Most of us have to take it on faith that germs exist and that they are responsible for infections up to weeks after transmission. To communicate and think about germs, we use pictures or mental images of blobs to symbolize an invasion of germs, but we don't expect to see the blobs. Consequently, the ability to use letters and numbers as symbols carries over to other domains such as health. Mothers who have attended school are therefore more likely to believe that modern medicine works because they understand the symbols.

Schooling also gives one a background of knowledge on which to build. When one hears new information, it is embellished by one's existing beliefs, which give a slightly new meaning to the information. In a homogeneous and traditional community, one learns the habits and knowledge of past generations. School habits and knowledge go beyond one's daily reality and thus provide an alternative framework for interpreting information. Because the information provided through health education fits this framework, it is more likely to be remembered and viewed as reasonable, even if it is not fully understood.

Finally, schooling alters the values of the whole family. Mothers and fathers who have attended school are more likely to send their children to school. This reflects a different value for children, one that places greater emphasis on a child's future potential than on responsibilities

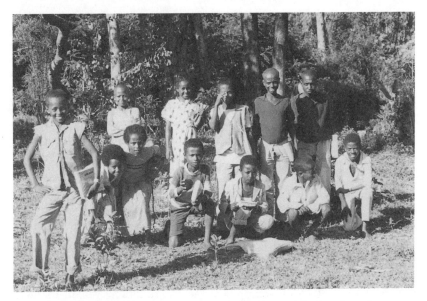

*Only 50% of children may continue to attend school beyond the fourth grade.*

for current household tasks. Not only does a mother lack her children's daily help when they attend school, she must also find money for their books and clothes and contend with the new morality and authority of the school. Wealth goes from parents to children in this case, rather than from children to parents as in the traditional family. Educated mothers may have more credence with their husbands when requesting money and time for children's needs. She may place more value on the quality rather than quantity of children, and so feed, clean, and talk more with her children to make sure that quality is realized in the future (Caldwell et al., 1988).

The behavioral pathways from these skills, knowledge, and values to healthier children (Cleland & van Ginneken, 1988) could therefore include:

immunization and better child feeding,
protection against infection through hygiene and sanitation,
better recovery from illness through home care and health services, and
reduced risk of accidents and injuries through closer supervision.

Universal **primary schooling** is far from a reality. The following countries have **enrollment** rates well under 50%: Niger, Somalia, Afghanistan, Liberia, Mali, Ethiopia, Bhutan, and Burkina Faso. In sub-Saharan Africa, enrollment in primary school is 50% of eligibles from that age group. Elsewhere, rates are more than 80%. In Africa, many parents delay their children's entry to school for up to 5 years; this used to be because of the distances to travel, although another explanation is that malnutrition stunts children, which makes them look younger to parents (Lloyd & Blanc, 1996). Many African countries were steadily increasing their student enrollments until recently when their debt repayments took such a large chunk of the budget that education and health spending declined.

Another indicator of schooling is the percentage of children who complete fourth grade, the level considered necessary for functional literacy. Lloyd and Blanc (1996) analyzed the figures for seven countries in Africa; approximately 50% to 60% of children in the 10 to 14 age group, ever enrolled, had completed fourth grade. This means that less than 50% of the children in that age group are functionally literate. This low rate is not due to dropouts but to children starting late and making slow progress. The authors suggest that parents largely make decisions about whether and when to enroll a child in school, whereas the low quality of schooling is responsible for the slow progress. Many schools operate two 4-hour sessions with 60 children per class to accommodate all the pupils. The schools often lack books, paper, pencils, and a usable chalkboard. It takes dedication and concentration to work in these conditions.

The "education gender gap" refers to the lower enrollment of girls in primary school and the lower literacy rates for women generally. In South Asia, the Middle East, and Africa, girls' enrollment is on average 20% below boys', and women's literacy is 25% below men's (UNICEF, 1996), although the seven-country African study found little advantage for either sex (Lloyd & Blanc, 1996). Girls are more likely to be kept home for a variety of reasons: Girls care for younger siblings, they have more household chores, they require adequate clothing, they are more vulnerable to sexual pressure from teachers and students, and they are not allowed to travel too far from home. Many new projects are attempting to accommodate the needs of parents and girls, and bring girls into the school system, by having women teachers in small community schools with flexible hours. These are not radical innovations, but they require buildings, books, and trained teachers. If it is difficult to encourage girls to complete fourth grade, imagine how challenging it is to get them through teacher training and into a rural school system where women teachers are looked on with suspicion. Because people know the power of education to change the course of life, they can be simultaneously fearful and hopeful about sending their children.

## STUDENT ACTIVITY

Select any of the published studies reported in this book, or any known health education project in your country, and analyze it the way we have here. If you were to do that project again, how would you improve it?

# 9

# MENTAL HEALTH AND ILLNESS

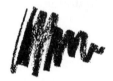

The World Health Organization defines health in terms of physical, mental, and social well-being. Because most developing countries operate with scarce resources, they have concentrated on physical health. However, mental illness substantially contributes to the loss of healthy productive years of life around the world. Expressed in terms of disability adjusted life years (DALYs) lost, neuropsychiatric diseases rank high, accounting for 6.8% of the worldwide total (World Bank, 1993). In sub-Saharan Africa and India, mental illness accounts for a loss equivalent to that caused by nutritional deficiencies. If we look at the burden of disease among adults 15 to 44 years of age, when they are most productive, mental illness accounts for 12%. The disability resulting from mental illness has many parallels with nutritional deficiencies: It often begins in youth when it is not particularly noticeable, but when it is perhaps most preventable; it has repercussions that last well into adulthood; and it rarely shows up in mortality statistics but can have long-lasting effects on well-being and productivity.

The pervasive impact of mental illness has become particularly apparent in developed countries, where it accounts for 25% of doctor visits (Goldberg, 1995). Recent surveys record a similar figure for health clinics in developing countries. In 15 health centers around the world, 21% of the patients had a definite psychiatric disorder (Ormel et al., 1994), ranging from a high of 53% in Santiago, Chile, and 34% in Rio de Janeiro, to a low of 8% in Shanghai, China. Most will have come to the clinic complaining of physical symptoms. The health workers have been trained to detect and treat physical problems but probably know little about psychological symptoms. Consequently, the patient's psychological distress is frequently overlooked and he or she is forced to return again and again seeking relief. As a result of studies such as this, more attention is being paid to mental illness in developing countries and to its prevention and treatment.

## DEFINITION AND CLASSIFICATION

**Mental health** refers to satisfactory functioning in cognitive, emotional, and social domains. Because it represents a continuum, mental health may be more or less satisfactory, and it is safe to say that most people have room for improvement.

Very impaired functioning _____ Fully functioning

Everyone can be located somewhere along this continuum of mental health. Some function more competently than others in the cognitive, emotional, and social domains of life. Presumably we all aim to function at a high level sometime during our adult years. At what point along this continuum do we place the threshold for mental illness? That is the task of those who develop and use assessment procedures.

Below a certain threshold, psychosocial functioning becomes a problem for the person and/or the community, and the person is said to be mentally ill or to have a mental disorder. **Mental disorders** are defined as behavioral or psychological syndromes (groups of associated features) that are associated with one or more of the following:

- Present distress
- Impairment in one or more important areas of functioning
- A significantly increased risk of suffering death, pain, or disability

It excludes an expectable and culturally sanctioned response to a particular event such as sadness at the death of a relative, deviant behavior of minorities in a society (e.g., religious minorities), and conflicts between an individual and society arising from the person's voluntary efforts to express individuality. Mental disorders may result from biological, developmental, or psychosocial factors, and fall on a continuum according to degree of impairment and distress (American Psychiatric Association, 1994).

Current systems for classifying mental disorders are based on the idea that there is a finite set of distinguishable disorders and that each one has identifiable symptoms. The *International Classification of Disease (ICD-10)* developed by the World Health Organization (1992) is the system used everywhere except North America (see Box 9.1). The *Diagnostic and Statistical Manual (DSM-IV)* for North America is very similar. These classifications cover organic mental disorders, substance-related disorders, schizophrenia, mood disorders, anxiety disorders, somatoform disorders, personality disorders, and developmental disorders. The disorders are described in terms of clinical symptoms, a certain number of which must be present; there are also exclusion criteria—for example, that the symptom not be due to temporary medication. A clinical interview is usually used for diagnosis. Casebooks show how the classification systems are applied to individual people (Ustun et al., 1996).

## COMMUNITY MEASUREMENT INSTRUMENTS

Research instruments have been developed to assess the prevalence of mental illness in large populations. There are several reasons that one might want to conduct large-scale studies of mental illness. One is to determine how many people suffer from mental disorders sometime during their lifetime or at any one point in time so as to plan for treatment facilities. Another reason is to examine conditions that foster

> **BOX 9.1.**
> **THE *ICD-10* CLASSIFICATION OF MENTAL AND BEHAVIORAL DISORDERS**
>
> Organic, including symptomatic, mental disorders (e.g., dementia)
> Mental and behavioral disorders due to substance use (e.g., acute alcohol intoxication and alcohol dependence)
> Schizophrenia and delusional disorders (e.g., acute and transient psychotic disorders)
> Mood (affective) disorders (e.g., manic episode, depression)
> Neurotic, stress-related, and somatoform disorders (e.g., phobic anxiety disorders, panic disorder, generalized anxiety disorder, somatization disorder, hypochondriacal disorder, neurasthenia)
> Disorders of adult personality and behavior
> Mental retardation
> Disorders of psychological development

mental health and illness so as to promote health and prevent illness. A third reason is to evaluate different treatment programs. Initially, the WHO developed short self-report questionnaires to identify "potential" cases of mental illness: the 24-item Self-Reporting Questionnaire for adults and the 10-item Reporting Questionnaire for Children. More recently, a second generation of tests have been developed to identify specific disorders such as depression and schizophrenia. This includes the *Composite International Diagnostic Interview (CIDI),* the *Diagnostic Interview Schedule* for adults and for children, and the *Child Behavior Checklist (CBCL).* These have been used to decide the kinds of treatment services needed in a community because schizophrenia, depression, organic disorders, and alcohol abuse require different services.

A number of important criteria have been considered when constructing these measures:

- The test must be simple enough to be administered by workers with minimal training.
- The symptoms must be relevant across cultures.
- The wording of symptoms must be simple and easily understood.

- Questions must produce reliable answers.
- Questions must produce valid answers, that is, measure mental illness.

The tests generally consist of a list of common symptoms of a disorder. Respondents are asked to indicate whether they have experienced the symptom, either with a Yes or No response or in terms of frequency (Often, Sometimes, Rarely). The respondent's score is simply the sum of symptoms he or she reports experiencing.

1. *The Self Reporting Questionnaire (SRQ)* was developed by the WHO as a screening instrument to detect mental disorders among patients using primary care facilities (Harding et al., 1983). It has also been used to estimate the prevalence of mental disorders in community settings. The first 20 items describe neurotic symptoms; the last 4 items describe psychotic symptoms (see Box 9.2). The items were selected from four existing instruments used in different countries such as Britain, Colombia, India, Jamaica, and the United States. The number of Yes answers to the 20 questions constitutes the person's score. A cutoff point for distinguishing between people who possibly have a disorder (potential cases) and people who do not have a disorder (noncases) is decided after comparing scores on the SRQ with the results of another method, such as an interview. Cutoff points have ranged from $4/5$ to $10/11$ and vary according to the country, whether the sample comes from a clinic or from the general population and whether they are literate or illiterate. On the four items used to detect psychosis, a score of 1 or more indicates that the person is a potential case. There has been considerable criticism of this subscale, so it is less frequently used. However, as a whole, the scale has good validity and reliability. A *User's Guide to the Self Reporting Questionnaire* compiled by Beusenberg and Orley (1994) contains information gathered from use of the test around the world.

2. *The Composite International Diagnostic Interview* includes more detailed questions that lead to a diagnosis. The questions form a decision tree, so that inclusion and exclusion criteria can be followed. The developers chose items that satisfy both *DSM* and *ICD* classification systems. Procedures to validate and, if necessary, revise items are under way in various field test locations around the world (Cottler et al., 1991; Robins et al., 1988; Wittchen et al., 1991).

> **BOX 9.2.**
> **SELF-REPORTING QUESTIONNAIRE (SRQ)**
>
> 1. Do you often have headaches?
> 2. Is your appetite poor?
> 3. Do you sleep badly?
> 4. Are you easily frightened?
> 5. Do your hands shake?
> 6. Do you feel nervous, tense, or worried?
> 7. Is your digestion poor?
> 8. Do you have trouble thinking clearly?
> 9. Do you feel unhappy?
> 10. Do you cry more than usual?
> 11. Do you find it difficult to enjoy your daily activities?
> 12. Do you find it difficult to make decisions?
> 13. Is your daily work suffering?
> 14. Are you unable to play a useful part in life?
> 15. Have you lost interest in things?
> 16. Do you feel that you are a worthless person?
> 17. Has the thought of ending your life been on your mind?
> 18. Do you feel tired all the time?
> 19. Do you have uncomfortable feelings in your stomach?
> 20. Are you easily tired?
> 21. Do you feel that somebody has been trying to harm you in some way?
> 22. Are you a much more important person than most people think?
> 23. Have you noticed any interference or anything else unusual with your thinking?
> 24. Do you ever hear voices without knowing where they come from or that other people cannot hear?

3. *The Reporting Questionnaire for Children (RQC)* for children 5 to 15 years of age was developed by the WHO as a screening instrument to identify moderate to severe mental retardation, significant degrees of emotional or behavioral disorders, and psychotic disorders (Harding et al., 1983). Parents answer simply Yes or No to indicate whether their child has

> **BOX 9.3.**
> **REPORTING QUESTIONNAIRE**
> **FOR CHILDREN (RQC)**
>
> 1. Is the child's speech in any way abnormal (retarded, incomprehensible, stammering)?
> 2. Does the child sleep badly?
> 3. Did the child ever have a fit or fall to the ground for no reason?
> 4. Does the child suffer from frequent headaches?
> 5. Does the child run away from home frequently?
> 6. Does the child steal things from home?
> 7. Does the child get scared or nervous for no good reason?
> 8. Does the child in any way appear backward or slow to learn as compared with other children of about the same age?
> 9. Does the child nearly never play with other children?
> 10. Does the child wet or soil him- or herself?

the symptom (see Box 9.3). At least one Yes answer indicates that the child possibly has a mental disorder. This cutoff point has been validated in comparison with a clinical interview and parent/teacher ratings (Abiodun, 1993a; Giel et al., 1981). Although useful as a screening instrument, the 10-item scale lacks the ability to provide information on a range of psychological problems such as aggression and withdrawal.

4. The need for more detailed diagnoses has led to greater interest in the *Child Behavior Checklist* (Achenbach & Edelbrock, 1983; Weisz, Sigman, Weiss, & Mosk, 1993). The checklist consists of 118 specific behavior problems to be answered by the parent as Not True, Somewhat/Sometimes True, or Very/Often True. Parents' answers have indicated that certain problems tend to go together in their children. For example, a child with a high total score who has trouble sleeping is also very likely to feel lonely and to demand attention. A statistical strategy that looks for clusters of problems found that these three occur together. Nine such clusters, or syndromes, appear in North American samples, the most common being hyperactive, delinquent, aggressive, socially withdrawn,

depressed, anxious, and somatic. Similar syndromes were found in an Ethiopian sample (Mulatu, 1995a).

5. *The Diagnostic Interview Schedule (DIS)* and the *Diagnostic Interview Schedule for Children (DISC)* have been developed and used extensively in the United States to assess mental illness in community and health center populations. Both are able to identify specific disorders, but the child form is still being revised (Piacentini et al., 1993; Regier et al., 1993).

## IS MENTAL ILLNESS UNIVERSAL OR CULTURE SPECIFIC?

People who develop and use instruments such as the *SRQ*, the *CIDI*, and the *RQC* assume that mental illness is a universal phenomenon. They assume that the concept of abnormal behavior is universal, that the core symptoms are universal, that the classification of these symptoms into specific diagnoses is universal, and that the experience is similar across cultures. The opposite position is taken by those who believe that all of these assumptions are wrong and that mental illness is culture specific. Underlying the latter position is the well-documented argument that one's culture influences how one thinks and feels, how one interacts with others, the norms that determine acceptable and abnormal behavior, the stresses one encounters, and the socially defined role of a sick person.

Patel (1995) has examined these assumptions by reviewing anthropological studies of mental illness in 11 sub-Saharan African cultures. Although there is no definitive answer in this controversy, each issue can be addressed with relevant data.

How Universal Is the
Concept of Abnormal Behaviors?

Although some cultures have a more holistic view of health, all studied cultures distinguish mind from body and distinguish abnormal from normal behavior. Most cultures have a separate category for "nonnormal" behavior that is voluntary and practiced within defined roles, for example, religious leaders and traditional healers who listen to the voices of spirits. Despite the distinction between mind and body, people around the world express their mental distress through physical states such as headaches, ulcers, and pain all over the body. Similarly, they locate mental phenomena in different sites, for example, in the brain, heart, and abdomen. Abnormal behavior may also be tolerated more by the sufferer's family in some cultures.

How Universal Are the Core Symptoms?

Symptoms of psychological distress show some universality and some culture specificity. Across cultures, people complain of sadness, feeling worthless, worry, fear of certain objects, and a heart pounding with fright. Thus certain symptoms of depression and anxiety are similar. Also, the symptoms of psychosis are similar: agitation, hallucinations, thought and speech disturbances, suspiciousness, laughing and talking to oneself, and saying bizarre things. Other symptoms are more common in certain cultures, such as pain all over, heat or crawling sensations in the head, burning in the stomach, weakness, dizziness, coldness, or thinking too much. These are typically not included in the WHO symptom checklists. It is sometimes said that sufferers in developing countries are more likely to express their mental distress as a physical symptom. However, Goldberg (1995) noted that somatization is common throughout the world; that is, 95% of disturbed patients seeking services from 15 health centers in different countries complained of physical rather than psychological distress.

How Universal Is the
Classification of Disorders?

Classification of mental disorders by ordinary people and traditional healers alike is often by cause as well as by subjective experience, as has been the case throughout the history of formal systems such as the *ICD* and *DSM* (see Kortmann's 1987 description of the Ethiopian system). Attributed causes are very different, some being natural—such as heredity, infection, and climate—but most being supernatural—such as family spirits and community ancestral spirits upset by the person breaking a taboo, the evil eye of a jealous person who intends no harm, or magic and witchcraft (see Box 9.4). The symptoms of psychosis appear to be commonly used to classify this disorder, and many cultures have a label to identify schizophrenia. In Africa, psychotics, who may appear disheveled or without clothes and wearing garbage, are most easily identified. Depression and anxiety are less easily identified; some of the core symptoms may be similar but many of the symptoms are somatic. A common psychological symptom for depression in sub-Saharan Africa is that the person is seen to "think too much," a state that could easily be equated with the Euro-American symptom of self-critical rumination. Other clusters of neurotic symptoms are less likely to be recognized by the general population. However, in all cultures there is a difference between the way the general population and the scientific community classify illness.

Patel points to two syndromes that are common in Africa but not found in Euro-American classifications. One is "brain fag syndrome" often reported by students and perhaps caused by the stress of schooling. The symptoms are headaches, heat and crawling sensations in the scalp, abdominal and chest pains, fatigue, palpitations, dizziness, faintness, inability to concentrate, falling asleep in class, impaired appetite and sleep, and social withdrawal. The second syndrome is "reactive psychosis" during which symptoms of intense overarousal, aggression, pressured speech, and disrobing last for 1 month with complete recovery.

How Universal Are the Course and Outcome?

The course and outcome of mental illness tend to differ in different cultures. Although certain disorders such as schizophrenia were thought to be chronic, many people in developing countries appear to be symptom-free 1 year later (see Box 9.5). After a large-scale study, Jablensky (1995) concluded that the profile of these people is not different from others at intake, so there would be no way to classify them differently. Research is currently being conducted to determine what conditions in developing countries facilitate the recovery of mentally ill people—conditions such as community attitudes, social roles, and emotions expressed by family members toward the ill person.

In summary, it is clear that there are different perceptions of mental illness and its causes in different cultures. But it is not yet clear whether these perceptions influence the experience of mental illness and require a different list of symptoms. It remains an open question as to whether there are certain syndromes with unique clusters of symptoms that are

## BOX 9.4.
## BEWARE THE EVIL EYE

The evil eye is commonly believed to cause misfortune and illness in many developing countries. Lisbeth Sachs (1983) studied beliefs about the evil eye among Turkish migrants in Sweden. *Nasar* is the Turkish name for the jealous look of someone who may consciously intend no harm but is responsible for misfortune, such as losing one's husband or an accident that causes injury. The evil spell may be cast by an envious look or by words of praise about someone who is beautiful or successful. It may cause a healthy child to become ill with fever, a husband to become disenchanted with his wife, or a teenager to become disobedient and aggressive. In Turkey, fair, blue-eyed persons in particular are able to activate the evil power of Nasar because their appearance is different from other Turks, but any admiring person poses a threat. To ward off the evil eye, children are kept concealed from outsiders for 40 days after birth and remain close to home for several years after. Women and children wear amulets—beads or a sac of metal or herbs worn around the neck. The amulet works by drawing into it any evil power that would otherwise be directed to the child. When a woman or her child receives a compliment or an admiring glance, the woman will say *Masallah* (in the name of God) to neutralize the evil influence. If the evil power is too strong, rather than seeking out the person who is the source of evil, the woman may try to use certain objects, such as salt, molten tin, or water, to counteract the evil force. Thus the person who is afflicted by illness or injury is not blamed for the misfortune because it was caused not by his or her own behavior but by another person. In Ethiopia, *buda* is the name for the evil eye cast by envious people against their will. It too may cause a person to have headaches or fits of madness. And it may be fatal if not cured. Distinctions are made between the evil eye of certain people and other evil forces that come from supernatural spirits that now inhabit streams, animals, or trees. The latter are called *cins* in Turkey and *djinis* in Ethiopia. If one wanders into a dark place at night, one may be led astray and mentally confused by one of these animate spirits. A more serious mental illness or family conflict may be caused by a magician who intends harm. It requires very strong positive magic from a person specially endowed with this power, or from an object, to exorcise the illness. Traditional healers and religious leaders often use holy water or special trances to cure a person afflicted with mental illness.

## BOX 9.5.
## IS SCHIZOPHRENIA
## THE SAME WORLDWIDE?

Schizophrenia remains somewhat of a mystery to mental health workers. Its causes, subjective experience, and treatment are not well known. Added to this is the surprising fact that schizophrenia appears to be less chronic in developing countries (Kulhara, 1994). Two key researchers, Nancy Waxler and Assen Jablensky, working independently, have confirmed this. Jablensky and his colleagues (1992) studied schizophrenia in 10 countries. They found twice as many first-contact psychotics from developing countries in complete remission 2 years later compared with those in developed countries (38% versus 16%). Waxler (1979) in Sri Lanka reported that 40% of patients hospitalized for schizophrenia had no additional episodes. Almost half worked continuously and a further 38% worked occasionally. According to their families, 58% took on normal social roles within their families. This may be due to differences in the type of psychosis being presented, in light of the fact that broad-band psychosis had double the incidence rate in developing countries (4% versus 2%) although schizophrenia had the same rate of 1%. Some of those diagnosed as psychotic may have a type of disorder that is acute and reactive, with only one episode. Jablensky (1995) considered the option of creating a special category for these people, called "nonaffective acute remitting psychosis." However, because their initial profile does not differ from others, the category is useless as a diagnosis. Patients could be identified only after remission. The *ICD-10* now has a category called Acute and Transient Psychotic Disorders, although if complete recovery does not occur within a few months, a change in classification is suggested. Why this is more common in developing than in developed countries is not known.

found specifically in one culture. A few syndromes have been identified that are more frequent in certain cultures, although they do not appear to violate the classification systems in existence. The fact that laypeople have their own system of causal attributions does not necessarily warrant revision of the scientific system of causes and classifications, although it might explain why traditional healers who share the lay system are more frequently sought for relief.

I suggest an empirical strategy to compare the Euro-American system of syndromes with a culture-based derivation of syndromes. The first step would be to find cases using community informants and health care workers. The cases would include people considered by the community to be mentally ill. The second step would be to collect a list of all the symptoms commonly reported by these people and their families; the ill people would likely describe internal experiences, and the family would likely describe external behaviors. A checklist of these plus the internationally compiled symptoms (from the *CIDI*) would then be used when interviewing mentally ill and mentally healthy people. The responses would be factor analyzed and normed to determine which symptoms actually occur together. One attempt to use this strategy (Mulatu, 1995a) found a great deal of overlap in syndromes between North America and Ethiopia. There were two major differences: Two new syndromes appeared, and the symptoms within clusters were not always the same. For example, somatic symptoms did not cluster separately but appeared commonly along with psychological descriptors in various syndromes. In North America, the somatic syndrome in children and the somatization disorder in adults reflects the fact that somatic complaints represent a qualitatively different category of mental disorder. However, although the lifetime prevalence of somatization disorder in the United States—requiring at least eight physical symptoms—is .13%, a much higher figure of 11.6% of the sample reported a slightly lower number of four to six physical symptoms (Robins et al., 1991). Thus the cultural differences do not always appear to be as great as we initially thought.

## PREVALENCE OF MENTAL ILLNESS

As stated previously, one of the purposes for developing cross-cultural measures of mental illness is to determine the number of people in a community who might need mental health services. Specifically, one of the goals is to find out if mental illness is universal; if it is, then there should be no need to survey each and every community. The results of a few surveys in each region should be sufficient to generalize to a wider population and to accurately assess the need for services.

**TABLE 9.1** One-Year Prevalence Rates in the United States and Taiwan

| Disorder | Five U.S. Sites | Three Taiwanese Sites |
|---|---|---|
| Mental retardation | 1.0% | — |
| Dementia (> 65 yrs) | 1.4% | 3.8% |
| Alcohol abuse | 3.8% | 7.2% |
| Schizophrenia | 1.0% | 0.3% |
| Mood (depression, bipolar) | 5.0% | 3.0% |
| Anxiety | 20.0% | 13.0% |
| Personality | 16.5% | — |
| Somatization | 0.13% | 0.08% |
| Any diagnosis | 15.3% | 21.56% |

Two types of people have been surveyed: community samples and people attending health services. Generally, the prevalence rates in community surveys of the general population range from 10% to 20% with higher figures if alcoholism is assessed. Large surveys in the United States (Regier et al., 1993) and Taiwan (Compton et al., 1991), using the *Diagnostic Interview Schedule (DIS)* described previously, found 1-year prevalence rates to be 15.3% and 21.5%, respectively. In both countries, anxiety disorders were the most common (see Table 9.1).

Only a portion of these people actually show up at a health clinic, and less than half of these are identified by health workers (Goldberg, 1995). Consequently, surveys have been conducted at health centers to determine how many seek help with physical or psychological complaints, and how many are identified by health workers. For example, a survey in Manchester, England, found the following: Out of 100 adults in the general population, 25 had a mental disorder according to the *DIS*, 21 showed up at a general health center, and 10 were identified as having psychological problems (Goldberg, 1995). In developing countries, health workers tend to detect mental illness in only 30% of their adult patients and 10% of their child patients (Harding et al., 1980). An awareness of these "missed opportunities" to treat people who come to a clinic, but are never identified, has provoked a surge of mental health training for general health workers.

If the focus of detection and treatment were to be the health clinic, one would want to know what percentage of patients who come with physical illness have a mental health problem. In this case, the denominator of the calculation is the number of patients tested. The rate found among a relatively unselected population at 15 health centers around the world was 24% (Goldberg, 1995), ranging from 8% in Shanghai, China, to 53% in Santiago, Chile. The most common diagnoses were depression (10.2%), generalized anxiety (8.2%), and alcohol use (5.8%), although 40% had more than one diagnosis. Practically all had somatic rather than psychological complaints.

In brief, community surveys of both adults and children report rates from 10% to 20%, and health center surveys range from 20% to 30% (Abiodun, 1993b; Giel et al., 1981; Harding et al., 1980; Mulatu, 1995a). The rates appear to be similar in developed and developing countries. Diagnoses may differ by culture, gender, and age. For example, acute and transient schizophrenia is at least double in developing compared with developed countries (Jablensky et al., 1992); boys are more likely to have hyperactivity and aggression, women more depression and anxiety (phobia and panic), and men more alcoholism and antisocial personality.

## SOCIAL AND PERSONAL CONSEQUENCES

The social impact of mental illness is high, although it may differ by culture. It depends on prevailing attitudes toward mental illness as well as the role demands of the society. In industrialized countries, mental illness is viewed as a major disability that interferes with normal functioning within the family and workplace. In many developing countries, mentally ill people are tolerated and expected to adopt family and community roles. For example, Waxler (1979) suggests that strong, supportive families in developing countries tolerate the abnormal behavior of their members, and traditional communities may integrate mentally ill people by providing them with economic and social roles. Thus, to the extent that attitudes are positive, the community will provide productive roles that minimize the financial and social costs of mental illness.

Studies of community attitudes toward mental illness (Wig et al., 1980), using key informants as their source, indicate that in some cultures, such as Sudan, people consider mental illness to be serious but to have few negative consequences for work and marriage. In others, such as India, informants said mentally ill people would have problems finding a marriage partner and a job, and even problems living with their families.

Attitudes toward epilepsy provide an interesting example. Although most epileptics are capable of performing social and occupational roles, in many cultures they do not; by implication, negative community attitudes prevent them from doing so. In places where epileptics do not receive medication to control their convulsions, people have seen their seizures and developed fearful attitudes toward epilepsy. In an Ethiopian community where the prevalence rate of epilepsy was 5.2 per 1,000, the mostly illiterate population preferred to avoid an epileptic adult, but fewer people were negative toward an epileptic child (Tekle-Haimanot et al., 1991). Although 14% had a family member with epilepsy, 45% thought it was contagious, 75% said they would not employ an epileptic, 74% would not let someone from their family marry an epileptic, and 60% would not befriend an epileptic. When asked how society should take care of people with epilepsy, 46% did not know and 34% said by giving alms. Marginalized in this way by community attitudes, many epileptic adults leave their communities and live by begging alms.

Whether due to social stigma or to problems in functioning, mental illness has a number of serious consequences for the community, the family, and the person. Briefly, they include the following:

- Economic underproductivity and inability to work regularly (Westermeyer, 1984)
- Marital breakdown
- Inadequate child rearing, abuse, neglect, and child pathology
- A burden on health services as the sufferer returns frequently because he or she does not get relief from the treatment that is based on a misdiagnosis of physical illness

The magnitude of disability caused by mental illness is not generally appreciated. Ormel and colleagues (1994) asked patients at 15 primary health care facilities, in different countries, about limitations in performing daily activities and roles required by the family and community (e.g., gainful employment, household chores). They found that psychological problems interfered more than physical illness with daily functioning and prevented patients from carrying out the activities that help support their family and community.

Within the family, we have important social and emotional roles as a spouse and as a parent. In the long term, these roles may be as important as the economic ones. In some cultures, young adults with a mental illness are not marriageable. In countries where they do marry, researchers have examined whether the marriage suffers. In the United States, it does (E. Kelly & Conley, 1987). American couples were followed from the time they were first engaged to 40 years after. Marital stability and satisfaction were most negatively affected if the husband or wife was neurotic or if the husband lacked impulse control (usually leading to aggression or alcohol abuse). Even if spouses remain together, conflict between husband and wife can lead to behavior problems in sons and emotional problems in daughters. Similarly, mental problems are associated with poor parenting. Abusive and alcoholic parents are at the extreme end of poor parenting. Even parents with less extreme forms of mental illness, such as those who are hostile, aggressive, alcoholic, and depressed, cannot adequately perform their social and emotional roles as parents (e.g., Offord, Boyle, & Racine, 1989; Phares & Compas, 1992). The consequence is that the physical, mental, and social health of their children suffers.

## RISK FACTORS

Certain disorders are more prevalent at particular ages or among males or females. This does not necessarily implicate age or gender as a cause. For example, young boys are more likely to be hyperactive, girls to be fearful or withdrawn, adults to be schizophrenic, women to be depressed or anxious, and men to be alcoholic or antisocial (e.g., Paltiel, 1987). Hormones, child rearing, and social roles may account for some of the gender differences; nonetheless, they are neither necessary nor sufficient causes of mental illness. Because no definitive answers are available for the question of what causes mental illness, we will instead discuss **risk factors,** which refers to characteristics of people or their environments that are associated with mental illness and therefore increase the likelihood that these people will suffer from mental illness. Identifying risk factors allows us to narrow the field of possible causes for further study and to target certain populations that need support and monitoring. Similarly, the concept of **protective factors** is defined as characteristics of people or their environments that are associated with mental health in the presence of adversity (Garmezy & Masten, 1991; Rutter, 1985).

A family history of mental illness is a strong risk factor, due either to genetic or to environmental reasons. For example, 17% of children with a schizophrenic mother are likely to become schizophrenic themselves. Concordance rates, or the risk of having the disorder if a twin has it, are higher for monozygotic than for dizygotic twins in several cases: schizophrenia (48% versus 17%), bipolar mood disorder (69% versus 19%), unipolar depression (54% versus 24%), dementia (50% versus 20%), panic (31% versus 0%), phobia (24% versus 15%), and generalized anxiety (28% versus 17%) (Oltmanns & Emery, 1995). Thus genetic factors appear to play a role in these disorders. Unfortunately, it is difficult to separate the role of genetic similarity and environmental similarity: Monozygotic twins have more genetic similarity than dizygotic twins, but, because they look alike, they may also have more environmental similarity. Twin adoption studies allow a better assessment of the separate effects of genes and environment, as do DNA linkage studies. Yet these studies will probably produce similar conclusions, namely, that schizophrenia and depression have a strong genetic link, but that social and psychological conditions contribute to the onset of as well as to the recovery from these and other mental illnesses. Schizophrenia, in particular, appears to have a family link although the connection is much stronger in developed than in developing countries (Jablensky et al., 1992).

Stress is another common risk factor for mental disorders. A **stressor** is an aspect of the environment that is perceived as threatening or that requires adaptation. **Stress** is the internal state of tension or disequilibrium that results from repeated or intense stressors. Measures of stress assess either acute and uncommon life events (Holmes & Rahe, 1967), daily hassles that are minor or major recurring irritations (Kanner, Coyne, Schaefer, & Lazarus, 1981), or chronic strains characterized as "enduring aspects of the social and/or physical environment which involve deprivation or disadvantage and create a continuous stream of threats and challenges for the individual" (Compas, 1987, p. 276).

In developed countries, acute stressors and daily hassles may precipitate psychosomatic symptoms and other mental illnesses such as depression and anxiety (e.g., DeLongis, Coyne, Dakof, Folkman, & Lazarus, 1982). In developing countries, such as India, chronic strains are common enough to constitute the major threat to people's mental health (Lapore, Palsane, & Evans, 1991). They include lack of a steady income, inadequate food and water, housing that does not protect one from the elements, and overcrowding. Those with more chronic strains often tend to have less social support, further depriving them of ways to cope with the stressors. In one study, we found that stressors were more numerous for males than females, for the educated, for those with chronic physical disabilities, for those in the 35 to 44 age group, and for women who were divorced, separated, or widowed (Tafari, Aboud, & Larson, 1991). These groups, then, are at greater risk of having psychological complaints.

Women experience many stressors in their roles as mother, wife, and household manager. This is compounded by chronic strains such as lack of control over personal and family decisions, inequality in their relationships, and economic disadvantage. Women are overworked in their social roles and undervalued by their families and communities. Perhaps for this reason, they are more subject to depression, manic depression (bipolar disorder), and anxiety (Paltiel, 1987).

Family stress is also associated with child psychopathology among children (Links, 1983). Werner (1989) in Hawaii and Mulatu (1995a) in Ethiopia found that children were more likely to have behavior and emotional problems if they lived in homes where there was substance abuse and other chronic illnesses, unemployment, illiteracy, and crowding. However, living with only one biological parent does not appear to be a risk factor in developing countries as much as in developed countries (e.g., Giel & van Luijk, 1968), unless, of course, the child loses his or her mother in the early years. A child who loses a mother at birth is deprived of breast milk and therefore is at risk for malnutrition and other illnesses.

Protective factors concern characteristics of the person or the environment that make the person resistant to illness. Personal characteristics include high and stable self-esteem, optimism, intelligence, and an active, outgoing temperament. Social support is the best example of an environmental factor. People who live in developing countries are often part of a close extended family that supports the parenting role of mothers. Grandmothers, for example, are available for child care when the mother is busy with household chores or a newborn or preoccupied with emotional distress. This may explain why children who were part of an extended family in Khartoum, Sudan, had fewer behavior problems than those in nuclear families (El Hassan & Sonuga-Barke, 1992). Likewise, three protective factors prevented Hawaiian children from succumbing to mental problems despite high levels of early family stress. One was the presence of a surrogate parent or mentor who provided the child with advice and emotional support. Another was an active temperament that led the child to explore and seek contacts outside the family. A third protective factor was birth spacing, meaning that children who were well spaced received more family resources and developed a more secure attachment than they would have had other children followed closely (Werner, 1989).

There are cross-cultural similarities and differences in the way parents raise their children (e.g., LeVine et al., 1994; Weisner, 1989; Whiting & Edwards, 1988) and in the way children raise children on the streets (Aptekar. 1988). In all cultures, one can find emotional support in the form of affection, informational support in terms of transmitting knowledge about skills and resources, and tangible support in the form of food and shelter. Differences are more problematic in that, at first glance, some "supportive gestures" appear to be anything but. Weisner describes how support is given by adults and children to a distressed child in Kenya: The child will be given a job to calm him or her and this will be accompanied by teasing and dominance (aggression). Giving food to an upset child is also a common supportive response, whether or not hunger is the cause of the distress. These gestures serve to distract the child, and perhaps other empathic family members, so as to minimize disruptions to the family's work and leisure. Teaching a child how to cope with emotional distress through distraction has its value, particularly if one has no control over the problem that led to the distress. Other cultures emphasize planful problem solving and emotional support, in the sense of building self-confidence, to tackle the problem directly. Cultures differ in the extent to which they emphasize problem-focused or emotion-focused coping and individual or collective strategies (e.g., Folkman & Lazarus, 1988; Triandis, Bontempo, Villareal, Asai, & Lucca, 1988).

## PREVENTION AND TREATMENT

The 10% to 20% point prevalence for mental illness and 1% lifetime prevalence for schizophrenia translate into many millions of people living with emotional pain. The availability of health professionals trained to deal with mental illness is so low in many developing countries that mental health care is virtually unavailable to all but a few urban dwellers. Consequently, people seek help from traditional healers and family members before going to a clinic. These three options for treatment will be discussed: traditional healers, community/clinic health workers, and the family. But first there is a reminder that prevention is the best cure.

Prevention

Prevention of mental illness is rarely addressed (except by Eisenberg, 1993) but may be implied by the list of risk and protective factors. When mothers are mentally ill, their children need to find parent surrogates, such as relatives and teachers, to whom they can become attached and from whom they can learn appropriate social and emotional skills. High-quality day care for preschoolers is effective, as a supplement to family life, in developing useful cognitive, social, and emotional skills. Community- and school-based programs targeted at certain groups of people, such as sons of alcoholics, teenage girls, and divorced or widowed women, could strengthen the skills needed by these groups to cope with the problems they may encounter. Programs that are part of UNICEF's promotion of immunization, good nutrition, injury prevention, and family planning also prevent many cases of mental illness. Immunization against measles, for example, prevents a form of mental retardation called measles encephalitis; good nutrition facilitates a secure attachment to the mother and positive social relations to peers; injury prevention eliminates sensory and motor disabilities; and family planning allows the child time to develop a strong bond with its mother and enough food and attention to develop mentally and physically. The UNICEF book called *Facts for Life* (Adamson, 1993) has a section on how to provide stimulation and emotional support to young children, which are as important as physical support, although they are often overlooked.

Treatment

The goal of treatment is not to cure the patient, because this is difficult to accomplish. Rather, it is to reduce relapses, reduce symptoms, and optimize the person's social and economic functioning. Two features of successful programs have caught the attention of mental health care planners. The first is that goals can best be achieved if the patient remains close to the family rather than in large urban institutions. The second is that lower level professionals cost less and can be adequately trained. Thus the new approach is to decentralize and deprofessionalize treatment. This entails primarily setting up community-based rehabilitation programs outside cities, integrating mental and physical disability services, and giving short training to primary health care workers. With these services in place, the treatment would consist of medication to prevent relapses along with family and patient education. Whether or not this new system will be attractive enough to compete with the popularity of traditional healers remains to be seen.

*Traditional healers.* Dating from long before the advent of modern medicine and existing now in parallel with it in most developing countries is a well-developed system of traditional beliefs and traditional healing practices (Kortmann, 1987). Many types of mental illness are thought to be caused by supernatural powers. There are family and community ancestral spirits who protect against illness unless angered by a broken taboo. There are evil spirits such as the devil and the evil eye that possess a person or cast a shadow. Sometimes the evil is cast by another person in the community who is jealous of a healthy child or a beautiful woman. People therefore try to protect themselves by wearing an amulet, staying close to other people, and avoiding risky acts such as neglecting responsibilities to one's family or walking alone in a forest. These animistic beliefs are tolerated and often condoned by the established religions of Christianity and Islam. Similarly, educated people continue to believe in spiritual as well as social and personal causes of illness and health. If the cause of the illness is thought to be external to the sufferer and supernatural, people will be more sympathetic to the sufferer. The treatment of choice in this case is a traditional or religious healer, one specializing in magical powers. The treatment may consist of holy water, sacrificial rites to appease the angry spirits, powerful suggestions directed at the evil eye, confessions, and a trance state to exorcise the spirit. For a substance abuse problem, the herbalist will be sought.

Despite their popularity, the success rate of traditional and religious healers is often no better than that of health professionals (Giel, Gezahegn, & van Luijk, 1968; Workneh & Giel, 1975). Perhaps this is because only chronic patients seek help from traditional healers, after they have received no relief from health workers and pharmacists. Yet others have concluded that traditional therapies are effective at managing symptoms of neurotic, psychotic, psychosomatic, and psychosocial disorders, along with alcohol/drug dependence and reactive depression (Jelik, 1993). Whatever side one takes in this debate, one must acknowledge that the popularity of traditional healers far outweighs their success.

Why is this so? One explanation is the accessibility of traditional healers. They are part of an informal network, and they share the people's beliefs about causes and cures of illness. They accept the patients' and their families' description of the problem and use procedures that people are familiar with. Some experts attribute the success of healers to their charismatic personality style, which gives them the power to reduce anxiety and guilt in the patient and family (Jelik, 1993). To the extent that negative emotions and family stress are part of the problem, this form of treatment may be successful, at least in the short term. Unfortunately, another reason for the popularity of healers is the conspicuous lack of success and frequent disinterest of health workers who are not trained to understand or manage mental illness. More often than not, mentally ill patients will receive treatment for their somatic complaints; when this brings no relief, they return again and again, only to acquire a reputation as a complainer or malingerer. To obtain treatment from a mental health professional, people are forced to leave home with a family member and travel to a large city—an expensive and disruptive burden.

*Families and communities.* In one Ethiopian study, respondents advocated family and home care over healers for all forms of mental illness except those caused by supernatural retribution. Family care was preferred for illnesses caused by stress, social disadvantage, and biological defects (Mulatu, 1995b). This is consistent with the well-known fact that families in developing countries have usually taken on the responsibility of looking after their sick members. Traditional values legitimate the strong influence of older family members as well as doing things in the same way they have been done in the past. According to a community attitude study of mental illness (Wig et al., 1980), key informants in three developing countries thought that there would be little or no problem for a neurotic, psychotic, or mentally retarded person living at home; problems might arise only if he or she ventured into the community to seek a job or marriage partner. Thus, although mentally ill people are well cared for by their families, they may be ostracized by the larger community. The community's response may seem at odds with our notion of collectivist cultures. It makes more sense when we realize that the collective refers to the family, not to the whole community. In fact, there is a sharper division between the in-group (extended family and friends) and the out-group in collectivist cultures than in individualist cultures (Triandis et al., 1988).

The social and economic impairment of schizophrenics and people suffering from other psychoses appears to be minimal when patients are cared for by their families. Because families are supportive and because productive work is often unskilled (livestock management, weeding and harvesting, crafts, collecting firewood and water), schizophrenics continue to maintain their social roles in the family and rarely require hospitalization.

There are differing explanations for the finding that schizophrenics in developing countries show higher rates of recovery and better functioning with the family. One is social labeling theory, which suggests that better outcomes result when negative labels are not attached to the schizophrenic. The negative connotation in developed countries constrains patients and families to expect negative outcomes and to behave in ways that fulfill the expectation. Perhaps more to the point are the external causes (supernatural or social stress) held responsible for mental illness in developing countries, so that family and community members feel sympathetic to the sufferer. With this attitude, it is easier to include patients in family life and tolerate a certain amount of unusual behavior. Another explanation focuses on a difference in the type of schizophrenia being diagnosed. Although the incidence of narrowly defined schizophrenia is similar throughout the world, the incidence of paranoid schizophrenia is lower and the incidence of acute, transient schizophrenia is (four times) higher in developing countries (Jablensky et al., 1992). The latter group may be the ones showing better functioning and recovery.

A final explanation is based on the concept of expressed emotion, which refers to criticism and other negative emotions communicated to the patient. Evidence from different countries, such as India, shows that patients recover better if their families express less negative emotion (e.g., Leff et al., 1990). In developed countries, treatment aimed at reducing expressed emotion in the families of schizophrenics has reduced relapses by half or more in comparison with a group who had drug treatment only (Hogarty et al., 1986; Langsley, Hodes, & Grimson, 1993). Thus the concept of expressed emotion within the family has important implications for cross-cultural differences as well as for treatment of schizophrenia and other disorders.

*Health workers.* Typically, health workers in developing countries receive little training in the nature and treatment of mental illness. Consequently, their ability to detect cases of mental illness at a clinic was very poor: They identified 33% of adult cases and under 10% of child cases (e.g., Abiodun, 1993b; Giel et al., 1981; Harding et al., 1980). In Nigeria, the health workers thought that 5% or less of their caseload had mental disorders, compared with the 21.3% identified by symptom checklists (Abiodun, 1993a). When presented with vignettes describing the symptoms of seven disorders, 71% identified the psychotic but only 36% identified the neurotic. Health workers therefore may be no more accurate than untrained community members in identifying mental illness. Recall that key informants in the Wig et al. (1980) study, despite their many social contacts, could identify only two to four people with a mental illness. Health workers also tend to share the population's views on the cause of mental illness and may be reluctant to tamper with ancestral or evil spirits.

Health workers also have an attitude problem; in one Nigerian study, 72% had a negative attitude toward mentally ill patients (Abiodun, 1991). The frustration of not understanding and not being able to find relief for their complaints may turn into hostility and rejection. Because of these problems, health workers have not in the past satisfactorily treated mental illness. Since the initial studies, attempts have been made to train rural health workers in the identification of mental disorders and to use psychiatric nurses in rural settings to dispense antipsychotic and antidepressant drugs (Saraceno, Tognoni, & Garattini, 1993).

Despite their shortcomings, health workers are considered to be the best partners to work along with families in treating mentally ill people. Short training of primary health workers and psychiatric nurses has been successful (Giel et al., 1988; Gittelman et al., 1989). A manual for community mental health workers produced by the Schizophrenic Research Foundation (SCARF) India (Thara, Padmavati, & Ayankaran, 1995) outlines ways to include family, employer, and community supports in the care of a mentally ill person. In some cases, health workers who deal with rehabilitation of physical disabilities are chosen to extend their responsibilities to rehabilitation of mental disabilities. The goal is to improve diagnoses, give low-dosage medication when needed, and provide education to families and patients on the course of the illness and the need to continue medication. The term *family psychoeducation* is used to refer to the periodic meetings held with a patient and his or her family to discuss information about the illness, noncritical communication, problem solving, and taking medication. Unlike therapy in developed countries, those who work in the mental health field in developing countries feel there is no need to schedule regular long-term visits with the patient because the family provides sufficient social support. The two major thrusts of this approach are to decentralize mental health services into community-based rehabilitation programs and to deprofessionalize the dispenser of services. There appears to be some optimism for the success of such programs (e.g., Gittelman et al., 1989; Langsley et al., 1993; Phillips, Pearson, & Wang, 1994).

## STUDENT ACTIVITY

At the end of their comprehensive book on world mental health, Desjarlais, Eisenberg, Good, and Kleinman (1995) rightly point out that, although health is defined in terms of physical, mental, and social well-being, too little attention is being paid to mental and social health. Their agenda for research proposes, among others, two priority areas that were not extensively discussed in this book. One is collective and interpersonal violence, and the second is women's mental health. What is known about these two issues around the world, such as their prevalence, outcomes, risk/protective factors, and prevention?

# A FINAL NOTE: WHERE DO YOU GO FROM HERE?

Forward-looking enthusiasm, tempered with caution and realistic expectations, has spiced this overview of international health. The enthusiasm to try harder is what motivates people who work in developing countries. Yet it is all too easy to pack a few facts in your head and some money in your pocket and launch a new campaign to eradicate ill health and poverty. As one of my colleagues tactfully put it to me, "Be careful you don't just fire up another wave of idealistic workers to go out and press contraceptives on reluctant women." I hope we have realized that problems and solutions are not as simple as they appear at first glance.

The catchphrase of UNICEF and other international agencies is "local problems generating global solutions." Problems, such as not enough food and exposure to HIV, are experienced at a local level—within the person, the family, and the community—with variations at each level. While recognizing that people have different emotional reactions to these problems, ranging from anger to acceptance, the community health approach focuses on their common experiences. People who share a culture often experience health and illness similarly. So it is reasonable to generate solutions within a cultural community. But, although we like to think of ourselves and our culture as unique, we share many health-related practices and problems with other cultures. The evil eye, attraction to injections, food taboos, withholding food and fluid from a sick child, and myths about condoms and AIDS are common across cultures. For this reason, it is important to learn about problems and solutions in other cultures, and to build on them and modify them when developing solutions for our own. Global solutions, such as the child immunization program and oral rehydration salts, have many components that are universal while allowing for cultural flexibility at the community level.

Other solutions have no universal appeal because they have not worked at the local level in many countries, although they might have worked in some. The system of community health workers has not worked in many places, although we have been able to learn lessons from these failures. We have learned that the health workers need regular and frequent supervision and a resource such as drugs to make them gain respectability in their communities. Community participation is a promising activity, but as implemented in many countries, it has not increased the use of health services. Many health education projects have not had the impact they hoped for because they changed knowledge but not behavior. From these experiences, we learn that change does not come about easily. Some people are receptive to the innovative practices proposed, but many others are not convinced enough to change their habits. Basic primary school education seems to be the one common resource that makes a difference. But even this is not universally acceptable in its present form.

Where you go from here depends on the kind of expertise you can offer. Several routes appear to be more promising than others. One route is with NGOs who work at the grassroots level. They can make a difference by promoting change through community involvement. NGOs often have job openings for people who are good at helping groups to

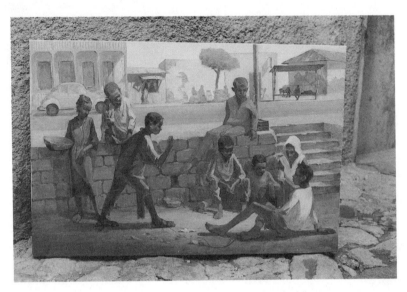

*A painting of Ethiopian street children gathering to play, by Yitagesu.*

organize and make decisions. Changes at the community level are sustainable if they are institutionalized through training managers, forming decision-making structures, and identifying sources of funds and human resources. Another route is work within local health and educational institutions and government structures to train people. Governments usually have a clear idea of the kinds of skills they are lacking, and these are most often at the mid- and lower level health worker positions. Specialists are not likely to be their priority.

A final route is by working with governments to bring about policy changes. A recent headline in the *Guardian Weekly* read, "Foreign Aid 'Has No Impact'" (Blustein, 1997). Reviewing an upcoming World Bank report, the article pointed out that billions of dollars in foreign aid have produced no appreciable impact on the overall economic performance of the Third World because governments have not developed and implemented new policies aimed at reforming old practices. Some countries, such as Ghana, have used aid to support policy reform, but many others have not. Good government, quality education, and involved communities are three important catalysts for change.

The most important lesson we have learned and relearned is that people and problems cannot be stereotyped. After reading Lewis Aptekar's (1988) book on street children, I realized that I had a stereotype of street children as forlorn, frightened, homeless boys. This description fits some, but not all, of them. Many are very competent and confident, and grow up to be productive, satisfied members of their society. Through research, we learn about the way different cultures give meaning to health and illness, as well as the way they raise their children. We may see problems in the way other people conduct their lives. Our ethnocentrism often hinders us from realizing that there are many different routes to the same goal of well-being.

I hope this book has helped you become informed about health problems and solutions in an international perspective. Research and personal experience have informed my own awareness. Only when we give others the research tools to inform themselves can we hope to achieve a workable partnership.

# *GLOSSARY*

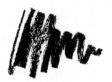

**Absolute poverty level:** The income level below which a minimum nutritionally adequate diet plus essential nonfood requirements is not affordable.

**Acceptability:** People's satisfaction with the health service in question.

**Access to adequate sanitation:** Percentage of the population that has household waste disposal facilities such as a latrine and garbage pit.

**Access to health services:** Percentage of the population that can reach appropriate local health services by the local means of transportation in no more than 1 hour; sometimes a distance of 10 km is used. Documents usually provide separate figures for urban and rural populations because of the disparity.

**Access to safe water:** Percentage of the population that can reach a protected source of drinking water that is uncontaminated by parasites and bacteria.

**Acute respiratory infection:** An infection of the tract from the nose to the lungs. The most fatal, pneumonia, is an infection of the lungs.

**Adult literacy rate:** Percentage of persons aged 15 and over who can read and write. This probably requires 4 years of formal schooling.

**Affordability:** The total cost to a client, including payment for service and transportation to the service.

**Aid:** Emergency, life-saving interventions that are not intended to be sustained; 80% of donor funds and resources are used for aid.

**Alcohol abuse or harmful use:** Harmfully excessive and recurrent use of alcohol resulting in physical, personal, or social problems. One or more of the following alcohol-related problems are experienced within a 12-month period: (a) failure to fulfill major role obligations at work, school, or home; (b) recurrent use in physically hazardous situations such as when using industrial equipment or driving an automobile; (c) legal problems such as arrests; and (d) continued use despite persistent social or interpersonal problems exacerbated by the effects of alcohol.

**Alcohol dependency:** Excessive and prolonged drinking, which affects the person at many levels and creates physiological dependency that manifests as withdrawal (symptoms of nonuse such as seizures and tremors) and tolerance (needing more alcohol to have an effect), craving alcohol, and curtailing normal activities so as to obtain alcohol.

**Alcohol intoxication:** A temporary state due to the recent consumption of alcohol resulting in maladaptive behavioral or psychological changes such as aggressive or argumentative behavior, disinhibition, and impaired social or occupational functioning. Other signs such as slurred speech and uncoordinated movements are apparent. Legal levels of intoxication may be under 0.10% blood alcohol concentration (BAC), which means 100 parts of alcohol per 10,000 parts of blood, or 100 mg of alcohol per 100 ml of blood.

**Alcoholism:** The excessive and regular use of alcohol leading to alcohol-related problems.

**Attitudes:** Predispositions to respond in a positive or negative manner toward a person, object, or event.

# Glossary

**Autonomy:** Having the resources necessary to think, decide, and act independently, using but not needing input from others.

**Availability:** The number of health workers serving 1,000 people.

**Behavioral diagnosis of a health problem:** The process by which we look at the causes of a health problem and find out whether human behavior is involved in its prevention or treatment.

**Biopsychosocial framework:** A systematic approach that seeks to understand health and illness in terms of three components: biological, psychological, and social.

**Births attended by a trained health worker:** Percentage of deliveries made by someone trained in obstetric care as opposed to deliveries made by relatives or traditional attendants who do not follow sterile procedures.

**Breast-feeding:** Percentage of children who are exclusively breast-fed from 0 to 3 months, breast-fed along with solid food (6-9 months), and breast-fed for up to 2 years (20-23 months).

**Children reaching grade 5 of primary school:** Percentage of the children entering the first grade of primary school who eventually reach grade 5. The difference from 100% is the dropout rate. Note that some children may not even enter first grade.

**CIDI-SAM:** The *Composite International Diagnostic Interview's Substance Abuse Module*, which assesses whether a person has a serious problem of substance abuse and dependency, including alcohol abuse and dependency.

**Cognition:** Interpreting the world, memory, learning, thinking, reasoning, problem solving, and knowledge.

**Communication:** The transmission of a message from one person to another. It can be face to face or mass media, auditory and visual; it can be informative and emotional and persuasive; it can be positive (what to do and the benefits) and negative (what not to do and the disadvantages).

**Community health workers (CHW):** People who are selected by their communities and given some training in health so that they can serve their community by performing basic preventive and curative services.

**Community participation:** A social process whereby specific groups with shared needs living in a defined geographic area actively pursue identification of their needs, make decisions, and establish mechanisms to meet these needs.

**Conduct disorder:** A childhood mental health problem, comparable to the term *antisocial personality* used for people 18 years and older. It describes people who are aggressive, destructive of property, deceitful, or who frequently violate rules.

**Contraceptive prevalence rate:** Percentage of married women aged 15-49 years currently using contraception.

**Coping:** Cognitive and behavioral efforts to manage specific external and/or internal demands that are appraised as taxing or exceeding the resources of the person. Coping strategies include, among others, social support seeking, planful problem solving, and escape/avoidance.

**Coverage:** The proportion of the population that received a particular health service, such as immunization or antenatal care.

**Crude birth rate:** Annual number of births per 1,000 population.

**Crude death rate:** Annual number of deaths per 1,000 population.

**Dehydration:** A loss of water and dissolved salts from the body that occurs, for instance, as a result of diarrhea.

**Dependency ratio:** The number of people under 15 years and over 49 years of age divided by the number of people aged 15 to 49 years.

**Dependent population:** Percentage of the population 0 to 15 years of age.

**Development:** Interventions that are intended to be sustainable, such as skill training and resource building; 20% of donor funds and resources are used for development. Health development activities are only one part of overall development, which also includes agriculture and education.

***Diagnostic and Statistical Manual (DSM-IV)* for mental disorders:** The classification system used in North America. It covers organic mental disorders, substance-related disorders, schizophrenia, mood disorders, anxiety disorders, somatoform disorders, sexual disorders, eating and sleep disorders, personality disorders, and developmental disorders.

**Diarrheal diseases:** An illness of the digestive system, caused by many microorganisms, the most common of which are rotavirus and Escherichia coli. A child with diarrhea passes three or more loose, watery stools in one day, and this continues for several days.

**Disability adjusted life years (DALYs) lost:** The product of two indicators. The first is the number of years lost, calculated by subtracting the age of death or onset of disability from the life expectancy of a healthy person, usually set between 65 and 75. The second is a value from 0 to 1, representing the degree of functional disability; death receives a maximum value of 1 and minor disabilities are closer to 0.

**Effectiveness:** An indicator of how well the service worked, such as the percentage of children who recovered from diarrhea after receiving ORT.

**Emic-etic dilemma:** Two extreme ways of incorporating cultural differences in a measure. Emic is the strategy of including items derived from and relevant to a particular culture with no intention of comparing responses from another culture. Etic is the strategy of importing a measure developed in one culture to another culture, for the sake of comparability. There are strategies in between these two extremes, for example, maintaining some constancy in the underlying concepts while varying the surface expression.

**Emotion:** States of affect (e.g., happiness, anger, fear), moods (a brief positive or negative emotion), and attitudes (long-term evaluations of people, objects, and events).

**Empowerment:** The gaining of power, influence, and control over one's life at personal, interpersonal, and community levels.

**Endemic:** A situation in which a disease commonly exists at very high levels in a particular locality.

**Epidemic:** A situation in which a disease that is normally not common experiences an outbreak and becomes very prevalent.

**Episodic heavy drinking:** Having six or more drinks per occasion at least weekly, similar to regular binge drinking.

**Estimate:** A close approximation of the true value of a variable based on the partial information available from a representative sample of the population.

**Focus group:** A method of collecting information on people's perceptions and opinions. A group of people with similar backgrounds are brought together to talk about a specific topic of interest under the guidance of a moderator.

**Fully immunized 1-year-old children:** Percentage of all 1-year-old children who have been immunized for tuberculosis, diphtheria, pertussis, tetanus, polio, and measles. More than 120 million babies born each year need to receive vaccinations on five occasions during their first year.

**GNP and GDP:** Gross national product and gross domestic product reflect the amount of money spent and earned on goods and services, which reflects the economic activity of a country.

**Goiter rate:** Percentage of children aged 6-11 with palpable or visible goiter. This is an indicator of iodine deficiency, which causes mental retardation.

**Habit:** A set of actions that has become automatic, fixed, and easily and effortlessly carried out as a result of repetition.

**Hazardous consumption:** Operationally defined as an average daily consumption of six or more drinks in a typical month for men and four or more drinks for women.

**Health:** Physical, mental, and social well-being—an important resource for a satisfying and productive life.

**Health behaviors:** Actions that directly influence one's own and others' health. They include behaviors that promote physical well-being, prevent illness, and manage or eliminate illness, and also those that demote or reduce health.

**Health education:** A process with intellectual, psychological, and social dimensions relating to activities that increase the abilities of people to make informed decisions affecting their personal, family, and community well-being. This process, based on scientific principles, facilitates learning and behavioral change in both health personnel and consumers, including children and youth.

**Health locus of control:** Generalized expectancies that either self (internal), powerful others (P), or chance (C) determine one's health and illness. A fourth source of health and illness for some cultures may be powerful spirits.

**Health promotion:** Political, social, and educational action that enhances public awareness of health, fosters healthy lifestyles and community action in support of health, and empowers people to exercise their rights and responsibilities in shaping environments, systems, and policies that are conducive to health and well-being.

**Incidence:** A measure of the occurrence of new cases over a specified time interval (frequently 1 year).

**Infant mortality rate:** Number of deaths of infants under 1 year of age per 1,000 live births.

***International Classification of Disease (ICD-10):*** Classification system for all disorders developed by the World Health Organization, which covers organic mental disorders, substance-related disorders, schizophrenia, mood disorders, anxiety disorders, somatoform disorders, sexual disorders, eating and sleep disorders, personality disorders, and developmental disorders.

**International health:** A multidisciplinary field of study that takes a multination perspective on the state of people's health, seeking knowledge and effective action strategies through a systematic examination of health problems, their determinants, and their solutions around the world.

**KAP questionnaire:** A structured set of questions that assess knowledge, attitudes, and practices relevant for a particular health problem. The items should be answered in the reverse order—PAK—so that describing what you do is not influenced by hearing the knowledge items.

**Key informant interviews:** Unstructured questioning of informed individuals to collect information quickly about events and people in a community or to gain a deeper understanding of how community members think about an event. A key informant has wide contacts, good communication skills, and a reflective attitude.

**Knowledge:** All the information possessed by a person or group, however it was acquired (i.e., a form of cognition).

**Kwashiorkor:** A form of malnutrition due to insufficient protein in one's diet. The child's legs and sometimes face are swollen with edema; the skin becomes flaky and the hair turns a red color.

**Leadership style:** The task-oriented or relation-oriented style one uses to influence and motivate other people.

**Learning:** The process of acquiring a relatively permanent mental or behavioral response as a result of rewarded practice or observation of someone performing the behavior. The reward may take the form of a biologically satisfying object or it may be social approval and recognition. The observed model is likely to be a parent, older sibling, or teacher.

**Leprosy:** A disease caused by the Mycobacterium leprae. A mild form results in depigmentation of a patch of skin that spontaneously heals, whereas a more severe form results in damage to nerves, bones, and muscles.

**Lessons learned:** A phrase that refers to reasons for a failure, which we identify after much reflection and evaluation and hope not to repeat in subsequent attempts.

**Level of confidence:** A numerical value that describes an interval within which one is certain the estimate exists. A narrow interval indicates certainty and unlikelihood of error.

**Life expectancy at birth:** The number of years newborn children would live if subject to the mortality risks prevailing for the cross section of population at the time of their birth.

**Locus of control:** In terms of health, it is the expectation that either oneself or others or chance factors determine one's health and illness.

**Low birth weight infants:** Newborns weighing less than 2,500 gm. If the child is a full-term newborn, the low birth weight is attributed to intrauterine growth retardation.

**Malaria:** An infection due to a parasite that is carried by the Anopheles mosquito. The main symptom is a fever.

**Malnutrition:** A state of deficiency in energy, protein, or other micronutrients such as vitamin A, iodine, and iron.

**Marasmus:** An extreme form of malnutrition, the result of insufficient calories due to diet or illness. The child's body lacks the layer of fat normally seen under the skin, and the muscles are wasted.

**Maternal depletion:** The decline in a woman's health as a result of giving birth to many children in countries where women experience ill health, malnutrition, and closely spaced births.

**Maternal mortality:** The number of women who die in pregnancy and childbirth is usually expressed as the number of deaths from pregnancy-related causes per 100,000 live births (which is a proxy for the number of pregnancies).

**McGill Pain Questionnaire:** Measures the subjective perception of tissue injury, extreme temperature, or pressure in terms of sensory and emotional experiences.

**Measles:** A very contagious viral disease transmitted from person to person through simple respiration. The main symptoms are rash and fever.

**Mental disorders:** Behavioral or psychological syndromes (groups of associated features) that are associated with one or more of the following: present distress, impairment in one or more important areas of functioning, a significantly increased risk of suffering death, pain, or disability.

**Mental health:** Satisfactory functioning in cognitive, emotional, and social domains.

**Motivation:** Energized, goal-directed behavior, influenced by need, value of the goal, and expectations of reward.

**Neonatal tetanus:** A disease acquired when the tetanus bacteria, present in the soil and dust, enter an open wound. In the case of newborns, the bacteria enter from unsterile razors or other sharp objects used to cut the umbilical cord or from improper dressing or cleaning of the stump. Tetanus manifests with rigidity of the mouth and lips and, finally, death.

**Nongovernmental organizations (NGOs):** Organizations or institutions that conduct activities in one or more countries on the basis of a written agreement with the host country. They are generally nonprofit groups that raise money from donors and government agencies in their own countries. Their goals are to promote development and training, and they often work at the grassroots level with local communities.

**Number of radio and television sets per 1,000 population:** Indicates the amount of public information received by a population.

**Official development assistance (ODA):** Annual amount of grants, in U.S. dollars, received from donor governments to be used for development. A target level of 0.7% of the donor's GNP was set in 1969, but few countries now meet this standard. This figure is also expressed as a percentage of the recipient country's GNP.

**Oral rehydration salts (ORS):** Specifically, the standard WHO/UNICEF-recommended formula, which consists of four constituents: sodium chloride, trisodium citrate (or sodium bicarbonate), potassium chloride, and glucose. Dissolved in 1 liter of clean drinking water, it is given to children to prevent or correct dehydration resulting from diarrhea.

**Oral rehydration therapy (ORT):** The administration of fluid by mouth to prevent or correct the dehydration that is a consequence of diarrhea, including use of porridge, drinks, and ORS.

**ORT use rate:** Percentage of all cases of diarrhea in children under 5 years of age treated with oral rehydration salts (the UNICEF sachet) or an appropriate household solution of salt, sugar, water, and sometimes porridge.

**Pandemic:** A situation in which a disease becomes common and spreads to many locations.

**Participant observation:** An in-depth case study of group life from the perspective of someone who has a prolonged, intense involvement in that life, that is based on naturalistic observations and information intentionally solicited.

**Per capita alcohol consumption:** An estimate of the amount of alcohol consumed in a country per person (sometimes excluding abstainers). Figures are usually based on what is commercially produced in the country plus whatever is imported minus whatever is exported during that year. The amounts are usually converted to quantities of 100% ethanol per capita population 15 years and over.

**Personality:** Relatively enduring ways of behaving, thinking, and feeling that characterize a person and that to a certain extent distinguish that person from others.

**Poliomyelitis:** A viral infection; only 1% of those infected have symptoms. Muscles may become sore and lower limbs paralyzed. In time, the paralyzed limb becomes wasted from lack of use and the person may need crutches.

**Population doubling time:** The number of years it will take for the population to double its current numbers, estimated by dividing the crude growth rate (as a percentage) into 75.

**Positive consequences:** The social, emotional, or material benefits that follow from an action, for example, receiving approval, social recognition, or any other rewarding event.

**Prevalence:** The proportion of the population currently ill; a crude measure of the burden of disease in a population.

**Primary health care (PHC):** Essential health care made available at a cost that countries and communities can afford with methods that are practical, scientifically sound, and socially acceptable. It is the first line of health service and includes promotive, preventive, and curative services. There are eight components, following the acronym MEDECINS.

**Primary school enrollment ratio (gross):** The total number of children enrolled in primary school, whether or not they are of the age for that level, expressed as a percentage of the total number of children of that age. This indicates how many eligible children are enrolled in primary school. Figures are also available for **secondary school enrollment.**

**Protective factors:** Characteristics of people or their environments that are associated with health in the presence of adversity and that therefore decrease the likelihood that these people will suffer from illness.

**Qualitative methods:** Ways of collecting rich descriptive information about a community or about individuals, usually accompanied by information about the context in which they function. Examples are focus group discussion, participant observation, and key informant interviews.

**Quantitative methods:** Ways of collecting information that can be given a numerical value for the purpose of estimating prevalence or average tendencies, or to conduct statistical analyses of the association between different variables. Examples are nonparticipant observation and structured survey questionnaires.

**Relational:** Actual interactions with other people that involve participation in friendship, family, and community life as well as the mental processes involved in relationships with others, such as emotional attachments and realistic interpretations of others.

**Risk factors:** Characteristics of people or their environments that are associated with illness and therefore increase the likelihood that people with the characteristics will suffer from illness.

**Salt and sugar solution:** The salt and sugar added to water to make a homemade fluid for oral rehydration.

**Sampling:** The procedure of selecting from a population those who will become participants in a survey or other method of data collection. Representative sampling means that the sample will have the same proportions of people from different age and sex groups as the general population from which they were selected, accomplished through random or systematic sampling.

**Self-efficacy:** Confidence that one can perform the actions considered necessary for the role (e.g., leader, organizer, health educator) or for the outcome (e.g., to persuade people to give resources).

**Self-esteem** (or self-confidence): A person's perception of his or her worth generally and in specific domains such as family, social, and work.

**Self-Reporting Questionnaire:** A 24-item measure of adult mental health problems developed by experts from the WHO and intended for use in developing countries.

**Skills:** Capacities for carrying out complex, well-organized patterns of behavior smoothly and adaptively to achieve a goal.

**Social Readjustment Rating Scale:** Measure of the psychological impact of major life events experienced in the past year.

**Stress:** An internal state of tension or disequilibrium that results from repeated or intense stressors.

**Stressor:** An aspect of the environment that is perceived as threatening or that requires adaptation.

**Structured self-report measures:** Usually an interview instrument that includes a standard set of questions about a person's health behavior, attitudes, beliefs, or whatever, the answers to which can be quantified and summed to create a composite score. The questions are written and read in the same way to all respondents.

**Stunting:** An index of chronic or long-term malnutrition because it implies that insufficient protein for bone growth (and energy) has existed for months or years. Children who are below minus two standard deviations from the median height for their age and gender reference population (formerly 90% of the median height for their age) are considered moderately to severely stunted.

**Subjective norm:** The perception that significant other people will approve of the action. In other words, it is one's view of the unwritten social rules specifying acceptable behaviors.

**Systematic observation:** Planned, methodical, objective observation of events in their sequence and in their natural context. The observations can be coded and quantified.

**Total fertility rate:** The number of children who would be born to a woman if she were to live to the end of her childbearing years and bear children at each age in accordance with prevailing age-specific fertility rates.

**Traditional birth attendants (TBA):** Usually women who serve as the midwife in their community and who are given extra training so that they can care for women during pregnancy and during the delivery of their babies. If given extra training, they are called trained traditional birth attendants (TTBA).

**Tuberculosis:** A disease caused by the bacillus Mycobacterium tuberculosis, which is transmitted from one person to another through coughing or sneezing. This infects the lungs.

**Under-5 mortality rate:** Number of deaths of children under 5 years of age per 1,000 live births. This is the probability of dying between birth and exactly 5 years of age, and it is one of the most important indicators of the health of a nation's children because it reflects many inputs from nutrition, immunization, use of oral rehydration solution, mothers' knowledge, and access to health services.

**Underweight:** Moderately and severely underweight children weigh less than two standard deviations below the median weight for their age. In the past, some definitions were stated in terms of weighing less than 80% of the median.

**Utilization of health services:** Percentage of the population that uses preventive or curative services offered by a local clinic or a community health worker.

**Values:** Relatively enduring preferences for certain end states such as health and social recognition and the means for achieving them such as through self-control or obedience. Rokeach measured the values of a person and culture by asking people to rank in the importance to them a list of 18 values. A traditional culture is one that values ways of living that have been passed down through many generations.

**Verbal autopsy:** A technique for identifying the cause of death by asking structured questions of an adult who cared for the deceased before death.

**Wasting:** Moderate and severe wasting refers to weighing less than two standard deviations below the median weight for that height (previously less than 80% of the median).

**Ways of Coping Questionnaire:** A 66-item questionnaire to measure cognitive and behavior efforts to manage specific external and/or internal demands that are appraised as taxing or exceeding the resources of that person.

**Weaning foods:** The semisolid foods that are given to children from 6 to 24 months of age, along with breast milk, to provide extra energy and other nutrients.

# REFERENCES

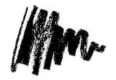

Abiodun, O. A. (1991). Knowledge and attitude concerning mental health of primary health care workers in Nigeria. *International Journal of Social Psychiatry, 37*, 113-120.

Abiodun, O. A. (1993a). Emotional illness in a pediatric population in Nigeria. *Journal of Tropical Pediatrics, 39*, 49-51.

Abiodun, O. A. (1993b). A study of mental morbidity among primary care patients in Nigeria. *Comprehensive Psychiatry, 34*, 10-13.

Aboud, F. E. (1997). Methods from social sciences: Overview of qualitative and quantitative methods. In J. Pickering (Ed.), *Health research for development: A manual* (pp. 101-131). Montreal: CUCHID and McGill Printing.

Aboud, F. E., & Alemu, T. (1995). Nutritional status, maternal responsiveness and mental development of Ethiopian children. *Social Science & Medicine, 41*, 725-732.

Aboud, F. E., Samuel, M., Hadera, A., & Addus, A. (1991). Cognitive, social and nutritional status of children in an Ethiopian orphanage. *Social Science & Medicine, 33*, 1275-1280.

AbouZahr, C., Wardlaw, T., Stanton, C., & Hill, K. (1996). Maternal mortality. *World Health Statistics Quarterly, 49*, 77-87.

Achenbach, T. M., & Edelbrock, C. S. (1983). *Manual for the Child Behavior Checklist and Revised Child Behavior Profile*. Burlington: University of Vermont, Department of Psychiatry.

Acuda, S. W. (1985). International review series: Alcohol and alcohol problems research. 1. East Africa. *British Journal of Addiction, 80*, 121-126.

Adair, L., Popkin, B. M., VanDerslice, J., Guilkey, D., Black, R., Briscoe, J., & Flieger, W. (1993). Growth dynamics during the first two years of life: A prospective study in the Philippines. *European Journal of Clinical Nutrition, 47,* 42-51.

Adamson, P. (1993). *Facts for life.* Benson, Oxfordshire: P & LA (for UNICEF).

Adamson, P. (1996). A failure of imagination. In *UNICEF: The progress of nations* (pp. 3-9). Wallengford, Oxen: P & LA.

Adler, N. E., Boyce, T., & Chesney, M. A. (1994). Socioeconomic status and health: The challenge of the gradient. *American Psychologist, 49,* 15-24.

Adler, P. A., & Adler, P. (1994). Observational techniques. In N. K. Denzin & Y. S. Lincoln (Eds.), *Handbook of qualitative research* (pp. 377-392). Thousand Oaks, CA: Sage.

Aggleton, P. (1996). Global priorities for HIV/AIDS intervention research. *International Journal of STD & AIDS, 7*(Suppl. 2), 13-16.

Ajzen, I. (1988). *Attitudes, personality, and behavior.* Chicago: Dorsey.

Allen, S., Serufilira, A., Bogaerts, J., Van de Perre, P., Nsengumuremyi, F., Lindan, C., Carael, M., Wolf, W., Coates, T., & Hulley, S. (1992). Confidential HIV testing and condom promotion in Africa: Impact on HIV and gonorrhea rates. *JAMA, 268,* 3338-3343.

American Psychiatric Association. (1994). *Diagnostic and statistical manual of mental disorders* (4th ed.). Washington, DC: Author.

Anderson, R. M., May, R. M., Ng, T. W., & Rowley, J. T. (1992). Age-dependent choice of sexual partners and the transmission dynamics of HIV in sub-Saharan Africa. *Philosophical Transactions of the Royal Society of London, 336*(Series B), 135-155.

Aplasca, M. R. A., Siegel, D., Mandel, J. S., Santana-Arciaga, R. T., Paul, J., Hudes, E. S., Monzon, O. T., & Hearst, N. (1995). Results of a model AIDS prevention program for high school students in the Philippines. *AIDS, 9,* S7-S13.

Aptekar, L. (1988). *Street children of Cali.* Durham, NC: Duke University Press.

Armstrong, S. (1991). Female circumcision: Fighting a cruel tradition. *New Scientist, 129,* 42-47.

Asthana, S., & Oostvogels, R. (1996). Community participation in HIV prevention: Problems and prospects for community-based strategies among female sex workers in Madras. *Social Science & Medicine, 43,* 133-148.

Ayele, F., Desta, A., & Larson, C. P. (1993). The functional status of community health agents: A trial refresher courses and regular supervision. *Health Policy and Planning, 8,* 379-384.

Bandura, A. (1982). Self-efficacy mechanism in human agency. *American Psychologist, 37,* 122-147.

Barker, C., & Green, A. (1996). Opening the debate on DALYs. *Health Policy & Planning, 11,* 179-183.

Barrett, D. E., & Radke-Yarrow, M. (1985). Effects of nutritional supplementation on children's responses to novel, frustrating and competitive situations. *American Journal of Clinical Nutrition, 42,* 102-120.

Becker, M. H., & Joseph, J. G. (1988). AIDS and the behavioral change to reduce risk: A review. *American Journal of Public Health, 78,* 394-410.

Bedi, K. S. (1987). Lasting neuroanatomical changes following undernutrition during early life. In J. Dobbing (Ed.), *Early nutrition and later achievement* (pp. 1-36). New York: Academic Press.

Bekele, A., Zewdi, W. G., & Kloos, H. (1993). Food, diet and nutrition. In H. Kloos & Z. A. Zein (Eds.), *The ecology of health and disease in Ethiopia* (pp. 85-102). Boulder, CO: Westview.

Bentley, M. E., Dickin, K. L., Mebrahtu, S., Kayode, B., Oni, G. A., Verzosa, C. C., Brown, K. H., & Idowu, J. R. (1991). Development of a nutritionally adequate and culturally appropriate weaning food in Kwara State, Nigeria: An interdisciplinary approach. *Social Science & Medicine, 33,* 1103-1111.

Bentley, M. E., Pelto, G. H., Straus, W. L., Schumann, D. A., Adegbola, C., de la Pena, E., Oni, G. A., Brown, K. H., & Huffman, S. L. (1988). Rapid ethnographic assessment: Applications in a diarrhea management program. *Social Science & Medicine, 27,* 107-116.

Bernhart, M. H., & Kamal, G. M. (1994). Management of community distribution programs in Bangladesh. *Studies in Family Planning, 25,* 197-210.

Bertrand, J. T., Pineda, M. A., Santiso, R., & Hearn, S. (1980). Characteristics of successful distributors in the community-based distribution of contraceptives in Guatemala. *Studies in Family Planning, 11,* 274-285.

Beusenberg, M., & Orley, J. (1994). *A user's guide to the Self Reporting Questionnaire (SRQ).* Geneva, Switzerland: WHO.

Bhatia, J. C., & Cleland, J. (1995). Self-reported symptoms of gynecological morbidity and their treatment in South India. *Studies in Family Planning, 26,* 203-216.

Bhave, G., Lindan, C. P., Hudes, E. S., Desai, S., Wagle, U., Tripathi, S. P., & Mandel, J. S. (1995). Impact of an intervention on HIV, sexually transmitted diseases, and condom use among sex workers in Bombay, India. *AIDS, 9,* S21-S30.

Bien, T. H., Miller, W. R., & Tonigan, J. S. (1993). Brief interventions for alcohol problems: A review. *Addiction, 88,* 315-336.

Bilqis, A. H., Zeitlyn, S., Ali, N., Yahya, F. S., & Shaheed, N. M. (1994). Promoting sanitation in Bangladesh. *World Health Forum, 15,* 358-362.

Binion, A., Miller, C. D., Beauvais, F., & Oetting, E. R. (1988). Rationales for the use of alcohol, marijuana, and other drugs by eighth grade Native American and Anglo youth. *International Journal of the Addictions, 23,* 47-64.

Blustein, P. (1997, June 1). Foreign aid "has no impact." *Guardian Weekly,* p. 16.

Boerma, J. T., Rustein, S. O., Sommerfelt, E., & Bicego, G. T. (1991). Bottle use for infant feeding in developing countries: Data from the demographic and health surveys. *Journal of Tropical Pediatrics, 37,* 116-120.

Bogdewic, S. P. (1992). Participant observation. In B. F. Crabtree & W. L. Miller (Eds.), *Doing qualitative research: Multiple strategies* (pp. 45-69). Newbury Park, CA: Sage.

Bonati, G., & Hawes, H. (1992). *Child-to-Child: A resource book.* London: Child-to-Child Trust.

Bongaarts, J. (1990). The measurement of wanted fertility. *Population and Development Review, 16,* 487-506.

Bongaarts, J. (1996). Global trends in AIDS mortality. *Population and Development Review, 22,* 21-45.

Bongaarts, J., Mauldin, W. P., & Phillips, J. F. (1990). The demographic impact of family planning programs. *Studies in Family Planning, 21,* 299-310.

Brady, M. (1990, Summer). Indigenous and government attempts to control alcohol use among Australian Aborigines. *Contemporary Drug Problems,* pp. 195-220.

Brown, J. E., Ayowa, O. B., & Brown, R. C. (1993). Dry and tight: Sexual practices and potential AIDS risk in Zaire. *Social Science & Medicine, 37,* 989-994.

Brown, P. (1997, May 25). And now for the bad news about AIDS. *Guardian Weekly,* p. 25.

Brun, T. A., Geissler, C., & Kennedy, E. (1991). The impact of agricultural projects on food, nutrition, and health. *World Review of Nutrition and Diet, 65,* 99-123.

Brunswick, A. F., Messeri, P. A., & Aidala, A. A. (1990). Changing drug patterns and treatment behavior: A longitudinal study of urban black youth. In R. R. Watson (Ed.), *Drug and alcohol abuse prevention* (pp. 263-311). Clifton, NJ: Humana.

Bry, B. H., & Greene, D. M. (1990). Empirical bases for integrating school- and family-based interventions against early adolescent substance abuse. In R. J. McMahon & R. D. Peters (Eds.), *Behavior disorders of adolescence: Research, intervention, and policy in clinical and school settings* (pp. 81-97). New York: Plenum.

Bucholz, K. K., & Robins, L. N. (1989). Sociological research on alcohol use, problems, and policy. *Annual Review of Sociology, 15,* 163-186.

Buehler, J. W., De Cock, K. M., & Brunet, J.-B. (1993). Surveillance definitions for AIDS. *AIDS, 7*(Suppl. 1), S73-S81.

Bushman, B. J., & Cooper, H. M. (1990). Effects of alcohol on human aggression: An integrative research review. *Psychological Bulletin, 107,* 341-354.

Caldwell, J. C. (1980). Mass education as a determinant of the timing of fertility decline. *Population & Development, 6,* 225-255.

Caldwell, J. C., Reddy, P. H., & Caldwell, P. (1988). *The causes of demographic change: Experimental research in South India.* Madison: University of Wisconsin Press.

Cameron, M., & Hofvander, Y. (1983). *Manual on feeding infants and young children.* Oxford: Oxford University Press.

Caprara, A., Seri, D., De Gregorio, G. C., Parenzi, A., Salazar, C. M., & Goze, T. (1993). The perception of AIDS in the Bete and Baoule of the Ivory Coast. *Social Science and Medicine, 36,* 1229-1235.

Carlin, E. M., & Boag, F. C. (1995). Women, contraception and STDs including HIV. *International Journal of STD & AIDS, 6,* 373-386.

Cartwright, D., & Zander, A. (Eds.). (1968). *Group dynamics: Research and theory.* New York: Harper & Row.

Cassidy, C. M. (1987). World-view conflict and toddler malnutrition: Change agent dilemmas. In N. Scheper-Hughes (Ed.), *Child survival* (pp. 293-324). Boston: D. Reidel.

Chaiken, M. R. (1990). Evaluation of Girl Clubs of America's Friendly PEERsuasion Program. In R. R. Watson (Ed.), *Drug and alcohol abuse prevention* (pp. 95-132). Clifton, NJ: Humana.

Chambwe, A., Slade, P., & Dewey, M. (1983). Behavior patterns of alcohol use among young children in Britain and Zimbabwe. *British Journal of Addiction, 78,* 311-316.

Chin, J. (1990). Global estimates of AIDS cases and HIV infections: 1990. *AIDS, 4*(Suppl. 1), S277-S283.

Cleland, J., & Mauldin, W. P. (1990). *The promotion of family planning by financial payments: The case of Bangladesh.* New York: Population Council.

Cleland, J. G., & van Ginneken, J. K. (1988). Maternal education and child survival in developing countries: The search for pathways of influence. *Social Science & Medicine, 27,* 1357-1368.

Coates, T. J., Chesney, M., Folkman, S., Hulley, S. B., Haynes-Sanstad, K., Lurie, P., VanOss Marin, B., Roos, L., Bunnett, V., & Du Wors, R. (1996). Designing behavioral and social science to impact practice and policy in HIV prevention and care. *International Journal of STD & AIDS, 7*(Suppl. 2), 2-12.

Coeytaux, F. M., Leonard, A. H., & Bloomer, C. M. (1993). Abortion. In M. Koblinsky, J. Timyan, & J. Gay (Eds.), *The health of women: A global perspective* (pp. 133-146). Boulder, CO: Westview.

Cohen, J. (1996). The marketplace of HIV/AIDS. *Science, 272,* 1880-1881.

Cohen, J. M., & Uphoff, N. T. (1980). Participation's place in rural development: Seeking clarity through specificity. *World Development, 8,* 213-235.

Compas, B. E. (1987). Stress and life events during childhood and adolescence. *Clinical Psychology Review, 7,* 275-302.

Compton, W. M., Helzer, J. E., Hwu, H. G., Yeh, E. K., McEvoy, L., Tipp, J. E., & Spitznagel, E. L. (1991). New methods in cross-cultural psychiatry: Psychiatric illness in Taiwan and the United States. *American Journal of Psychiatry, 148,* 1697-1704.

Coombs, D. W., & Lowe, J. B. (1987). Alcohol abuse and economic underdevelopment in Guatemala. *Alcohol Health and Research World, 12,* 52-55.

Coreil, J. (1987). Maternal-child supplementary feeding programmes in Haiti. *Journal of Tropical Pediatrics, 33,* 203-207.

Cottler, L. B., Robins, L. N., Grant, B. F., Blaine, J., Towle, L. H., Wittchen, H. U., & Sartorius, N. (1991). The CIDI-core substance abuse and dependence questions: Cross-cultural and nosological issues. *British Journal of Psychiatry, 159,* 653-658.

Covell, K., Dion, K. L., & Dion, K. K. (1994). Gender differences in evaluations of tobacco and alcohol advertisements. *Canadian Journal of Behavioural Science, 26,* 404-420.

Cowan, B., & Dhanoa, J. (1983). The prevention of toddler malnutrition by home-based nutrition health education. In D. S. McLaren (Ed.), *Nutrition in the community: A critical look at nutrition policy, planning, and programmes* (pp. 339-356). New York: John Wiley.

Dasen, P. R., Berry, J. W., & Sartorius, N. (Eds.). (1988). *Health and cross-cultural psychology: Toward applications.* Thousand Oaks, CA: Sage.

Davidson, R. S. (1985). Behavioral medicine and alcoholism. In N. Schneiderman & J. T. Tapp (Eds.), *Behavioral medicine: The biopsychosocial approach* (pp. 379-404). Hillsdale, NJ: Lawrence Erlbaum.

DeLongis, A., Coyne, J. C., Dakof, G., Folkman, S., & Lazarus, R. S. (1982). Relationship of daily hassles, uplifts and major life events to health status. *Health Psychology, 1,* 119-136.

Des Jarlais, D. C., & Friedman, S. R. (1996). HIV epidemiology and interventions among injecting drug users. *International Journal of STD & AIDS, 7*(Suppl. 2), 57-61.

Desjarlais, R., Eisenberg, L., Good, B., & Kleinman, A. (1995). *World mental health: Problems and priorities in low-income countries.* Oxford: Oxford University Press.

DeVellis, R. F., DeVellis, B. M., Blanchard, L. W., Klotz, M. L., Luchok, K., & Voyce, C. (1993). Development and validation of the Parent Health Locus of Control scales. *Health Education Quarterly, 20,* 211-225.

Dhillon, H. S., & Philip, L. (1994). *Health promotion and community action for health in developing countries.* Geneva, Switzerland: WHO.

Donovan, J. E., & Jessor, R. (1985). Structure of problem behavior in adolescence and young adulthood. *Journal of Consulting & Clinical Psychology, 53*, 890-904.

Dorkenoo, E. (1996). Combating female genital mutilation: An agenda for the next decade. *World Health Statistics Quarterly, 49*, 142-145.

Downs, E. (1993). NGOs and the transfer of cultural values. *Development, 1*, 61-64.

Dwyer, J. M. (1996). Behavioral interventions required in South East Asia to minimize infections with HIV. *International Journal of STD & AIDS Research, 7*(Suppl. 2), 71-74.

Eagly, A. H., & Chaiken, S. (1993). *The psychology of attitudes.* Orlando, FL: Harcourt Brace Jovanovich.

Eisemon, T. O., Patel, V. L., & Ole Sena, S. (1987). Uses of formal and informal knowledge in the comprehension of instructions for oral rehydration therapy in Kenya. *Social Science & Medicine, 25*, 1225-1234.

Eisenberg, L. (1993). Relationship between treatment and prevention policies. In N. Sartorius, G. de Girolamo, G. Andrews, G. A. German, & L. Eisenberg (Eds.), *Treatment of mental disorders: A review of effectiveness* (pp. 35-57). Washington, DC: American Psychiatric Press.

Elder, J. P., & Estey, J. D. (1992). Behavior change strategies for family planning. *Social Science and Medicine, 35*, 1065-1076.

Elder, J. P., Geller, E. S., Hovell, M. F., & Mayer, J. (1994). *Motivating health behavior.* Albany, NY: Delmar.

El Hassan Al Awad, A. M., & Sonuga-Barke, E. J. S. (1992). Childhood problems in a Sudanese city: A comparison of extended and nuclear families. *Child Development, 63*, 906-914.

Eliany, M. (1992, Autumn). Alcohol and drug consumption among Canadian youth. *Statistics Canada: Canadian Social Trends,* pp. 10-13.

Eng, E., Briscoe, J., & Cunningham, A. (1990). Participation effect from water projects on EPI. *Social Science and Medicine, 30*, 1349-1358.

Eschen, A., & Whittaker, M. (1993). Family planning: A base to build on for women's reproductive health services. In M. Koblinsky, J. Timyan, & J. Gay (Eds.), *The health of women: A global perspective* (pp. 105-131). Boulder, CO: Westview.

Espinosa, M. P., Sigman, M. D., Neumann, C. G., Bwibo, N. O., & McDonald, M. A. (1992). Playground behaviors of school-age children in relation to nutrition, schooling and family characteristics. *Developmental Psychology, 28*, 1188-1195.

Everett, S. A., & Telljohann, S. K. (1996). The elementary health teaching self-efficacy scale. *American Journal of Health Behavior, 20*, 90-97.

Fauvreau, V., Yunus, M., & Zaman, K. (1991). Diarrhea mortality in rural Bangladesh children. *Journal of Tropical Pediatrics, 37*, 31-36.

Fillmore, K. M., Hartka, E., Johnstone, B. M., Laino, E. V., Motoyoshi, M., & Temple, M. T. (1991). A meta-analysis of life course variation in drinking. *British Journal of Addiction, 86*, 1221-1268.

Folkman, S., & Lazarus, R. S. (1988). *Manual for the Ways of Coping Questionnaire.* Palo Alto, CA: Consulting Psychologists Press.

Fontana, A., & Frey, J. H. (1994). Interviewing: The art of science. In N. K. Denzin & Y. S. Lincoln (Eds.), *Handbook of qualitative research* (pp. 361-376). Thousand Oaks, CA: Sage.

Food & Agricultural Organization/WHO/U.N. University. (1985). *Energy and protein requirements* (Technical Report Series No. 724). Geneva, Switzerland: WHO.

Ford, K., Wirawan, D. N., Fajans, P., Meliawan, P., MacDonald, K., & Thorpe, L. (1996). Behavioral interventions for reduction of sexually transmitted disease/HIV transmission among female commercial sex workers and clients in Bali, Indonesia. *AIDS, 10,* 213-222.

Foreit, K. G., de Castro, M. P. P., & Franco, E. F. D. (1989). The impact of mass media in advertising on a voluntary sterilization program in Brazil. *Studies in Family Planning, 20,* 107-116.

Foster, G. (1982). Community development and primary health care: Their conceptual similarities. *Medical Anthropology, 6*(3), 183-195.

Frankel, D. G., & Roer-Bornstein, D. (1982). Traditional and modern contributions to changing infant-rearing ideologies of two ethnic communities. *Monographs of SRCD, 47*(4).

Freedman, L. P., & Maine, D. (1993). Women's mortality: A legacy of neglect. In M. Koblinsky, J. Timyan, & J. Gay (Eds.), *The health of women: A global perspective* (pp. 147-170). Boulder, CO: Westview.

Freyens, P., Mbakuliyemo, N., & Martin, M. (1993). How do health workers see community participation? *World Health Forum, 14,* 253-257.

Fryer, M. L. (1991). Health education through interactive radio: A Child-to-Child project in Bolivia. *Health Education Quarterly, 18,* 65-77.

Galler, J. R., & Ramsey, F. (1987). A follow-up study of the influence of early malnutrition on development: V. Delayed development of conservation. *Journal of the American Academy of Child and Adolescent Psychiatry, 26,* 23-27.

Galvez-Tan, J. Z. (1983). We are for the people: Reflections of a community health worker in the Philippines. In D. Morely, J. Rohde, & G. Williams (Eds.), *Practising health for all* (pp. 154-167). Oxford: Oxford University Press.

Garmezy, N., & Masten, A. S. (1991). Stress, competence, and resilience: Common frontiers for therapist and psychopathologist. *Behavior Therapy, 17,* 500-521.

Geen, R. G. (1990). *Human aggression.* Pacific Grove, CA: Brooks/Cole.

Gerein, N. M., & Ross, D. A. (1991). Is growth monitoring worthwhile? An evaluation of its use in three child health programmes in Zaire. *Social Science & Medicine, 32,* 667 675.

Giel, R., De Arango, M. V., Climent, C. E., Harding, T. W., Wig, N. N., & Younis, Y. O. A. (1981). Childhood mental disorders in primary health care: Results of observation in four developing countries. *Pediatrics, 68,* 677-683.

Giel, R., Gezahegn, Y., & van Luijk, J. N. (1968). Psychiatric morbidity in 200 Ethiopian medical outpatients. *Psychiatric Neurological Neurochemistry, 71,* 169-176.

Giel, R., Harding, T. W., Ten Horn, G. H. M. M., Ladrido-Ignacio, L., Murthy, R. S., Sirag, A. O., Suleiman, M. A., & Wig, N. N. (1988). The detection of childhood mental disorders in primary care in some developing countries. In A. S. Henderson & G. D. Burrows (Eds.), *Handbook of social psychiatry* (Chap. 18, pp. 233-244). Amsterdam: Elsevier Science.

Giel, R., & van Luijk, J. N. (1968). On the significance of a broken home in Ethiopia. *British Journal of Psychiatry, 114,* 957-961.

Gilchrist, V. J. (1992). Key informant interviews. In B. G. Crabtree & W. L. Miller (Eds.), *Doing qualitative research: Multiple strategies* (pp. 70-89). Newbury Park, CA: Sage.

Gillies, P. A. (1994). Sex education and HIV/AIDS prevention. *Sexual and Marital Therapy, 9,* 159-170.

Giovino, G. A., Henningfield, J. E., Tomar, S. L., Escobedo, L. G., & Slade, J. (1995). Epidemiology of tobacco use and dependence. *Epidemiologic Reviews, 17,* 48-65.

Gittelman, M., Dubuis, J., Nagaswami, V., Asuni, T., Fallon, I. R. H., & Publico, L. (1989). Mental health promotion through psychosocial rehabilitation. *International Journal of Mental Health, 18,* 99-116.

Goldberg, D. (1995). Epidemiology of mental disorders in primary care settings. *Epidemiologic Reviews, 17,* 182-190.

Golden, L. L., & Anderson, W. T. (1992). AIDS prevention: Myths, misinformation and health policy perceptions. *Journal of Health & Social Policy, 3,* 37-50.

Goldin, C. S. (1994). Stigmatization and AIDS: Critical issues in public health. *Social Science & Medicine, 39,* 1359-1366.

Good, C. M. (1995). Incentives can lower the incidence of HIV/AIDS in Africa. *Social Science & Medicine, 40,* 419-424.

Gorman, K. S. (1995). Malnutrition and cognitive development: Evidence from experimental/quasi-experimental studies among the mild-to-moderately malnourished. *Journal of Nutrition, 125*(Suppl.), 2239S-2244S.

Gorman, K. S., & Pollitt, E. (1996). Does schooling buffer the effects of early risk? *Child Development, 67,* 314-326.

Graeff, J. A., Elder, J. P., & Booth, E. M. (1993). *Communication for health and behavior change: A developing country perspective.* San Francisco: Jossey-Bass.

Graeff, J. A., & Waters, H. (1994). *Behavior change and maintenance for child survival.* Washington, DC: HealthCom.

Grantham-McGregor, S. M., Powell, C. A., Walker, S. P., & Himes, J. H. (1991). Nutritional supplementation, psychosocial stimulation, and mental development of stunted children: The Jamaican study. *Lancet, 38,* 1-5.

Grantham-McGregor, S. M., Schofield, W., & Powell, C. A. (1987). Development of severely malnourished children who received psychosocial stimulation: Six-year follow-up. *Pediatrics, 79,* 247-254.

Green, A., & Matthias, A. (1996). How should governments view non-governmental organization? *World Health Forum, 17,* 42-45.

Green, E. C., Zokwe, B., & Dupree, J. D. (1995). The experience of an AIDS prevention program focused on South African traditional healers. *Social Science and Medicine, 40,* 503-515.

Green, L. W., Kreuter, M. W., Deeds, S. G., & Partridge, K. B. (1980). *Health education planning: A diagnostic approach.* Palo Alto, CA: Mayfield.

Green, L. W., & Lewis, F. M. (1986). *Measurement and evaluation in health education and health promotion.* Palo Alto, CA: Mayfield.

Greenough, W. B., & Khin-Maung-U [full name]. (1991). Oral rehydration therapy. In M. Field (Ed.), *Diarrheal diseases* (pp. 485-499). New York: Elsevier.

Guba, E. G., & Lincoln, Y. S. (1994). Competing paradigms in qualitative research. In N. K. Denzin & Y. S. Lincoln (Eds.), *Handbook of qualitative research* (pp. 105-117). Thousand Oaks, CA: Sage.

Gureje, O., Obikoya, B., & Ikuesan, B. A. (1992). Alcohol abuse and dependence in an urban primary care clinic in Nigeria. *Drug and Alcohol Dependence, 30,* 163-167.

Hamilton, R. (1997). The need for centres of health research excellence in the developing world. *Policy Sciences, 30,* 25-46.

Harding, T. W., Climent, C. E., Giel, R., Ibrahim, H. H. A., Murthy, R. S., Suleiman, M. A., & Wig, N. N. (1983). The WHO collaborative study on strategies for extending mental health care. II: The development of new research methods. *American Journal of Psychiatry, 140,* 1474-1480.

Harding, T. W., De Arango, M. V., Baltazar, J., Climent, C. E., Ibrahim, H. H. A., Ladrido-Ignacio, L., Murthy, R. S., & Wig, N. N. (1980). Mental disorders in primary health care: A study of their frequency and diagnosis in four developing countries. *Psychological Medicine, 10,* 231-241.

Harvey, P. D. (1994). The impact of condom prices on sales in social marketing programs. *Studies in Family Planning, 25,* 52-58.

Hauge, R., & Irgens-Jensen, O. (1986). The relationship between alcohol consumption, alcohol intoxication and negative consequences of drinking in four Scandinavian countries. *British Journal of Addiction, 81,* 513-524.

Haverkos, H. W., & Quinn, T. C. (1995). The third wave: HIV infection among heterosexuals in the United States and Europe. *International Journal of STD & AIDS, 6,* 227-232.

Hawes, H., & Scotchmer, C. (1993). *Children for health.* London: Child-to-Child Trust.

Haworth, A. (1989). Alcohol-related casualties in Africa. In N. Giesbrecht, R. Gonzalez, M. Grant, E. Osterberg, R. Room, I. Rootman, & L. Towle (Eds.), *Drinking and casualties: Accidents, poisonings, and violence in an international perspective* (pp. 83-111). London: Routledge.

Heise, L. (1993). Violence against women: The missing agenda. In M. Koblinsky, J. Timyan, & J. Gay (Eds.), *The health of women: A global perspective.* Boulder, CO: Westview.

Heise, L. L., & Elias, C. (1995). Transforming AIDS prevention to meet women's needs: A focus on developing countries. *Social Science & Medicine, 40,* 931-943.

Helzer, J. E., Canino, G. J., Yeh, E. K., Bland, R. C., Lee, C. K., Howes, H. G., & Newman, S. (1990). Alcoholism: North America and Asia. *Archives of General Psychiatry, 47,* 313-319.

Hilton, D. (1983). "Tell us a story": Health teaching in Nigeria. In D. Morely, J. Rohde, & G. Williams (Eds.), *Practising health for all* (pp. 145-153). Oxford: Oxford University Press.

Hirschhorn, N., & Greenough, W. B. (1991). Progress in oral rehydration therapy. *Scientific American, 264,* 50-56.

Hoffman, L. W. (1988). Cross-cultural differences in child-rearing goals. In R. A. LeVine, P. M. Miller, & M. M. West (Eds.), *Parental behavior in diverse societies* (New Directions for Child Development No. 40, pp. 99-122). San Francisco: Jossey-Bass.

Hogarty, G. E., Anderson, C. M., Russ, D. J., Kornblith, S. J., Greenwald, D. P., Javna, C. D., & Madonia, M. J. (1986). Family psychoeducation, social skills training, and maintenance chemotherapy in the aftercase treatment of schizophrenia. *Archives of General Psychiatry, 43,* 633-642.

Holmes, T. H., & Rahe, R. H. (1967). The Social Readjustment Rating Scale. *Journal of Psychosomatic Research, 11,* 213-218.

Huberman, A. M., & Miles, M. B. (1994). Data management and analysis methods. In N. K. Denzin & Y. S. Lincoln (Eds.), *Handbook of qualitative research* (pp. 428-444). Thousand Oaks, CA: Sage.

Hubley, J. (1993). *Communicating health.* London: Macmillan (TALC).

Hudson, C. P. (1996). AIDS in rural Africa: A paradigm for HIV-1 prevention. *International Journal of STD & AIDS, 7,* 236-243.

Hull, V. J., Thapa, S., & Wiknjosastro, G. (1989). Breast-feeding and health professionals: A study in hospitals in Indonesia. *Social Science and Medicine, 28,* 355-364.

Huntington, D., & Schuler, S. R. (1993). The simulated client method: Evaluating client-provider interactions in family planning clinics. *Studies in Family Planning, 24,* 187-193.

Hurley, J., & Horowitz, J. (1990). *Alcohol and health.* New York: Hemisphere.

Idjradinata, P., & Pollitt, E. (1993). Reversal of developmental delays in iron-deficient anaemic infants treated with iron. *Lancet, 34,* 1-4.

Irwin, K., Bertrand, J., Mibandumba, N., Mbuyi, K., Muremeri, C., Mukoka, M., Munkolenkole, K., Nzilambi, N., Bosenge, N., Ryder, R., Peterson, H., Lee, N. C., Wingo, P., O'Reilly, K., & Rufo K. (1991). Knowledge, attitudes and beliefs about HIV infection and AIDS among healthy factory workers and their wives, Kinshasa, Zaire. *Social Science & Medicine, 32,* 917-930.

Jablensky, A. (1995). Schizophrenia: Recent epidemiologic issues. *Epidemiologic Review, 17,* 10-20.

Jablensky, A., Sartorius, N., Ernberg, G., Anker, M., Korten, A., Cooper, J. E., Day, R., & Bertelson, A. (1992). Schizophrenia: Manifestations, incidence and course in different cultures: A WHO ten-country study. *Psychological Medicine,* Mono. Suppl. 20, pp. 1-97.

Jager, J. C., Heisterkamp, S. H., & Brookmeyer, R. (1993). AIDS surveillance and prediction of the HIV and AIDS epidemic: Methodological developments. *AIDS,* 7(Suppl. 1), S67-S71.

Jamison, D. T., Mosley, W. H., Measham, A. R., & Bobadilla, J. L. (1993). *Disease control priorities in developing countries.* Oxford: Oxford University Press.

Janz, N. K., & Becker, M. (1984). The health belief model: A decade later. *Health Education Quarterly, 11,* 1-47.

Janz, N. K., Zimmerman, N. A., Wren, P. A., Israel, B. A., Freudenberg, N., & Carter, R. J. (1996). Evaluation of 37 AIDS prevention projects: Successful approaches and barriers to program effectiveness. *Health Education Quarterly, 23,* 80-97.

Jelik, W. G. (1993). Traditional medicine relevant to psychiatry. In N. Sartorius, G. de Girolamo, G. Andrews, G. A. German, & L. Eisenberg (Eds.), *Treatment of mental disorders: A review of effectiveness* (pp. 341-390). Washington, DC: American Psychiatric Press.

Johnson, K. E., Kisubi, W. K., Mbugua, J. K., Lackey, D., Stanfield, P., & Osuga, B. (1989). Community-based health care in Kibewezi, Kenya: 10 years in retrospect. *Social Science and Medicine, 28,* 1039-1051.

Jones, J., & Hunter, D. (1995). Consensus methods for medical and health services research. *British Medical Journal, 311,* 376-380.

Kamali, A., Seeley, J. A., Nunn, A. J., Kengeya-Kayondo, J. F., Ruberantwari, A., & Mulder, D. W. (1996). The orphan problem: Experience of a sub-Saharan Africa rural population in the AIDS epidemic. *AIDS Care, 8,* 509-515.

Kamali, A., Wagner, H. U., Nakiyingi, J., Sabiiti, I., Kengeya-Kayondo, J. F., & Mulder, D. W. (1996). Verbal autopsy as a tool for diagnosing HIV-related adult deaths in rural Uganda. *International Journal of Epidemiology, 25,* 679-684.

Kandel, D. B., & Logan, J. A. (1984). Patterns of drug use from adolescence to young adulthood: I. Periods of risk for initiation, continued use, and discontinuation. *American Journal of Public Health, 74,* 660-666.

Kandel, D. B., & Yamaguchi, K. (1985). Developmental patterns of the use of legal, illegal, and medically prescribed psychotropic drugs from adolescence to young adulthood. In C. L. Jones & R. J. Battjes (Eds.), *Etiology of drug abuse: Implications for prevention.* Washington, DC: Government Printing Office.

Kanner, A. D., Coyne, J. C., Schaefer, C., & Lazarus, R. S. (1981). Comparison of two modes of stress management: Daily hassles and uplifts versus major life events. *Journal of Behavioral Medicine, 4,* 1-39.

Kay, B. J., & Kabir, S. M. (1988). A study of costs and behavioral outcomes of menstrual regulation services in Bangladesh. *Social Science and Medicine, 26,* 597-604.

Keller, W., & Fillmore, C. M. (1983). Prevalence of protein-energy malnutrition. *World Health Statistics Quarterly, 36,* 129-167.

Kelly, E. L., & Conley, J. J. (1987). Personality and compatibility: A prospective analysis of marital stability and marital satisfaction. *Journal of Personality and Social Psychology, 52,* 27-40.

Kelly, K. J., & Van Vlaenderen, H. (1996). Dynamics of participation in a community health project. *Social Science and Medicine, 42,* 1235-1246.

Keusch, G. T. (1990). Malnutrition, infection, and immune function. In R. M. Suskind & L. Lewinter-Suskind (Eds.), *The malnourished child* (Nestle Nutrition Workshop Series, Vol. 19, pp. 37-55). New York: Vevey/Raven.

Khanna, J., VanLook, P. F. A., & Griffin, P. D. (Eds.). (1992). *Reproductive health: A key to a brighter future. Biennial Report 1990-1991.* Geneva, Switzerland: WHO.

Kimball, A. M., Berkley, S., Ngugi, E., & Gayle, H. (1995). International aspects of the AIDS/HIV epidemic. *Annual Review of Public Health, 16,* 253-282.

Kim-Farley, R. J. (1993). Expanded program on immunization: Achievements and challenges. *World Health, 46,* 14-16.

Kirby, M. D. (1985). Sexuality education: A more realistic view of its effects. *Journal of School Health, 55,* 421-424.

Kirby, M. D. (1996). HIV/AIDS: The twenty injunctions of London. Summary of the conference. *International Journal of STD & AIDS, 7*(Suppl. 2), 83-90.

Kloos, H., & Lindtjorn, B. (1993). Famine and malnutrition. In H. Kloos & Z. A. Zein (Eds.), *The ecology of health and disease in Ethiopia* (pp. 103-120). Boulder, CO: Westview.

Korten, D. C. (1987). Third generation NGO strategies: A key to people-centered development. *World development, 15*(Suppl.), 145-159.

Kortmann, F. (1987). Popular, traditional, and professional mental health care in Ethiopia. *Transcultural Psychiatric Research Review, 24,* 255-274.

Kortteinen, T. (1989). State monopoly systems and alcohol prevention in developing countries: Report on a collaborative international study. *British Journal of Addiction, 84,* 413-425.

Kramer, M. S. (1987). Determinants of low birth weight: Methodological assessment and meta-analysis. *Bulletin of the World Health Organization, 65,* 663-737.

Krause, R. M. (1996). Reflections on the first decade of the HIV/AIDS pandemic: Opportunities and priorities for international behavioral research and interventions. *International Journal of STD & AIDS, 7*(Suppl. 2), 47-51.

Kulhara, P. (1994). Outcome of schizophrenia: Some transcultural observations with particular reference to developing countries. *European Archives of Psychiatry & Clinical Neuroscience, 244,* 227-235.

Labonte, R. (1996). *The language of community development for evaluating participation in community development: Future directions.* Paper presented in Kingston, Ontario, Canada.

LaFond, A. (1994). UNICEF. *Health Policy & Planning, 9,* 343-346.

Lagarde, E., Pison, G., & Enel, C. (1996). Knowledge, attitudes and perception of AIDS in rural Senegal: Relationship to sexual behavior and behavior change. *AIDS, 10,* 327-334.

Laleman, G., & Annys, S. (1989). Understanding community participation: A health programme in the Philippines. *Health Policy and Planning, 4,* 251-256.

Lancaster, J. (1996, December 8). Egyptians stand by female circumcision. *Guardian Weekly,* p. 17.

Langsley, D. G., Hodes, M., & Grimson, W. R. (1993). Psychosocial intervention. In N. Sartorius, G. De Girolamo, G. Andrews, G. A. German, & L. Eisenberg (Eds.), *Treatment of mental disorders: A review of effectiveness* (pp. 253-288). Washington, DC: American Psychiatric Press.

Lapham, R., & Mauldin, W. P. (1985). Contraceptive prevalence: The influence of organized family planning programs. *Studies in Family Planning, 16,* 117-137.

Lapido, O. A., McNamara, G. E. D., Weiss, E., & Otolorin, E. O. (1990). Family planning in traditional markets in Nigeria. *Studies in Family Planning, 21,* 314-321.

Lapore, S. J., Palsane, M. N., & Evans, G. E. (1991). Daily hassles and chronic strains: A hierarchy of stressors? *Social Science & Medicine, 33,* 1029-1036.

Latham, M. C. (1983). The control of vitamin A deficiency and xerophthalmia in the Philippines. In D. S. McLaren (Ed.), *Nutrition in the community: A critical look at nutrition policy, planning, and programmes* (pp. 439-449). New York: John Wiley.

Launer, L. J., & Habicht, J. P. (1989). Concepts about infant health, growth, and weaning: A comparison between nutritional scientists and Madurese mothers. *Social Science and Medicine, 29,* 13-22.

Lee, K. (1994). The UNFPA: Twenty-five years and beyond. *Health Policy and Planning, 9,* 223-228.

Leff, J., Wig, N. N., Bedi, H., Menon, D. K., Kuipers, L., Korten, A., Ernberg, G., Day, R., Sartorius, N., & Jablensky, A. (1990). Relatives' expressed emotion and the course of schizophrenia in Chandigarh. A two-year follow-up of a first-contact sample. *British Journal of Psychiatry, 156,* 351-356.

Lepowsky, M. (1987). Food taboos and child survival: A case study from the Coral Sea. In N. Scheper-Hughes (Ed.), *Child survival* (pp. 71-92). Boston: D. Reidel.

LeVine, R. A., Dixon, S., LeVine, S., Richman, A., Leiderman, P. H., Keefer, C. H., & Brazelton, T. B. (1994). *Child care and culture: Lessons from Africa.* New York: Cambridge University Press.

Levinger, B. (1986). *School feeding programs in developing countries: An analysis of actual and potential impact.* Washington, DC: USAID.

Lindtjorn, B., & Alemu, T. (1997). Intra-household correlations of nutritional status in rural Ethiopia. *International Journal of Epidemiology, 26,* 160-165.

Link, P. G., & Phelan, J. C. (1996). Editorial: Understanding sociodemographic differences in health—the role of fundamental social causes. *American Journal of Public Health, 86,* 471-473.

Links, P. S. (1983). Community surveys of the prevalence of childhood psychiatric disorders: A review. *Child Development, 54,* 531-548.

Lloyd, C. B., & Blanc, A. K. (1996). Children's schooling in sub-Saharan Africa: The role of fathers, mothers, and others. *Population & Development Review, 22,* 265-298.

Lonner, W. J., & Berry, J. W. (Eds.). (1986). *Field methods in cross-cultural research.* Newbury Park, CA: Sage.

Lubben, J. E., Chi, I., & Kitano, H. H. L. (1988). Exploring Filipino American drinking behavior. *Journal of Studies on Alcohol, 49,* 26-29.

Lynch, M., West, S. K., Munoz, B., Kayongoya, A., Taylor, H. R., & Mmbaga, B. B. O. (1994). Testing a participatory strategy to change hygiene behaviour: Face washing in central Tanzania. *Transactions of the Royal Society of Tropical Medicine & Hygiene, 88,* 513-517.

Macklin, R. (1996). Ethics and reproductive health: A principled approach. *World Health Statistics Quarterly, 49,* 148-153.

Malepe, T. B. (1989). Alcohol problems in Swaziland. *Contemporary Drug Problems, 16,* 43-58.

Manderson, L., & Aaby, P. (1992). An epidemic in the field? Rapid assessment procedures and health research. *Social Science & Medicine, 35,* 839-850.

Mann, J. M. (1991). Global AIDS: Critical issues for prevention in the 1990s. *International Journal of Health Services, 21,* 553-559.

Marshall, M. (1988). Alcohol consumption as a public health problem in Papua New Guinea. *International Journal of the Addictions, 23,* 573-589.

Marshall, M. (1991). Beverage alcohol and other psychoactive substance use by young people in Chuuk, Federated States of Micronesia. *Contemporary Drug Problems, 18,* 331-372.

Mason, K. O., & Taj, A. M. (1987). Differences between women's and men's reproductive goals in developing countries. *Population and Development Review, 13,* 611-638.

Mathews, J. (1994, April 10). Population control that really works. *Guardian Weekly,* the Washington Post section, p. 15.

Mauldin, W. P., & Ross, J. A. (1991). Family planning programs: Efforts and results 1982-89. *Studies in Family Planning, 22,* 350-367.

Mauldin, W. P., & Segal, S. J. (1988). Prevalence of contraceptive use: Trends and issues. *Studies in Family Planning, 19,* 335-353.

McCauley, A. P., Lynch, M., Pounds, M. B., & West, S. (1990). Changing water-use patterns in a water-poor area: Lessons from a trachoma intervention project. *Social Science & Medicine, 31,* 1233-1238.

McGrath, J. W., Rwabukwali, C. B., Schumann, D. A., Pearson-Marks, J., Nakayiwa, S., Namande, B., Nakyobe, L., & Mukasa, R. (1993). Anthropology and AIDS: The cultural context of sexual risk behavior among urban Baganda women in Kampala, Uganda. *Social Science and Medicine, 36,* 429-439.

McPake, B., Hanson, K., & Mills, A. (1993). Community financing of health care in Africa: An evaluation of the Bamako initiative. *Social Science and Medicine, 36,* 1383-1395.

Medina-Mora, M. E., & Gonzalez, L. (1989). Alcohol-related casualties in Latin America: A review of the literature. In N. Giesbrecht, R. Gonzalez, M. Grant, E. Osterberg, R. Room, I. Rootman, & L. Towle (Eds.), *Drinking and casualties: Accidents, poisonings, and violence in an international perspective* (pp. 67-82). London: Routledge.

Meeks Gardner, J. M., Grantham-McGregor, S. M., Chang, S. M., Himes, J. H., & Powell, C. A. (1995). Activity and behavioral development in stunted and nonstunted children and response to nutritional supplementation. *Child Development, 66,* 1785-1797.

Melzack, R. (1975). The McGill Pain questionnaire: Major properties and scoring methods. *Pain, 1,* 277-299.

Melzack, R. (1987). The short-form McGill Pain questionnaire. *Pain, 30,* 191-197.

Merchant, K. M., & Kurz, K. M. (1993). Women's nutrition through the life cycle: Social and biological vulnerabilities. In M. Koblinsky, J. Timyan, & J. Gay (Eds.), *The health of women: A global perspective* (pp. 63-90). Boulder, CO: Westview.

Mertens, T. E., & Low-Beer, D. (1996). HIV and AIDS: Where is the epidemic going? *Bulletin of the World Health Organization, 74,* 121-129.

Meursing, K., & Morojele, N. (1989). Use of alcohol among high school students in Lesotho. *British Journal of Addiction, 84,* 1337-1342.

Millar, W. (1991). A trend to a healthier life. *Health Reports, 3,* 363-370.

Miller, W. R., Heather, N., & Hall, W. (1991). Calculating standard drink units: International comparisons. *British Journal of Addiction, 86,* 43-47.

Millwood, P., & Gezelius, H. (1985). *Good aid: A study of quality in small projects.* Stockholm: Swedish International Development Authority.

Miyazaki, M. (1995). Epidemiological characteristics of human immunodeficiency virus type-2 infection in Africa. *International Journal of STD & AIDS, 6,* 75-80.

Molamu, L. (1989). Alcohol in Botswana: A historical overview. *Contemporary Drug Problems, 16,* 3-42.

Moremoholo, R. A. (1989). The use and abuse of alcohol in Lesotho. *Contemporary Drug Problems, 16,* 59-69.

Morgan, D. L. (1992). Doctor-caregiver relationships: An exploration using focus groups. In B. F. Crabtree & W. L. Miller (Eds.), *Doing qualitative research: Multiple strategies* (pp. 205-227). Newbury Park, CA: Sage.

Moser, J. (1980). *Prevention of alcohol-related problems: An international review of preventive measures, policies, and programmes.* Geneva, Switzerland: WHO (ARF, Toronto).

Moses, P. F. (1989). The use and abuse of alcohol in Zimbabwe. *Contemporary Drug Problems, 16,* 71-80.

Mosley, W. H. (1994). Population change, health planning and human resource development in the health sector. *World Health Statistics Quarterly, 47,* 26-30.

Mott, F. L., & Mott, S. A. (1985). Household fertility in West Africa: A comparison of male and female survey results. *Studies in Family Planning, 16,* 88-99.

Moulton, J., & Roberts, A. H. (1993). Adapting the tools to the field: Training in the use of focus groups. In R. E. Seidel (Ed.), *Notes from the field in communication for child survival* (pp. 31-37). Washington, DC: USAID.

Mulatu, M. S. (1995a). The prevalence and risk factors of psychopathology in Ethiopian children. *American Academy of Child and Adolescent Psychiatry, 34,* 100-109.

Mulatu, M. S. (1995b). *Lay causal beliefs about psychological and physical illnesses in Ethiopia.* Paper presented at Canadian Psychological Association, Charlottetown, PEI.

Mull, D. S. (1991). Traditional perceptions of marasmus in Pakistan. *Social Science & Medicine, 32,* 175-191.

Muller, F. (1983). Contrast in community participation: Case studies from Peru. In D. Morely, J. Rohde, & G. Williams (Eds.), *Practising health for all* (pp. 190-207). Oxford: Oxford University Press.

Murdoch, D., Pihl, R. O., & Ross, D. (1990). Alcohol and crimes of violence: Present issues. *International Journal of Addictions, 25,* 1065-1081.

Mustafa, M. A. B., & Mumford, S. D. (1984). Male attitudes towards family planning in Khartoum, Sudan. *Journal of Biosocial Science, 16,* 437-449.

Negrette, J. C. (1976). Alcoholism in Latin America. *Annals of the New York Academy of Sciences, 273,* 9-23.

Negrette, J. C. (1985). *Primary prevention of alcohol abuse: Latin American perspectives.* Paper presented at the seminar, Alcohol Use in Latin America: Cultural Realities and Policy Implications.

Nelson, K. R., Jenkins, R. M., et al. (1989). A Third World supplemental feeding project: Expectations and realities—a dichotomy. *Nutrition Today, 24,* 19-24.

Nichter, M. (1989). *Anthropology and international health: South Asian case studies.* London (Boston): Kluwer.

Nielsen, M. F. J., Resnick, C. A., & Acuda, S. W. (1989). Alcoholism among outpatients of a rural district general hospital in Kenya. *British Journal of Addiction, 84,* 1343-1351.

Ntozi, J. P. M., & Kabera, J. B. (1991). Family planning in rural Uganda: Knowledge and use of modern and traditional methods in Ankole. *Studies in Family Planning, 22,* 116-123.

Oakley, P. (1989). *Community involvement in health development.* Geneva, Switzerland: WHO.

Odebiyi, A. I. (1989). Food taboos in maternal and child health: The views of traditional healers in Ile-Ife, Nigeria. *Social Science & Medicine, 28,* 985-996.

Oetting, E. R., & Beauvais, F. (1990). Adolescent drug use: Findings of national and local surveys. *Journal of Consulting & Clinical Psychology, 58,* 385-394.

Offord, D. R., Boyle, M. H., & Racine, Y. (1989). Ontario child health study: Correlates of disorders. *Journal of the American Academy of Child and Adolescent Psychiatry, 28,* 856-860.

Oltmanns, T. F., & Emery, R. E. (1995). *Abnormal psychology.* Englewood Cliffs, NJ: Prentice Hall

O'Nell, T. D., & Mitchell, C. M. (1996). Alcohol use among American Indian adolescents: The role of culture in pathological drinking. *Social Science & Medicine, 42,* 565-578.

Ormel, J., VonKorff, M., Ustun, T. B., Pini, S., Korten, A., & Oldehinkel, T. (1994). Common mental disorders and disability across cultures. *Journal of the American Medical Association, 272,* 1741-1748.

Orubuloye, I. O., Caldwell, J. C., & Caldwell, P. (1993). African women's control over their sexuality in an era of AIDS: A study of the Yoruba of Nigeria. *Social Science and Medicine, 37,* 859-872.

Otieno, B., Owola, J. A., & Oduo, P. (1979). A study of alcoholism in a rural setting in Kenya. *East African Medical Journal, 56,* 665-670.

Pacqué-Margolis, S., Pacqué, M., Dukuly, Z., Boateng, J., & Taylor, H. R. (1990). Application of the verbal autopsy during a clinical trial. *Social Science & Medicine, 31,* 585-591.

Paltiel, F. L. (1987). Women and mental health: A post-Nairobi perspective. *World Health Statistics Quarterly, 40,* 233-266.

Pan-American Health Organization (PAHO). (1990). *Drug abuse.* Washington, DC: WHO.

Pant, C. R., Pokharel, G. P., Curtale, F., Pokhrel, R. P., Grosse, R. N., Lepkowski, J., Muhilal [full name], Bannister, M., Gorstein, J., Pak-Gorstein, S., Atmarita [full name], Tilden, R. L. (1996). Impact of nutrition education and mega-dose vitamin A supplementation on the health of children in Nepal. *Bulletin of the World Health Organization, 74,* 533-545.

Parker, R. G. (1996). Behavior in Latin American men: Implications for HIV/AIDS interventions. *International Journal of STD & AIDS, 7*(Suppl. 2), 62-65.

Patel, V. (1995). Explanatory models of mental illness in sub-Sahara Africa. *Social Science & Medicine, 40,* 1291-1298.

Patel, V. L., Eisemon, T. O., & Arocha, J. F. (1988). Causal reasoning and the treatment of diarrheal disease by mothers in Kenya. *Social Science & Medicine, 27,* 1277-1286.

Patil, V., Solanki, M., Kowli, S. S., Naik, V. A., Bhalerao, V. R., & Subramanian, P. (1996). Long-term follow-up of school health education programmes. *World Health Forum, 17,* 81-82.

Pauw, J., Ferrie, J., Villegas, R. R., Martinez, J. M., Gorter, A., & Egger, M. (1996). A controlled HIV/AIDS-related health education program in Managua, Nicaragua. *AIDS, 10,* 537-544.

Peltzer, K. (1989). Causative and intervening factors of harmful alcohol consumption and cannabis use in Malawi. *International Journal of the Addictions, 24,* 79-85.

Perry, C. L., Baranowski, T., & Parcel, G. S. (1990). How individuals, environments, and health behavior interact: Social learning theory. In K. Glanz, F. M. Lewis, & B. K. Rimer (Eds.), *Health behavior and health education* (pp. 161-180). San Francisco: Jossey-Bass.

Perry, C. L., & Grant, M. (1988). Comparing peer-led to teacher-led youth alcohol education in four countries. *Alcohol Health and Research World, 12,* 322-326.

Peterson, J. B., Rothfleisch, J., Zelazo, P. D., & Pihl, R. O. (1990). Acute alcohol intoxication and cognitive functioning. *Journal of Studies on Alcohol, 51,* 114-122.

Phares, V., & Compas, B. E. (1992). The roles of fathers in child and adolescent psychopathology: Make room for daddy. *Psychological Bulletin, 111,* 387-412.

Phillips, J. F., Hossain, M. B., Simmons, R., & Koenig, M. A. (1993). Worker-client exchanges and contraceptive use in rural Bangladesh. *Studies in Family Planning, 24,* 329-342.

Phillips, M. R., Pearson, V., & Wang, R. (1994). Psychiatric rehabilitation in China: Models for change in a changing society. *British Journal of Psychiatry, 165*(Suppl. 24).

Piacentini, J., Shaffer, D., Fisher, P., Schwab-Stone, M., Davies, M., & Gioia, P. (1993). The Diagnostic Interview Schedule for Children-Revised Version (DISC-R): III. Concurrent criterion validity. *Journal of the American Academy of Child and Adolescent Psychiatry, 32,* 658-665.

Pihl, R. O., & Peterson, J. B. (1992). Etiology. *Annual Review of Addictions Research and Treatment, 2,* 153-175.

Pihl, R. O., Peterson, J. B., & Finn, P. R. (1990). The inherited predisposition to alcoholism: Characteristics of sons of male alcoholics. *Journal of Abnormal Psychology, 9,* 291-301.

Ping, T. (1995). IUD discontinuation patterns and correlates in four counties in north China. *Studies in Family Planning, 26,* 169-179.

Ping, T., & Smith, H. L. (1995). Determinants of induced abortion and their policy implications in four counties in north China. *Studies in Family Planning, 26,* 278-286.

Piot, P., Kapita, B. M., Ngugi, E. N., Mann, J. M., Colebunders, R., & Wabitsch, R. (1992). *AIDS in Africa: A manual for physicians.* Geneva, Switzerland: WHO.

Piotrow, P. T., & Kincaid, D. L. (1988). How should vasectomy be promoted in Guatemala? *Studies in Family Planning, 19,* 248-249.

Piotrow, P. T., Rimon, J. G., II, Winnard, K., Kincaid, D. L., Huntington, D., & Convisser, J. (1990). Mass media family planning promotion in three Nigerian cities. *Studies in Family Planning, 21,* 265-274.

Pollitt, E., Gorman, K. S., Engle, P. L., Martorell, R., & Rivera, J. (1993). Early supplementary feeding and cognition. *Monographs of the SRCD, 58*(Whole No. 7).

Preble, E. A. (1990). Impact of HIV/AIDS on African children. *Social Science and Medicine, 31,* 671-680.

Preble, E. A., & Foumbi, J. (1991). The African family and AIDS: A current look at the epidemic. *AIDS, 5,* S263-S267.

Ramalingaswami, V., Jonsson, U., & Rohde, J. (1996). The Asian enigma. In *UNICEF: The progress of nations* (pp. 11-17). Wellinford, Oxon: P & LA.

Rasmuson, M. R., Seidel, R. E., Smith, W. A., & Booth, E. M. (1988). *Communication for child survival.* Washington, DC: USAID.

Reber, A. S. (1985). *The Penguin dictionary of psychology.* New York: Penguin.

Regier, D. A., Farmer, M. E., Rae, D. S., Myers, J. K., Kramer, M., Robins, L. N., George, L. K., Karmo, M., & Locke, B. Z. (1993). One-month prevalence of mental disorders in the United States and sociodemographic characteristics: The Epidemiologic Catchment Area study. *Acta Psychiatrica Scandinavica, 88,* 35-47.

Richards, T. J., & Richards, L. (1994). Using computers in qualitative research. In N. K. Denzin & Y. S. Lincoln (Eds.), *Handbook of qualitative research* (pp. 445-462). Thousand Oaks, CA: Sage.

Rifkin, S. B. (1990). *Community participation in maternal and child health/family planning programmes.* Geneva, Switzerland: WHO.

Rifkin, S. B. (1996). Paradigms lost: Toward a new understanding of community participation in health programmes. *Acta Tropica, 61,* 79-92.

Rifkin, S. B., Muller, F., & Bichmann, W. (1988). Primary health care: On measuring participation. *Social Science and Medicine, 26,* 931-940.

Rigdon, S. M. (1996). Abortion law and practice in China: An overview with comparisons to the United States. *Social Science & Medicine, 42,* 543-560.

Roberts, A., Pareja, R., Shaw, W., & Boyd, B. (1996). *A tool box for building health communication capacity.* Washington, DC: Academy for Educational Development & BASICS.

Robertson, A., & Minkler, M. (1994). New health promotion movement: A critical examination. *Health Education Quarterly, 21,* 295-312.

Robins, L. N., Locke, B. Z., & Regier, D. A. (1991). An overview of psychiatric disorders in America. In L. N. Robins & D. A. Regier (Eds.), *Psychiatric disorders in America: The Epidemiologic Catchment Area Study* (pp. 328-366). New York: Free Press.

Robins, L. N., Wing, J., Wittchen, H. U., Helzer, J. E., Babor, T. F., Burke, J., Farmer, A., Jablensky, A., Pickens, R., Regier, D. A., Sartorius, N., & Towle, L. H. (1988). The Composite International Diagnostic Interview. *Archives of General Psychiatry, 45,* 1069-1077.

Robinson, S. A., & Larsen, D. E. (1990). The relative influence of the community and the health system on work performance: A case study of community health workers in Colombia. *Social Science and Medicine, 30,* 1041-1048.

Rogers, E. M. (1983). *Diffusion of innovations.* New York: Free Press.

Roizen, J. (1989). Alcohol and trauma. In N. Giesbrecht, R. Gonzalez, M. Grant, E. Osterberg, R. Room, I. Rootman, & L. Towle (Eds.), *Drinking and casualties: Accidents, poisonings, and violence in an international perspective* (pp. 21-66). London: Routledge.

Rootman, I., & Moser, J. (1984). *Guidelines for investigating alcohol problems and developing appropriate responses* (Offset Publication No. 81). Geneva, Switzerland: WHO.

Rosenstock, I. M. (1990). The health belief model: Explaining health behavior through expectancies. In K. Glanz, F. M. Lewis, & B. K. Rimer (Eds.), *Health behavior and health education* (pp. 39-62). San Francisco: Jossey-Bass.

Ross, J. A., & Isaacs, S. L. (1988). Costs, payments, and incentives in family planning programs: A review for developing countries. *Studies in Family Planning, 19,* 270-283.

Roy, S. K., Rahman, M. M., Mitra, A. K., Ali, M., Alam, A. N., & Akbar, M. S. (1993). Can mothers identify malnutrition in their children? *Health Policy and Planning, 8,* 143-149.

Ruggiero, K. M. (1993). *International development agencies: Is our money being well spent?* Unpublished manuscript, McGill University.

Rutter, M. (1985). Resilience in the face of adversity: Protective factors and resistence to psychiatric disorders. *British Journal of Psychiatry, 147,* 598-611.

Sachs, L. (1983). *Evil eye or bacteria.* Stockholm: Stockholm Studies in Social Anthropology.

Sandala, L., Lurie, P., Sunkutu, M. R., Chani, E. M., Hudes, E. S., & Hearst, N. (1995). "Dry sex" and HIV infection among women attending a sexually transmitted diseases clinic in Lusaka, Zambia. *AIDS, 9,* S61-S68.

Saraceno, B., Tognoni, G., & Garattini, S. (1993). Critical questions in clinical psychopharmacology. In N. Sartorius, G. De Girolamo, G. Andrews, G. A. German, & L. Eisenberg (Eds.), *Treatment of mental disorders: A review of effectiveness* (pp. 63-90). Washington, DC: American Psychiatric Press.

Sarason, I. G., Johnson, J. H., & Siegel, J. M. (1978). Assessing the impact of life changes: Development of the life experiences survey. *Journal of Consulting and Clinical Psychology, 46,* 932-946.

Sauerborn, S. (1989). Low utilization of community health workers: Results from a household interview survey in Burkina Faso. *Social Science and Medicine, 29,* 1163-1174.

Saunders, J. B., Aasland, O. G., Amundsen, A., & Grant, M. (1993). Alcohol consumption and related problems among primary health care patients: WHO collaborative project on early detection of persons with harmful alcohol consumption—I. *Addiction, 88,* 349-362.

Scheier, L. M., & Newcomb, M. D. (1991). Psychosocial predictors of drug use initiation and escalation: An exposure of the multiple risk factors hypothesis using longitudinal data. *Contemporary Drug Problems, 18,* 31-73.

Schneiderman, N., & Tapp, J. T. (Eds.). (1985). *Behavioral medicine: The biopsychosocial approach.* Hillsdale, NJ: Lawrence Erlbaum.

Schoepf, B. G. (1993). AIDS action-research with women in Kinshasa, Zaire. *Social Science and Medicine, 37,* 1401-1413.

Schopper, D., Doussantousse, S., & Orav, J. (1993). Sexual behaviors relevant to HIV transmission in a rural African population. *Social Science & Medicine, 37,* 401-412.

Schuler, S. R., McIntosh, N., Goldstein, M. C., & Pande, B. R. (1985). Barriers to effective family planning in Nepal. *Studies in Family Planning, 16,* 260-270.

Scrimshaw, S. C. M., Carballo, M., Ramos, L., & Blair, B. A. (1991). The AIDS rapid anthropological assessment procedures: A tool for health education planning and evaluation. *Health Education Quarterly, 18,* 111-123.

Sepehri, A., & Pettigrew, J. (1996). Primary health care, community participation and community financing: Experience of two middle hill villages in Nepal. *Health Policy and Planning, 11,* 93-100.

Shack, K., Grivetti, L. E., & Dewey, K. G. (1990). Cash cropping, subsistence agriculture, and nutritional status among mothers and children in lowland Papua New Guinea. *Social Science and Medicine, 3,* 61-68.

Sigman, M., Neumann, C., Baksh, M., Bwibo, N., & McDonald, M. A. (1989). Relationship between nutrition and development in Kenyan toddlers. *Journal of Pediatrics, 115,* 357-364.

Sigman, M., Neumann, C., Carter, E., Cattle, D. J., D'Souza, S., & Bwibo, N. (1988). Home interactions and the development of Embu toddlers in Kenya. *Child Development, 59,* 1251-1261.

Sigman, M., Neumann, C., Jansen, A., & Bwibo, N. (1989). Cognitive abilities of Kenyan children in relation to nutrition, family characteristics, and education. *Child Development, 60,* 1463-1474.

Simeon, D. T., & Grantham-McGregor, S. M. (1990). Nutritional deficiencies and children's behavior and mental development. *Nutrition Research Reviews, 3,* 1-24.

Simmons, G. B. (1986). Reproductive mortality in developing countries. *American Journal of Public Health, 76,* 131-132.

Simmons, R., Baqee, L., Koenig, M. A., & Phillips, J. F. (1988). Beyond supply: The importance of family planning workers in Bangladesh. *Studies in Family Planning, 19,* 29-38.

Simmons, R., Koblinsky, M. A., & Phillips, J. F. (1986). Client relations in South Asia: Programmatic and societal determinants. *Studies in Family Planning, 17,* 257-268.

Standing, H. (1992). AIDS: Conceptual and methodological issues in researching sexual behavior in sub-Saharan Africa. *Social Science & Medicine, 34,* 475-483.

Steckler, A., McLeroy, K. R., Goodman, R. M., Bird, S. T., & McCormick, L. (1992). Toward integrating qualitative and quantitative methods: An introduction. *Health Education Quarterly, 19,* 1-8.

Stephenson, L. S. (1994). Helminth parasites, a major factor in malnutrition. *World Health Forum, 15,* 169-172.

Streeten, P. (1987). The contribution of non-governmental organizations to development. *Development: Seeds of Change, 4,* 92-95.

Super, C. M., Clement, J., Vuori, L., Christiansen, N., Mora, J. O., & Herrera, M. G. (1981). Infant and caregiver behaviors as mediators of nutritional and social interaction in the barrios of Bogota. In T. Field (Ed.), *Culture and early interaction* (pp. 171-188). Hillsdale, NJ: Lawrence Erlbaum.

Super, C. M., Herrera, M. G., & Mora, J. O. (1990). Long-term effects of food supplementation and psychological intervention on the physical growth of Colombian infants at risk of malnutrition. *Child Development, 61,* 29-49.

Tafari, S., Aboud, F. E., & Larson, C. P. (1991). Determinants of mental illness in a rural Ethiopian adult population. *Social Science & Medicine, 32,* 197-201.

Taha, T. E. T., Canner, J. K., Chiphangwi, J. D., Dallabetta, G. A., Yang, L.-P., Mtimavalye, L. A. R., & Miotti, P. G. (1996). Reported condom use is not associated with incidence of sexually transmitted diseases in Malawi. *AIDS, 10,* 207-212.

Tekle-Haimanot, R., Abebe, M., Forsgren, L., Gebre-Mariam, A., Heijbel, J., Holmgren, G., & Ekstedt, J. (1991). Attitudes of rural people in central Ethiopia toward epilepsy. *Social Science & Medicine, 32,* 203-209.

Terefe, A., & Larson, C. P. (1993). Modern contraception use in Ethiopia: Does involving husbands make a difference? *American Journal of Public Health, 83,* 1567-1571.

Thara, R., Padmavati, R., & Ayankaran, J. R. (1995). *Manual for community mental health workers.* Madras, India: Schizophrenia Research Foundation (SCARF) India.

Ticao, C. J., & Aboud, F. E. (in press). A problem-solving approach to nutrition education with Filipino mothers. *Social Science & Medicine.*

Torrey, E. F. (1967). *An introduction to health education in Ethiopia.* Addis Ababa, Ethiopia: Artistic Printers.

Triandis, H. C., Bontempo, R., Villareal, M. J., Asai, M., & Lucca, N. (1988). Individualism and collectivism: Cross-cultural perspectives on self-ingroup relationships. *Journal of Personality & Social Psychology, 54,* 323-338.

Trussell, J., & Pebley, A. R. (1984). The potential impact of changes in fertility on infant, child, and maternal mortality. *Studies in Family Planning, 15,* 267-280.

Tucker, G. M. (1986). Barriers to modern contraceptive use in rural Peru. *Studies in Family Planning, 17,* 308-316.

Ulin, P. R. (1992). African women and AIDS: Negotiating behavioral change. *Social Science and Medicine, 34,* 63-73.

UNAIDS. (1995). *HIV variability.* Geneva, Switzerland: UNAIDS and WHO.

UNAIDS. (1996a). *The HIV/AIDS situation in mid 1996: Global and regional highlights.* Geneva, Switzerland: UNAIDS and WHO.

UNAIDS. (1996b). *HIV/AIDS: The global epidemic, December 1996.* Geneva, Switzerland: UNAIDS and WHO.

UNICEF. (1993). *The state of the world's children.* Oxford: Oxford University Press.

UNICEF. (1996). *The state of the world's children.* Oxford: Oxford University Press.

U.S. Centers for Disease Control. (1996). Community-level prevention of human immunodeficiency virus infection among high-risk populations: The AIDS community demonstration projects. *Morbidity & Mortality Weekly Report, 45,* 1-24.

Ustun, T. B., Bertelsen, A., Dilling, H., van Drimmelen, J., Pull, C., Okasha, A., & Sartorius, N. (1996). *ICD-10 casebook: The many faces of mental disorders: Adult case histories according to ICD-10.* Washington, DC: American Psychiatric Press.

Valenzuela, M. (1990). Attachment in chronically underweight young children. *Child Development, 61,* 1984-1996.

Vallance, M. (1965). Alcoholism: A two-year follow-up study of patients admitted to the psychiatric department of a general hospital. *British Journal of Psychiatry, 111,* 348-356.

van de Vijver, F., & Leung, K. (1997). *Methods and data analysis for cross-cultural research.* Thousand Oaks, CA: Sage.

Visrutaratna, S., Lindan, C. P., Sirhorachai, A., & Mandel, J. S. (1995). "Superstar" and "model brothel": Developing and evaluating a condom promotion program for sex establishments in Chiang Mai, Thailand. *AIDS, 9,* S69-S75.

Vobejda, B. (1996, March 17). U.S. aid cut "will increase abortions." *Guardian Weekly*, the Washington Post Section, p. 16.

Wachs, T. D. (1995). Relation of mild-to-moderate malnutrition to human development: Correlational studies. *Journal of Nutrition, Supplement, 125*, 2245S-2254S.

Wachs, T. D., Sigman, M., Bishry, Z., Moussa, W., Jerome, N., Neumann, C., Bwibo, N., & McDonald, M. A. (1992). Caregiver-child interaction patterns in two cultures in relation to nutritional intake. *International Journal of Behavioral Development, 15*, 1-18.

Walker, A. F. (1990). The contribution of weaning foods to protein-energy malnutrition. *Nutrition Research Reviews, 3*, 25-47.

Walker, R. D., Lambert, M. D., Walker, P. S., & Kivlahan, D. R. (1993). Treatment implications of comorbid psychopathology in American Indians and Alaska Natives. *Culture, Medicine, & Psychiatry, 16*, 555-572.

Wallace, J. (1989). A biopsychosocial model of alcoholism. *Social Casework: The Journal of Contemporary Social Work, 70*, 352-332.

Wallston, K. A., Wallston, B. S., & DeVellis, R. (1978). Development of the multidimensional health locus of control (MHLC) scales. *Health Education Monographs, 6*, 160-170.

Walsh, B., & Grant, M. (1985). International trends in alcohol production and consumption: Implications for public health. *World Health Statistics Quarterly, 38*, 130-136.

Walt, G., Perera, M., & Heggenhougen, K. (1989). Are large-scale volunteer community health worker programmes feasible? The case of Sri Lanka. *Social Science and Medicine, 29*, 599-608.

Warren, C. W., Hiyari, F., Wingo, P. A., Abdel-Aziz, A. M., & Morris, L. (1990). Fertility and family planning in Jordan: Results from the 1985 Jordan husbands' fertility survey. *Studies in Family Planning, 21*, 33-39.

Waterlow, J. C. (1992). *Protein energy malnutrition*. London: Edward Arnold.

Waxler, N. E. (1979). Is outcome for schizophrenia better in non-industrialized countries? The case of Sri Lanka. *Journal of Nervous and Mental Disease, 167*, 144-158.

Weick, K. E. (1968). Systematic observational methods. In G. Lindzey & E. Aronson (Eds.), *The handbook of social psychology* (Vol. 2, pp. 357-451). Reading, MA: Addison-Wesley.

Weisner, T. S. (1989). Cultural and universal aspects of social support for children: Evidence from the Abaluyia of Kenya. In D. Belle (Ed.), *Children's social networks and social supports* (pp. 70-90). New York: John Wiley.

Weisz, J. R., Sigman, M., Weiss, B., & Mosk, J. (1993). Parent reports of behavioral and emotional problems among children in Kenya, Thailand, and the United States. *Child Development, 64*, 98-109.

Werner, E. E. (1989). Children of the Garden Island. *Scientific American, 260*, 106-111.

West, S., Munoz, B., Lynch, M., Kayongoya, A., Chilangwa, Z., Mmbaga, B. B. O., & Taylor, H. R. (1995). Impact of face-washing on trachoma in Kongwa, Tanzania. *Lancet, 345*, 155-158.

Westermeyer, J. (1984). Economic losses associated with chronic mental disorder in a developing country. *British Journal of Psychiatry, 144*, 475-481.

Whiting, B. B., & Edwards, C. P. (1988). *Children of different worlds: The formation of social behavior*. Cambridge: Harvard University Press.

Wig, N. N., Suleiman, M. A., Routledge, R., Murthy, R. S., Ladrido-Ignacio, L., Ibrahim, H. H. A., & Harding, T. W. (1980). Community reactions to mental disorders: A key

informant study in three developing countries. *Acta Psychiatrica Scandinavia, 61,* 111-126.
Wilkins, A., Hayes, R., Alonso, P., Baldeh, S., Berry, N., Cham, K., Hughes, A., Jaiteh, K., Oelman, B., Tedder, R., & Whittle, H. (1991). Risk factors for HIV-2 infection in the Gambia. *AIDS, 5,* 1127-1132.
Williams, A. O. (1992). *AIDS: An African perspective.* Ann Arbor: CRC Press.
Winikoff, B., & Laukaran, V. H. (1989). Breast feeding and bottle feeding controversies in the developing world: Evidence from a study in four countries. *Social Science & Medicine, 29,* 859-868.
Winikoff, B., & Sullivan, M. (1987). Assessing the role of family planning in reducing maternal mortality. *Studies in Family Planning, 18,* 128-143.
Winett, R. A. (1995). A framework for health promotion and disease prevention programs. *American Psychologist, 50,* 341-350.
Wittchen, H. U., Robins, L. N., Cottler, L. B., Sartorius, N., Burke, J. D., & Regier, D. (1991). Cross-cultural feasibility, reliability and source of variance of the Composite International Diagnostic Interview (CIDI). *British Journal of Psychiatry, 159,* 645-653.
Workneh, F., & Giel, R. (1975). Medical dilemma: A survey of the healing practice of a Coptic priest and an Ethiopian sheik. *Tropical and Geographical Medicine, 27,* 431-439.
World Bank. (1993). *World development report 1993: Investing in health.* Oxford: Oxford University Press.
World Health Organization (WHO). (1952). *Expert committee on mental health: Alcoholism subcommittee* (Technical Report Series 48). Geneva, Switzerland: Author.
World Health Organization (WHO), Scientific Group. (1980). *Problems related to alcohol consumption* (Technical Report Series 650). Geneva, Switzerland: Author.
World Health Organization (WHO). (1983). *Measuring change in nutritional status.* Geneva, Switzerland: Author.
World Health Organization (WHO). (1988). *Education for health: A manual on health education in primary healthcare.* Geneva, Switzerland: Author.
World Health Organization (WHO). (1992). *The international classification of diseases—10.* Geneva, Switzerland: Author.
World Health Organization (WHO). (1995). Progress towards health for all: Third monitoring report. *World Health Statistics Quarterly, 48,* 174-199.
Yamamoto, J., Silva, J. A., Sasao, T., Wang, C., & Nguyen, L. (1993). Alcoholism in Peru. *American Journal of Psychiatry, 150,* 1059-1062.
Young, D. R., Haskell, W. L., Taylor, C. B., & Fortmann, S. P. (1996). Effect of community health education on physical activity knowledge, attitudes, and behavior: The Stanford Five-City Project. *American Journal of Epidemiology, 144,* 264-274.

# AUTHOR INDEX

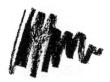

Aaby, P., 36
Aasland, O. G., 186, 187, 191, 192, 196, 197, 199
Abdel-Aziz, A. M., 77
Abebe, M., 259
Abiodun, O. A., 250, 258, 268
Aboud, F. E., 30, 42, 45, 166, 171, 178, 223, 262
AbouZahr, C., 73
Achenbach, T. M., 250
Acuda, S. W., 190, 196, 198, 199
Adair, L., 165
Adamson, P., 72, 73, 221, 264
Adegbola, D., 33
Adler, N. E., 239
Adler, P., 47
Adler, P. A., 47
Aggleton, P., 106, 118
Aidala, A. A., 198
Ajzen, I., 212, 235
Akbar, M. S., 168

Alam, A. N., 168
Alemu, T., 42, 45, 165, 166, 171, 178
Ali, M., 168
Ali, N., 226
Allen, S., 117
Alonso, P., 100, 115
American Psychiatric Association, 246
Amundsen, A., 186, 187, 191, 192, 196, 197, 199
Anderson, C. M., 268
Anderson, R. M., 101
Anderson, W. T., 109
Anker, M., 255, 258, 261, 268
Annys, S., 143
Aplasca, M. R. A., 116
Aptekar, L., 263, 274
Armstrong, S., 4, 112
Arocha, J. F., 240
Asai, M., 263, 267
Asthana, S., 107, 109, 115

311

Asuni, T., 269
Atmarita, 181
Ayankaran, J. R., 269
Ayele, F., 137
Ayowa, O. B., 111

Babor, R. F., 191, 248
Baksh, M., 166, 171, 177, 178
Baldeh, S., 100, 115
Baltazar, J., 257, 258, 268
Bandura, A., 63
Bannister, M., 181
Baqee, L., 89
Baranowski, T., 235
Barker, C., 20
Barrett, D. E., 176, 177
Beauvais, F., 197, 198
Becker, M. H., 106, 213, 235
Bedi, H., 268
Bedi, K. S., 176
Bekele, A., 167
Bentley, M. E., 33, 157, 166, 168, 184
Berkley, S., 97, 102-104, 106, 110, 112, 118
Bernhart, M. H. 89
Berry, J. W., 36, 59
Berry, N., 100, 115
Bertelson, A., 246, 255, 258, 261, 268
Bertrand, J., 107, 109, 110, 115
Bertrand, J. T., 90
Beusenberg, M., 248
Bhalerao, V. R., 220
Bhatia, J. C., 81
Bhave, G., 107, 109, 110, 115
Bicego, G. T., 165
Bichmann, W., 126, 141, 143
Bien, T. H., 205
Bilqis, A. H., 226
Binion, A., 198
Bird, S. T., 33
Bishry, Z., 157, 179
Black, R., 165
Blaine, J., 191, 193, 248
Blair, B. A., 33, 37
Blanc, A. K., 231, 239, 242
Blanchard, L. W., 62
Bland, R. C., 190, 194, 195, 203
Bloomer, C. M., 74
Blustein, P., 273

Boag, F. C., 97
Boateng, J., 63
Bobadilla, J. L., 11
Boerma, J. T., 165
Bogaerts, J., 117
Bogdewic, S. P., 47
Bonati, G., 220
Bongaarts, J., 69, 71, 100, 103
Bontempo, T., 263, 267
Booth, E. M., 33, 35, 37, 42, 45, 47, 213, 222, 227, 233, 236, 237
Bosenge, N., 107, 109, 110, 115
Boyce, T., 239,
Boyd, B., 37
Boyle, M. H., 260
Brady, M., 198
Brazelton, T. B., 179, 263
Briscoe, J., 129, 143, 152, 169
Brookmeyer, R., 99, 100
Brown, J. E., 111
Brown, K. H., 33, 157, 166, 168, 184
Brown, P., 122
Brown, R. C., 111
Brun, T. A., 163
Brunet, J-B., 99
Brunswick, A. F., 198
Bry, B. H., 209
Bucholz, K. K., 206
Buehler , J. W., 99
Bunnett, V., 95
Burke, J. D., 191, 248
Bushman, B. J., 202
Bwibo, N. O., 157, 166, 171, 176-179


Caldwell, J. C., 80, 109-111, 113, 115, 239, 241
Caldwell, P., 80, 109-111, 113, 115, 241
Cameron, M., 158, 159, 183
Canino, G. J., 190, 194, 195, 203
Canner, J. K., 110
Caprara, A., 109
Carael, M., 117
Carballo, M., 33, 37
Carlin, E. M., 97
Carter, E., 178
Carter, R. J., 117
Cartwright, D., 127
Cassidy, C. M., 4

## Author Index

Cattle, D. J., 178
Chaiken, M. R., 208
Chaiken, S., 235
Cham, K., 100, 115
Chambwe, A., 199
Chang, S. M., 177
Chani, E. M., 112
Chesney, M., 95
Chesney, M. A., 239
Chi, I., 195
Chilangwa, Z., 218
Chin, J., 100
Chiphangwi, J. D., 110
Christiansen, N., 178
Cleland, J., 81, 88, 239, 241
Clement, J., 178
Climent, C. E., 61, 248-250, 257, 258, 268
Coates, T. J., 95, 117
Coeytaux, F. M., 74
Cohen , J., 99
Cohen, J. M., 125, 128, 140
Colebunders, R., 99, 104
Compas, B. E., 260, 261
Compton, W. M., 194, 257
Conley, J. J., 260
Convisser, J., 88
Coombs, D. W., 195, 205, 208
Cooper, H. M., 202
Cooper, J. E., 255, 258, 261, 268
Coreil, J., 182
Cottler, L. B., 191, 193, 248
Covell, K., 207
Cowan, B., 166, 167, 183
Coyne, J. C., 261, 262,
Cunningham, A., 129, 143, 152
Curtale, F., 181


Dakof, G., 262
Dallabetta, G. A., 110
Dasen, P. R., 36
Davidson, R. S., 189, 201, 203, 204, 206
Davies, M., 251
Day, R., 255, 258, 261, 268
De Arango, M. V., 250, 257, 258, 268
de Castro, M. P. P., 89
De Cock, K. M., 99
De Gregorio, G. C., 109
de la Pena, E., 33

Deeds, S. G., 212
DeLongis, A., 262
Desai, S., 107, 109, 110, 115
Des Jarlais, D. C., 120
Desjarlais, R., 269
Desta, A., 137
DeVellis, B. M., 62
DeVellis, R. F., 62
Dewey, K. G., 163
Dewey, M., 199
Dhanoa, J., 166, 167, 183
Dhillion, H. S., 211
Dickin, K. L., 157, 166, 168, 184
Dilling, H., 246
Dion, K. K., 207
Dion, K. L., 207
Dixon, S., 179, 263
Donovan, J. E., 205
Dorkenoo, E., 4
Douossantousse, S., 110
Downs, E., 151
D'Souza, S., 178
Du Wors, R., 95
Dubuis, J., 269
Dukuly, Z., 63
Dupree, J. D., 106, 109, 110, 118, 119
Dwyer, J. M., 103, 104, 116


Eagly, A. H., 235
Edelbrock, C. S., 250
Edwards, C. P., 179, 263
Egger, M., 107, 109, 110, 119
Eisemon, T. O., 240
Eisenberg, L., 264, 269
Ekstedt, J., 259
El Hassan Al Awad, A. M., 263
Elder, J. P., 33, 37, 42, 45, 86, 87, 213, 215, 222, 233, 236, 237
Eliany, M., 198
Elias, C., 107, 109, 110, 113-115
Emery, R. E., 261
Enel, C., 107-109
Eng, E., 129, 143, 152
Engle, P. L., 172, 174
Ernberg, G., 255, 258, 261, 268
Eschen, A., 83, 85
Escobedo, L. G., 193, 194
Espinosa, M. P., 176

Estey, J. D., 86, 87
Evans, G. E., 216
Everett, S. A., 262

Fajans, P., 63
Falloon, I. R. H., 109, 110, 115
Farmer, A., 269
Farmer, M. E., 191, 248
Fauvreau, V., 163
Ferrie, J., 107, 109, 110, 119
Fillmore, C. M., 160
Fillmore, K. M., 186, 191, 193, 197, 198
Finn, P. R., 205
Fisher, P., 251
Flieger, W., 265
Folkman, S., 63, 95, 262, 263
Fontana, A., 35, 52
Food and Agricultural Organization, 157
Ford, K., 109, 110, 115
Foreit, K. G., 89
Forsgren, L., 259
Fortmann, S. P., 210
Foster, G., 128-131
Foumbi, J., 114
Franco, E. F. D., 89
Frankel, D. G., 180
Freedman, L. P., 73
Freudenberg, N., 117
Frey, J. H., 35, 52
Freyens, P., 134
Friedman, S. R., 120
Fryer, M. L., 220

Galler, J. R., 170
Galvez-Tan, J. Z., 136
Garattini, S., 269
Garmezy, N., 261
Gayle, H., 97, 102-104, 106, 110, 112, 118
Gebre-Mariam, A., 259
Geen, R. G., 201
Geissler, C., 163
Geller, E. S., 237
George, L. K., 251, 257
Gerein N. M., 160
Gezahegn, Y., 266
Gezelius, H., 151

Giel, R., 61, 248-250, 258, 262, 266, 268, 269
Gilchrist, V. J., 52
Gillies, P. A., 116
Gioia, P., 251
Giovino, G. A., 193, 194
Gittelman, M., 269
Goldberg, D., 193, 245, 252, 257, 258
Golden, L. L., 109
Goldin, C. S., 102
Goldstein, M. C., 83, 91
Gonzalez, L., 199, 201
Good, B., 269
Goodman, R. M., 33
Gorman, K. S., 172, 174, 179
Gorstein, J., 181
Gorter, A., 107, 109, 110, 119
Goze, T., 109
Graeff, J. A., 33, 37, 42, 45, 213, 222, 230, 233, 236, 237
Grant, B. F., 191, 193, 248
Grant, M., 185-187, 191-193, 196, 197, 199, 208
Grantham-McGregor, S. M., 170-172, 175, 177, 184
Green, A., 20, 151
Green, E. C., 106, 109, 110, 118, 119
Green, L. W., 33, 212
Greene, D. M., 209
Greenough, W. B., 6
Greenwald, D. P., 268
Griffin, P. D., 75, 77
Grimson, W. R., 268, 269
Grivetti, L. E., 163
Grosse, R. N., 181
Guba, E. G., 59
Guilkey, D., 165
Gureje, O., 196

Habicht, J. P., 168
Hall, W., 185
Hamilton, R., 6
Hanson, K., 124, 139, 150
Harding, T. W., 52, 54, 61, 248-250, 257, 258, 267-269
Hartka, E., 186, 191, 193, 197, 198
Harvey, P. D., 87
Haskell, W. L., 210

Hauge, R., 194
Haverkos, H. W., 92, 112
Hawes, H., 220, 221
Haworth, A., 199, 201
Hayes, R., 100, 115
Haynes-Sanstad, K., 95
Hearn, S., 90
Hearst, M., 112
Hearst, N., 116
Heather, N., 185
Heggenhougen, K., 137
Heijbel, J., 259
Heise, L., 107, 109, 110, 113-115
Heisterkamp, S. H., 99, 100
Helzer, J. E., 190, 191, 194, 195, 203, 248, 257
Henningfield, J. E., 193, 194
Herrera, M. G., 172, 178, 182, 184
Hill, K., 73
Hilton, D., 136
Himes, J. H., 171, 172, 175, 177, 184
Hirschhorn, N., 6
Hiyari, F., 77
Hodes, M., 268, 269
Hoffman, L. W., 75
Hofvander, Y., 158, 159, 183
Hogarty, G. E., 268
Holmes, T. H., 62, 65, 261
Holmgren, G., 259
Horowitz, J., 199, 200
Hossain, M. B., 89
Hovell, M. F., 237
Howes, H. G., 190, 194, 195, 203
Huberman, A. M., 35
Hubley, J., 9, 211, 213, 234
Hudes, E. S., 107, 109, 112, 115, 116
Hudson, C. P., 113
Huffman, S. L. 33
Hughes, A., 100, 115
Hull, V. J., 166
Hulley, S. B., 95, 117
Hunter, D., 35
Huntington, D., 88, 92
Hurley, J., 199, 200
Hwu, H. G., 194, 257

Ibrahim, H. H. A., 52, 54, 61, 248, 249, 257, 258, 267, 268

Idowu, J. R., 157, 166, 168, 184
Idjradinata, P., 173
Ikuesan, B. A., 196
Irgens-Jensen, O., 194
Irwin, K., 107, 109, 110, 115
Israel, B. A., 117
Isaacs, S. L., 86

Jablensky, A., 191, 248, 253, 255, 258, 261, 268
Jager, J. C., 99, 100
Jaiteh, K., 100, 115
Jamison, D. T., 11
Jansen, A., 171, 177
Janz, N. K., 106, 117, 235
Javna, C. D., 268
Jelik, W. G., 266
Jerome, N., 157, 179
Jenkins, R. M., 182
Jessor, R., 205
Johnson, K. E., 137
Johnson, J. H. 62, 65
Johnstone, B. M., 186, 191, 193, 197, 198
Jones, J., 35
Jonsson, U., 168

Kabera, J. B., 78, 82, 83
Kabir, S. M., 86
Kamal, G. M., 89
Kamali, A., 63, 114
Kandel, D. B., 186, 197
Kanner, A. D., 261
Kapita, B. M., 99, 104
Karmo, M., 251, 257
Kay, B. J., 86
Kayode, B., 157, 166, 168, 184
Kayongoya, A., 218
Keefer, C. H., 179, 263
Keller, W., 160
Kelly, E. L., 260
Kelly, K. J., 128
Kengeya-Kayondo, J. F., 63, 114
Kennedy, E., 163
Keusch, G. T., 163
Khanna, J., 75, 77
Khin-Maung-U, 6
Kim-Farley, R. J., 26, 27

Kimball, A. M., 97, 102-104, 106, 110, 112, 118
Kincaid, D. L., 88, 89
Kirby, M. D., 115-117
Kisubi, W. K., 137
Kitano, H. H. L., 195
Kivlahan, D. R., 204
Kleinman, A., 269
Kloos, H., 162, 167
Klotz, M. L., 62
Koblinsky, M. A., 89
Koenig, M. A., 89
Kornblith, S. J., 268
Korten, A., 245, 255, 258, 259, 261, 268
Korten, D. C., 151
Kortmann, F., 252, 265
Kortteinen, T., 186, 194, 203, 207
Kowli, S. S., 220
Kramer, M. S., 162
Kramer, M., 251, 257
Krause, R. M., 116
Kreuter, M. W., 212
Kuipers, L., 268
Kulhara, P., 255
Kurz, K. M., 162

Labonte, R., 152
Lackey, D., 137
Ladrido-Ignacio, L., 52, 54, 257, 258, 267-269
LaFond, A., 2, 26
Lagarde, E., 107-109
Laino, E. V., 186, 191, 193, 197, 198
Laleman, G., 143
Lambert, M. D., 204
Lancaster, J., 112
Langsley, D. G., 268, 269
Lapham, R., 86
Lapido, O. A., 90
Lapore, S. J., 262
Larsen, D. E., 137
Larson, C. P., 14, 90, 137, 214, 262
Latham, M. C., 167, 181
Laukaran, V. H., 165
Launer, L. J., 168
Lazarus, R. S., 63, 261-263
Lee, C. K., 190, 194, 195, 203
Lee, K., 68

Lee, N. C., 107, 109, 110, 115
Leff, J., 268
Leiderman, P. H., 179, 263
Leonard, A. H., 74
Lepkowski, J., 181
Lepowsky, M., 168
Leung, K., 57, 61
LeVine, R. A., 179, 263
LeVine, S., 179, 263
Levinger, B., 172, 231
Lewis, F. M., 33
Lincoln, Y. S., 59
Lindan, C. P., 107, 109, 110, 115, 117, 120
Lindtjorn, B., 162, 165
Link, P. G., 239
Links, P. S., 262
Lloyd, C. B., 231, 239, 242
Locke, B. Z., 194, 251, 256, 257
Logan, J. A., 197
Lonner, W. J., 36, 59
Low-Beer, D., 98
Lowe, J. B., 195, 205, 208
Lubben, J. E., 195
Lucca, N., 263, 267
Luchok, K., 62
Lurie, P., 95, 112
Lynch, M., 218

MacDonald, K., 109, 110, 115
Macklin, R., 4
Madonia, M. J., 268
Maine, D., 73
Malepe, T. B., 199
Mandel, J. S., 107, 109, 110, 115, 116, 120
Manderson, L., 36
Mann, J. M., 99, 104, 105
Marshall, M., 199, 200-202
Martin, M., 134
Martinez, J. M., 107, 109, 110, 119
Martorell, R., 172, 174
Mason, K. O., 76, 77
Masten, A. S., 261
Mathews, J., 230
Matthias, A., 151
Mauldin, W. P., 69, 71, 78, 85, 86, 88
May, R. M., 101
Mayer, J., 237
Mbakuliyemo, N., 134

Mbugua, J. K., 137
Mbuyi, K., 107, 109, 110, 115
McCauley, A. P., 218
McCormick, L., 33
McDonald, M. A., 157, 166, 171, 176-179
McEvoy, L., 194, 257
McGrath, J. W., 107, 109, 113, 115
McIntosh, N., 83, 91
McLeroy, K. R., 33
McNamara, G. E. D., 90
McPake, B., 124, 139, 150
Measham, A. R., 11
Mebrahtu, S., 157, 166, 168, 184
Medina-Mora, M. E., 199, 201
Meeks Gardner, J. M., 177
Meliawan, P., 109, 110, 115
Melzack, R., 62
Menon, D. K., 268
Merchant, K. M., 162
Mertens, T. E., 98
Messeri, P. A., 198
Meursing, D., 199, 203
Mibandumba, N., 107, 109, 110, 115
Miles, M. B., 35
Millar, W., 194
Miller, C. D., 198
Miller, W. R., 185, 205
Mills, A., 124, 139, 150
Millwood, P., 151
Minkler, M., 128
Miotti, P. G. 110
Mitchell, C. M., 192
Mitra, A. K., 168
Miyazaki, M., 97
Mmbaga, B. B. O., 218
Molamu, L., 186, 194, 201
Monzon, O. T., 116
Mora, J. O., 172, 178, 182, 184
Moremoholo, R. A., 196
Morgan, D. L., 35, 39
Morojele, N., 199, 203
Morris, L., 77
Moser, J., 192, 194, 195, 203, 206, 207
Moses, P. F., 196
Mosk, J., 250
Mosley, W. H., 11, 14
Motoyoshi, M., 186, 191, 193, 197, 198
Mott, F. L., 77
Mott, S. A., 77

Moulton, J., 35
Moussa, W., 157, 179
Mtimavalye, L. A., 110
Muhilal, 181
Mukasa, R., 107, 109, 113, 115
Mukoka, M., 107, 109, 110, 115
Mulatu, M. S., 251, 256, 258, 262, 267
Mulder, D. W., 63, 114
Mull, D. S., 168
Muller, F., 126, 132, 133, 141, 143
Mumford, S. D., 76, 82
Munkolenkole, K., 107, 109, 110, 115
Munoz, B., 218
Murdoch, D., 202
Muremeri, C., 107, 109, 110, 115
Murthy, R. S., 52, 54, 61, 248, 249, 257, 258, 267-269
Mustafa, M. A. B., 76, 82
Myers, J. K., 251, 257

Nagaswami, V., 269
Naik, V. A., 220
Nakayiwa, S., 107, 109, 113, 115
Nakiyingi, J., 63
Nakyobe, L., 107, 109, 113, 115
Namande, B., 107, 109, 113, 115
Negrette, J. C., 186, 195, 207
Nelson, K. R., 182
Neumann, C. G., 157, 166, 171, 176-179
Newcomb, M. D., 204
Newman, S., 190, 194, 195, 203
Ng, T. W., 101
Ngugi, E. N., 97, 99, 102-104, 106, 110, 112, 118
Nguyen, L., 195
Nichter, M., 83, 235
Nielsen, M. F. J., 190, 196
Nsengumuremyi, F., 117
Ntozi, J. P. M., 78, 82, 83
Nunn, A. J., 114
Nzilambi, N., 107, 109, 110, 115

O'Nell, T. D., 192
O'Reilly, K., 107, 109, 110, 115
Oakley, P., 130, 132, 134, 135
Obikoya, B., 196
Odebiyi, A. I., 168

Oduo, P., 196
Oelman, B., 100, 115
Oetting, E. R., 197, 198
Offord, D. R., 260
Okasha, A., 246
Oldehinkel, T., 245, 259
Ole Sena, S., 240
Oltmanns, T. F., 261
Oni, G. A., 33, 157, 166, 168, 184
Oostvogels, R., 107, 109, 115
Orav, J., 110
Orley, J., 248
Ormel, J., 245, 259
Orubuloye, I. O., 109-111, 113, 115
Osuga, B., 137
Otieno, B., 196
Otolorin, E. O., 90
Owola, J. A., 196

Pacqué, M., 63
Pacqué-Margolis, S., 63
Padmavati, R., 269
Pak-Gorstein, S., 181
Palsane, M. N., 262
Paltiel, F. L., 260, 262
Pan-American Health Organization, 195
Pande, B. R., 83, 91
Pant, C. R., 181
Parcel, G. S., 235
Pareja, R., 37
Parenzi, A., 109
Parker, R. G., 103, 109, 115
Partridge, K. B., 212
Patel, V. L., 240, 251, 253
Patil, V., 220
Paul, J., 116
Pauw, J., 107, 109, 110, 119
Pearson, V., 269
Pearson-Marks, J., 107, 109, 113, 115
Pebley, A. R., 74, 75
Pelto, G. H., 33
Peltzer, K., 186
Perera, M., 137
Perry, C. L., 208, 235
Peterson, H., 107, 109, 110, 115
Peterson, J. B., 202-205
Pettigrew, J., 142

Phares, V., 260
Phelan, J. C., 239
Philip, L., 211
Phillips, J. F., 70, 71, 89
Phillips, M. R., 269
Piacentini, J., 251
Pickens, R., 191, 248
Pihl, R. O., 202-205
Pineda, M. A., 90
Ping, T., 74, 81
Pini, S., 245, 259
Piot, P., 99, 104
Piotrow, P. T., 88, 89
Pison, G., 107-109
Pokharel, G. P., 181
Pokhrel, R. P., 181
Pollitt, E., 172-174, 179
Popkin, B. M., 165
Pounds, M. B., 218
Powell, C. A., 170-172, 175, 177, 184
Preble, E. A., 114
Publico, L., 269
Pull, C., 246

Quinn, T. C., 97, 112

Racine, Y., 260
Radke-Yarrow, M., 176, 177
Rae, D. S., 251, 257
Rahe, R. H., 62, 65, 261
Rahman, M. M., 168
Ramalingaswami, V., 168
Ramos, L., 33, 37
Ramsey, F., 170
Rasmuson, M. R., 35, 42, 47, 227
Reber, A. S., 10
Reddy, P. H., 80, 241
Regier, D. A., 191, 194, 248, 251, 256, 257
Resnick, C. A., 190, 196
Richards, L., 35, 45
Richards, T. J., 35, 45
Richman, A., 179, 263
Rifkin, S. B., 126, 127, 130, 141, 143, 148, 152, 153
Rigdon, S. M., 81
Rimon, J. G. II, 88
Rivera, J., 172, 174

Roberts, A. H., 35, 37
Robertson, A., 128
Robins, L. N., 191, 193, 194, 206, 248, 251, 256, 257
Robinson, S. A., 137
Roer-Bornstein, D., 180
Rogers, E. M., 234
Rohde, J., 168
Roizen, J., 199, 201
Roos, L., 95
Rootman, I., 191
Rosenstock, I. M., 213, 235, 236
Ross, D., 202
Ross, D. A., 160
Ross, J. A., 71, 85, 86
Rothfleisch, J., 202
Routledge, R., 52, 54, 258, 267, 268
Rowley, J. T. 101
Roy, S. K., 168
Ruberantwari, A., 114
Rufo, K., 107, 109, 110, 115
Ruggiero, K. M., 152
Russ, D. J., 268
Rustein, S. O., 165
Rutter, M., 261
Rwabukwali, C. B., 107, 109, 113, 115
Ryder, R., 107, 109, 110, 115

Sabiiti, I., 63
Sachs, L., 254
Salazar, C. M., 109
Sandala, L., 112
Santana-Arciaga, R. T., 116
Santiso, R., 90
Saraceno, B., 269
Sarason, I. G., 62, 65
Sartorius, N., 36, 191, 193, 246, 248, 255, 258, 261, 268
Sasao, T., 195
Sauerborn, S., 137
Saunders, J. B., 186, 187, 191, 192, 196, 197, 199
Schaefer, C., 261
Scheier, L. M., 204
Schneiderman, N., 7, 36
Schoepf, B. G., 115, 117
Schofield, W., 170
Schopper, D., 110

Schuler, S. R., 83, 91, 92
Schumann, D. A., 33, 107, 109, 113, 115
Schwab-Stone, M., 251
Scotchmer, C., 220, 221
Scrimshaw, S. C. M., 33, 37
Seeley, J. A., 114
Segal, S. J., 78
Seidel, R. E., 35, 42, 47, 227
Sepehri, A., 142
Seri, D., 109
Serufilira, A., 117
Shack, K., 163
Shaffer, D., 251
Shaheed, N. M., 226
Shaw, W., 37
Siegel, D., 116
Siegel, J. M., 62, 65
Sigman, M. D., 157, 166, 171, 176-179, 250
Silva, J. A., 195
Simeon, D. T., 172
Simmons, G. B., 74
Simmons, R., 89
Sirag, A. O., 269
Sirhorachai, A., 115, 120
Slade, J., 193, 194
Slade, P., 199
Smith, H. L., 74, 81
Smith, W. A., 35, 42, 47, 227
Solanki, M., 220
Sommerfelt, E., 165
Sonuga-Barke, E. J. S., 263
Spitznagel, E. L., 194, 257
Standing. H., 113
Stanfield, P., 137
Stanton, C., 73
Steckler, A., 33
Stephenson, L. S., 163
Straus, W. L., 33
Streeten, P., 151
Subramanian, P., 220
Suleiman, M. A., 52, 54, 61, 248, 249, 258, 267-269
Sullivan, M., 74
Sunkutu, M. R., 112
Super, C. M., 172, 178, 182, 184

Tafari, S., 262

Taha, T. E. T., 110
Taj, A. M., 76, 77
Tapp, J. T., 7, 36
Taylor, H. R., 62, 218
Taylor, C. B., 210
Tedder, R., 100, 115
Tekle-Haimanot, R., 259
Telljohann, S. K., 63
Temple, M. T., 186, 191, 193, 197, 198
Ten Horn, G. H. M. M., 269
Terefe, A., 90, 214
Thapa, S., 166
Thara, R., 269
Thorpe, L., 109, 110, 115
Ticao, C. J., 223, 224
Tilden, R. L., 181
Tipp, J. E., 194, 257
Tognoni, G., 269
Tomar, S. L., 193, 194
Tonigan, J. S., 205
Torrey, E. F., 84
Towle, L. H., 191, 193, 248
Triandis, H. C., 263, 267
Tripathi, S. P., 107, 109, 110, 115
Trussell, J., 74, 75
Tucker, G. M., 82, 83

Ulin, P. R., 110, 111, 115
UNAIDS, 95, 97, 98, 101-103, 110, 115
UNICEF, 24, 71, 72, 78, 161, 162, 164, 166, 169, 180, 242
United States Centers for Disease Control, 120
Uphoff, N. T., 125, 128, 140-142, 153
Ustun, T. B., 245, 246, 259

Valenzuela, M., 173, 177
Vallance, M., 188
van de Vijver, F., 57, 61
Van de Perre, P., 117
VanDerslice, J., 165
van Drimmelen, J., 246
van Ginneken, J. K., 239, 241
VanLook, P. F. A., 75, 77
van Luijk, J. N., 262, 266
VanOss Marin, B., 95
Van Vlaenderen, H., 128

Verzosa, C. C., 157, 166, 168, 184
Villareal, M. J., 263, 267
Villegas, R. R., 107, 109, 110, 119
Visrutaratna, S., 115, 120
Vobejda, B., 93
VonKorff, M., 245, 259
Voyce, C., 62
Vuori, L., 178

Wabitsch, R., 99, 104
Wachs, T. D., 157, 172, 179
Wagle, U., 107, 109, 110, 115
Wagner, H. U., 63
Walker, A. F., 158, 166
Walker, P. S., 204
Walker, R. D., 204
Walker, S. 171, 172, 175, 184
Wallace, J., 204
Wallston, B. S., 62
Wallston, A. K., 62
Walsh, B., 185, 186, 192, 193
Walt, G., 137
Wang, C., 195
Wang, R., 269
Wardlaw, T., 73
Warren, C. W., 77
Waterlow, J. C., 160, 161, 163
Waters, H., 230
Waxler, N. E., 255, 258
Weick, K. E., 42
Weisner, T. S., 263
Weiss, B., 250
Weiss, E., 90
Weisz, J. R., 250
Werner, E. E., 179, 262, 263
West, S. K., 218, 220
Westermeyer, J., 259
Whiting, B. B., 179, 263
Whittaker, M., 83, 85
Whittle, H., 100, 115
Wig, N. N., 52, 54, 61, 248-250, 257, 258, 267-269
Wiknjosastro, G., 166
Wilkins, A., 100, 115
Williams, A. O., 110
Winett, R. A., 211
Wing, J., 191, 248
Wingo, P., 107, 109, 110, 115

Wingo, P. A., 77
Winikoff, B., 74, 165
Winnard, K., 88
Wirawan, D. N., 109, 110, 115
Wittchen, H. U., 191, 193, 248
Wolf, W., 117
Workneh, F., 266
World Bank, 14, 244
World Health Organization, 11, 159, 188, 201, 203, 213, 246
Wren, P. A., 117

Yahya, F. S., 226
Yamaguchi, K., 186
Yamamoto, J., 195
Yang, L-P., 110
Yeh, E. K., 190, 194, 195, 203, 257
Young, D. R., 210
Younis, Y. O. A., 250, 258, 268
Yunus, M., 163

Zaman, K., 163
Zander, A., 127
Zeitlyn, S., 226
Zelazo, P. D., 202
Zewdi, W. G., 167
Zimmerman, N. A., 117
Zokwe, B., 106, 109, 110, 118, 119

# SUBJECT INDEX

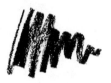

Abortion, 74, 79, 81, 93
Acquired immunodeficiency syndrome. *See* AIDS
Acute respiratory infection, 11, 276
Adapters and Activists, 4-5,
Adolescents, 186, 197-199, 208-209, 225-227
Aggression, 201-202
AIDS, 37, 64, 94-122
    perception of risk, 107-109
    prevalence, 99-104
    prevention programs, 116-122
    safe sex, 107-111, 115-120
    symptoms, 95
    transmission, 96-98, 111-115
    types, 96
Alcoholism, 185-209, 276
    alcohol, 185-186
    alcohol consumption, 192-199, 284
    measurement, 187-192
    prevalence, 193-199
    prevention, 206-209
    risk factors, 203-205
    treatment, 205
Attachment in children, 173-175
Attitudes, 7, 10, 83, 134-135, 212, 258-259, 276
    attitude change, 89, 208, 220-223, 234-235
    methods of measurement. *See also* KAP
Australia, 104, 193-197, 203, 208

Bamako initiative, 124, 139-140
Bangladesh, 5, 69, 72, 85, 89-90, 161, 225-227
Behavior, 7, 109-111
    methods of measurement
    *See also* Health behavior; KAP
Beliefs:
    about contraception, 83-84
    about food, 168

Subject Index

Calories (energy), 156-161, 166-167
Canada, 194
Caribbean. *See* Latin America and the Caribbean
Children, 18, 75-78, 94-95, 98, 102, 114, 204-205, 216-225, 249-251, 258, 262-263. *See also* Diarrhea; Education; Immunization; Malnutrition
China, 67-68, 78-79, 81, 245
Colombia, 69, 79, 85, 165, 172, 182, 231
Communication, 88-89, 92, 214-215, 220-223, 277
Community participation, 123-153, 278
   benefits and costs, 128-130
   evaluation of, 140-153
   facilitating conditions, 131-135
Community health worker (CHW), 124, 136-140, 143-145, 277
Condoms, 79, 84, 87, 110-111, 117-121. *See also* Contraception
Contraception, 23, 40-41, 67-92, 278
   methods, 78-82
   prevalence, 70, 78-81, 278
   programs, 85-92, 214-216
   reasons for, 69-78
Coping, 63, 278, 288
Costa Rica, 79
Culture, 179, 251-256, 263

Demography, 15, 68-72
Developed countries, 9, 29, 68, 70, 72, 78, 186, 207, 210, 258. *See also* Australia; Europe; Japan; North America
Developing countries, 9, 70, 72, 78, 122, 161-162, 203, 210-211, 258. *See also* East Asia and the Pacific; Latin America and the Caribbean; Middle East and North Africa; South Asia; Sub-Saharan Africa
Diarrhea, 5-6, 11, 19, 30, 37, 161, 163, 220-221, 227-230, 279. *See also* Oral rehydration salts; Oral rehydration therapy
Disability adjusted life years lost (DALY), 20, 244, 279
Drugs, 14, 122, 139-140

East Asia and the Pacific, 24, 70-72, 79, 86, 103-105, 165, 193, 195. *See also* China, Indonesia, Philippines, Thailand
Education, 230-232, 239-243, 276
   of children, 70, 172, 175, 230-232, 242-243, 277, 285
   of mothers, 31, 83, 174, 230, 239-241
   *See also* Health Education
Emic-etic, 4, 58-59, 279
Epilepsy, 259
Ethiopia, 72, 78, 90-91, 134, 136-137, 154, 161-162, 171, 214-216, 256
Europe, 103-104, 193-197. *See also* Britain, Developed countries, Scandinavia
Evil eye, 218, 252, 254
Exercise, 210

Family planning, 67-75, 214-216. *See also* Contraception
Female circumcision, 4, 112
Fertility, 16, 68-72, 287
Focus groups, 35-41, 279
Food taboos, 168

Gender, 7, 78, 157, 203, 242
Genetic, 7, 204-205
Gross national product (GNP), 70, 280
Guatemala, 79, 90, 161, 172-176, 205, 208

Haiti, 182, 231
Healers. *See* Traditional healers
Health behavior, 8, 10, 31, 216-223, 225-230, 236-238, 280
   antecedents, 31, 238
   consequences, 31-32, 233, 237-238, 285
Health education, 3, 14, 37, 88-89, 116-118, 207-209, 210-239, 280
   applied behavior analysis, 213, 227-230, 236-238
   health belief model, 234-236, 238
   persuasive communication, 213, 215, 234-235, 238
Health promotion. *See* Health education
Health services, 20-22
   accessibility, 20, 83, 89-91, 139, 275

coverage, 21-22
utilization, 21, 138, 140, 142-143, 288
See also Primary Health Care
Health workers, 91-92, 268-269. See Community health workers
Human immunodeficiency virus (HIV), 94-122. See also AIDS
Hygiene, 216-220

Immunization, 2, 14, 23, 26-27, 280
Incentives, 86-88, 231, 233
Incidence, 19, 100, 281
India, 6, 67, 72, 80-81, 87, 103, 107, 161, 183, 231, 269
Indonesia, 143, 152, 161, 165
Industrialized countries. See Developed countries
Infants, 17, 64-65, 75, 165-166, 281
International health, 1-5, 281
Iodine, 158, 161, 181
Iron, 159, 162, 173, 181

Japan, 186, 193

KAP, 57, 64-65, 82-83, 107-111, 116, 281
See also Knowledge; Attitudes
Kenya, 27, 71, 102, 139, 161, 165, 171, 186-187, 190, 196-198, 201, 231
Key informant, 51-57, 281
Knowledge, 11, 89, 107-109, 212, 220-223, 281. See also KAP

Latin America and the Caribbean, 24, 69-72, 79, 83, 86, 99, 102-103, 105, 165, 182, 193, 195-197, 201, 207. See also Colombia, Guatemala, Haiti, Mexico, Peru, South America

Leadership, 132, 144, 147, 149-150, 281
Learning, 8-10, 169, 236-238, 282
Least developed countries, 24, 70, 72, 78
Leprosy, 12, 282
Literacy. See Education
Locus of Control, 62, 280, 282

Low birth weight, 162, 170, 282

Malaria, 12, 282
Malnutrition, 4, 12, 14, 154-184, 282
and mental development, 169-180
causes, 162-169
consequences, 169-180
diet, 157-159, 164-169, 183, 223-225
measurement, 156-160
nutrient deficiencies, 158-159, 161-162
prevalence, 160-162
prevention programs, 180-184, 230-232
supplementation, 172-176, 181-183
treatment, 180
Maternal health, 14, 282, 283
Measles, 12
Mental health, 8, 32, 245, 283
Mental illness, 244-269, 283
classification systems, 246-248, 278, 281
cultural factors, 251-256
measurement, 246-251
prevalence, 256-258
prevention, 264
risk factors, 260-263
schizophrenia, 247, 253, 255, 267-268
treatment, 265-269
Methods of measurement, 29-66
of AIDS and HIV, 99-101
of alcohol use and abuse, 187-192
of contraception use
of malnutrition, 156-160
of mental development, 170-171
of mental illness
See also Qualitative methods; Quantitative methods
Mexico, 69, 85, 182, 186, 193, 196-197, 201
Middle East and North Africa, 24, 70-72, 86, 104
Morbidity, 18-20, 169
Mortality, 17, 72-75, 94-95, 169, 281, 283, 287
Mothers, 72-75, 98, 162, 165-168, 171, 177-178, 184, 216-220, 223-230, 239-241
Motivation, 7, 11, 216, 226-230, 233, 283

Neonatal tetanus, 13, 283

Nepal, 142-143
Nigeria, 72, 77, 88-89, 111, 139, 161, 183, 269
Nongovernmental organizations (NGO), 1, 27-28, 132-135, 143, 151-152, 181, 272, 283
Nonparticipant observation, 42-47
Norms, 78, 106-107, 111-116, 121, 186, 216-220, 235-236, 287
North Africa. *See* Middle East and North Africa
North America, 103, 120, 193-199. *See also* Canada, Developed countries, United States
Nutrients, 157-159, 161-162
Nutrition. *See* Malnutrition

Official development assistance (ODA), 24
Oral rehydration salts (ORS), 5-6, 164, 284
Oral rehydration therapy, 23, 164, 227-230, 284
Orphans, 75, 114

Pacific Islands, 200. *See also* East Asia and the Pacific
Pain, 62, 283
Pakistan, 69, 72
Participation. *See* Community Participation
Participant observation, 47-51, 284
Personality, 11, 205, 278, 284
Peru, 69, 133, 161, 195
Philippines, 116, 143-144, 161, 223-225, 231
Pneumonia, 11
Poliomyelitis, 13, 284
Practice. *See* KAP; Health behavior
Prevalence, 19, 285
  of AIDS and HIV, 100-104
  of alcohol use and abuse, 193-199
  of contraception use, 178-182
  of malnutrition, 160-162
  of mental illness, 256-258
Prevention, 138-139
  of AIDS and HIV, 116-122
  of alcohol abuse, 206-209
  of malnutrition, 180-184
  of mental illness, 264-
Primary health care (PHC), 114, 124, 269, 285. *See also* Health services
Problem-solving, 127, 213, 223-225
Protective factors, 262-263, 285
Protein, 156-158

Qualitative methods, 32-41, 47-57, 285
  *See also* Focus groups; Key informant; Participant observation
Quantitative methods, 32-37, 42-47, 57-66, 285, 287
Questionnaires, 57-66, 190-192, 247-251

Radio and television, 88-89, 220-223, 283
Reliability, 34, 43
Risk factors, 286
  for AIDS and HIV, 97
  for alcohol abuse, 203-205
  for mental illness, 260-263

Safe sex, 97
Safe water, 14, 23, 143, 164, 275
Salt:
  iodized, 161-162, 181
  salt-sugar solution, 5-6, 227-230, 286
  *See also* Oral rehydration salts
Sampling, 34-36, 286
Sanitation, 14, 23, 164, 225-227, 275
Scandinavia, 151, 186, 194, 196-197, 154
Schizophrenia. *See* Mental illness
School. *See* Education
School feeding programs, 172, 230-232
Self-efficacy, 63, 235-236, 286
Sex, 97, 102-107, 111-113
Sex workers, 98, 101-103, 106, 115-117, 120-121
Sexually-transmitted diseases (STD), 79, 97, 101, 119. *See also* AIDS
Skills, 11, 92, 134, 212-213, 229, 286
Socioeconomic status (SES), 31, 36, 55-57, 71-72, 91-92, 172, 175
South Asia, 24, 70-72, 76, 82-83, 86, 103, 105, 161-162, 168. *See also* Bangladesh; India; Nepal; Pakistan

South Africa, 27, 111, 114, 118-119
South America, 173, 220-223, 245. *See also* Latin America and the Caribbean
Soviet-bloc countries (former), 70
Sterilization, 78-81, 87-88
Street children, 273-274
Stress, 62, 65-66, 261-262, 286
Stunted children, 159-162, 287
Sub-Saharan Africa, 24, 27, 69-73, 76, 79, 82-83, 86, 99, 101-102, 105, 110, 139-140, 155, 161-162, 165, 193-194, 196, 242, 251-253. *See also* Ethiopia, Kenya, Nigeria, South Africa, Tanzania, Uganda

Tanzania, 102, 216-220
Thailand, 87, 103, 120-121, 165
Trachoma, 216-220
Traditional healers, 118-119, 168, 265-266
Traditional birth attendant, 23, 76, 136, 277, 287
Tuberculosis, 13, 287

Uganda, 82, 102, 107, 139
Underweight, 159-162, 288
UNICEF, 2, 6, 25-27, 123, 166, 264
United Nations (U.N.), 25
United Nations Children's Fund. *See* UNICEF
United States, 114, 122, 159, 194-198, 200-201, 203, 208, 256, 257
Utilization of health services. *See* Health services

Validity, 34
Verbal autopsy, 63, 288
Violence, 198-202
Vitamins, 158, 161, 184

Wasted children, 160-162, 288
Weaning, 166-168, 183-184, 288
Women, 68-92, 102-104, 112-115, 117-118, 169, 258, 262
World Health Organization (WHO), 6, 25, 32, 99-100, 123

# ABOUT THE AUTHOR

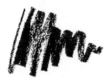

**Frances E. Aboud** is Professor in the Department of Psychology at McGill University in Montreal, Canada. She has been teaching there for 22 years, offering courses on personality and social psychology, social development, and international health psychology. She has conducted research on the development of ethnic prejudice in children and ways of reducing it, and has published a book on this topic called *Children and Prejudice*. For several years, she worked in Ethiopia as a member of the McGill-Ethiopia Community Health Project. At that time, she taught a behavioral science course to master's students in the public health program at the University of Addis Ababa and the Jimma Institute of Health Sciences. In collaboration with staff and students, she conducted and published research on malnutrition in children, mental illness, mothers' management of children's diarrhea, and community health workers.

# About the Contributors

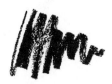

**Micheala Hynie** is currently Assistant Professor of psychology at York University in Toronto, Canada. She received her PhD from McGill University, where she conducted research on social psychological aspects of women's sexuality. In addition to continuing this research, she teaches community mental health and social psychology.

**Charles P. Larson** is Associate Professor in the Department of Epidermiology and Biostastics and the Department of Pediatrics at McGill University. He was Director of the McGill-Ethiopia Community Health Project and has been involved with projects in Vietnam and Russia. He has published extensively on topics related to public health in developing countries, some of which include randomized field trials of family planning promotion, functional status of community health workers, and oral rehydration therapies. He is currently co-chair of the Canadian Society for International Health.